D1557389

Western Diseases:

their emergence and prevention

Western Diseases:

their emergence and prevention

Edited by

H. C. Trowell OBE, MD, FRCP
Formerly Consultant Physician, Uganda

D. P. Burkitt CMG, MD, FRCSEd, DSc(Hon), FRCSI(Hon), FRS
Department of Geographical Pathology, St. Thomas's Hospital, London

Both formerly of Makerere University Medical School and Mulago
Hospital, Kampala, Uganda

Foreword by

John R. K. Robson MD, BS, DPH, DTMH
Professor of Medicine and Nutrition
Medical University of South Carolina

Harvard University Press
Cambridge, Massachusetts
1981

Printed in the United States of America

Library of Congress Cataloging in Publication Data
Main entry under title:

Western diseases, their emergence and prevention.

 Includes bibliographies and index.
 1. Nutritionally induced diseases.   2. Chronic diseases.   3. Epidemiology.
 4. Medical geography.
I. Trowell, Hubert Carey.   II. Burkitt, Denis Parsons.
[DNLM: 1. Disease—History.   2. History of medicine. WZ 40 W527]
RA645.N87W47   616.07′1   80–28917
ISBN 0-674-95020-8

Contributors

James W. Anderson, MD, Professor of Medicine and Clinical Nutrition, University of Kentucky, Lexington, Kentucky, USA

Bruce K. Armstrong, DPhil, BMedSc, Director, Health Research and Planning, Western Australia, Australia

Roberto G. Baruzzi, MD, Professor of Preventive Medicine and Epidemiology, Escola Paulista de Medicina, São Paulo, Brazil

Peter Beighton, MD, PhD, DTMH, DCH, FRCP, Professor of Human Genetics, University of Cape Town Medical School, Cape, South Africa

Norman J. Blacklock, OBE, MB ChB, FRCS, Professor of Urological Surgery, University Hospital of South Manchester, Manchester, England

Geoffrey Dean, MD, FRCP(I), FFCM(I), Director, Medico-Social Research Board, Lower Baggot Street, Dublin, Ireland

Hans A. Diehl, DrHealthSc, MPH (Nutrition), Research Director, Longevity Center, Santa Barbara and Post-Doctoral Scholar, University of California, School of Public Health, Division of Epidemiology, Los Angeles, California, USA

Paul M. Dodson, MB BS, MRCP, MRCS, Research Fellow in Diabetes, St. Bartholomew's Hospital, London, England

Sir Richard Doll, OBE, MD, FRS, Formerly Regius Professor of Medicine, University of Oxford, Oxford, England

Laercio J. Franco, MD, Assistant Professor in Preventive Medicine, Escola Paulista de Medicina, São Paulo, Brazil

Michael Gelfand, CBE, MD, FRCP, Formerly Professor of Medicine, University of Zimbabwe, Salisbury, Zimbabwe

Gary A. Glober, MD, Associate Professor of Medicine, John A. Burns School of Medicine, University of Hawaii, Hawaii

Kenneth W. Heaton, MA, MD, FRCP, Reader in Medicine, University Department of Medicine, Department of Medicine, Bristol Royal Infirmary, Bristol, England

Daphne M. Humphreys, MB BS, MRCP, Senior Registrar in Medicine, Royal Berkshire Hospital, Reading, England

David Landsborough, MD, FRCP, Physician, Changhua Christian Hospital, Chang-hua, Taiwan, Republic of China

Conrad Latto, FRCSE, FRCS, Senior Consultant Surgeon, Royal Berkshire Hospital, Reading, England

Don Mannerberg, MD, Formerly Medical Director, Longevity Center, Santa Barbara, California, USA

Baruch Modan, MD, Professor and Head, Department of Clinical Epidemiology, Chaim Sheba Medical Center, Tel Aviv University Medical School, Tel Hashoma, Israel

Peter M. Moodie, MD, BS, DTMH, Assistant Professor, Commonwealth Institute of Health, University of Sydney, New South Wales, Australia

Ian A. M. Prior, MD, FRCP, FRACP, Director, Epidemiology Unit, Wellington Hospital, Wellington, New Zealand

Otto Schaefer, MD, FRCP(C), Director, Northern Medical Research Unit, Medical Services, Health and Welfare Canada, Charles Camsell Hospital, Edmonton, Alberta, Canada

Emer Shelley, MB, MRCPI, Research Assistant, Medico-Social Research Board, Lower Baggot Street, Dublin, Ireland

Peter Sinnett, MB BS, MD, FRACP, Foundation Professor of Geriatrics, Faculty of Medicine, University of New South Wales, Australia

Louis Solomon, MD, FRCS, Professor of Orthopaedic Surgery, University of the Witwatersrand, Medical School, Johannesburg, South Africa

Grant N. Stemmermann, MD, Laboratory Director, Kuakini Medical Center, Hawaii

Clifford Tasman-Jones, MB ChB, FRCP, FRACP, Associate Professor, Department of Medicine, University of Auckland, New Zealand

Alexander R. P. Walker, DSc, Head, Medical Research Council Human Biochemistry Research Unit, South African Institute for Medical Research, Johannesburg, South Africa

Kelly M. West, MD. Professor of Biostatistics and Epidemiology, University of Oklahoma, Health Sciences Center, Oklahoma City, Oklahoma, USA

Sunny Whitehouse, Computer Fellow, Department of Metabolic Medicine and Epidemiology, Royal Southern Memorial Hospital, Melbourne, Australia

Malcolm Whyte, BSc, DPhil(Oxon), FRCP, FRACP, Emeritus Professor (formerly Professor of Clinical Science, Australian National University); Co-ordinator of Alcohol and Drug Dependence Unit, Canberra, Australia

Edward H. Williams, CBE, MB BS, MRCS, LRCP, Formerly Physician, Kuluva Hospital, West Nile District, Uganda

Peter H. Williams, MRCS, LRCP, DO, Formerly Physician, Kuluva Hospital, West Nile District, Uganda

Shun-ichi Yamamoto, MD, Professor of Hygiene and Preventive Medicine, Faculty of Medicine, Tokyo, Japan

Paul Zimmet, MB BS, PhD, FRACP, Director, Department of Metabolic Medicine and Epidemiology, Royal Southern Memorial Hospital, Melbourne, Australia

To Peggy and Olive our wives for they shared
the burden and the joy of the book

Foreword

John Robson
Professor of Medicine and Nutrition, Medical University of South
Carolina

Historically, diseases of tropical and temperate climates have been considered to be separate branches of medicine. The former being mainly concerned with communicable diseases and malnutrition, has now largely become a speciality for parasitology. Similar advances in the temperate scene have resulted in a shift of emphasis from the treatment of acute communicable disease to the treatment and control of chronic and degenerative diseases. Although atherosclerosis, diabetes, hypertension and cancer primarily affect the industrialized nations, a real increase in prevalence of these diseases is being observed in the developing tropical countries.

My fifteen years of work in medicine and clinical nutrition among hunter-gatherers, subsistence level farmers and the urban poor in Africa, and the Far and Middle East, stimulated an interest in the medical significance of the dietary changes that take place during his cultural, social and economic development. In Africa and elsewhere, development and the accompanying changes in diet have occurred over a relatively short period of time, but the modifications to the diet are very similar to the alterations in food patterns experienced by modern man as he passed through the Agricultural Evolution and the Industrial Revolution of the last 8000–10 000 years. Because of the similarities of these changes, research in developing countries would seem very important for the understanding of the genesis of Western diseases. While working with anthropologists at the University of Michigan I had opportunities to study the archaeological and contemporary records of man in varying stages of development and I became convinced that in some circumstances the simplification of the varied diet of the hunter-gatherer can adversely affect health. For example, the decrease in the varieties of food resources exploited by the subsistance farmer impairs the mothers' ability to provide her infant with an adequate weaning food. Thus the high prevalence of kwashiorkor in the children of peasant farmers is not surprising.

There is widespread concern among nutritionists also over the effects of high salt and sugar intakes from processed foods. Although cause and effect relationships between dietary, social, economic, and environmental changes and the prevalence of Western diseases are not yet clear, this possibility needs to be examined in greater detail.

In conducting research on global diseases several problems arise; for example, investigators are scattered far and wide. They publish their findings in numerous journals and books and the subject matter may cover diverse subjects such as epidemiology, parasitology, endocrinology or immunology and they may be published in a variety of languages. It is important for scientists to integrate their own knowledge with that of their colleagues in other disciplines or sciences. Past experience has shown that the anthropologist, epidemiologist and biochemist, among others, can contribute to clarifying the cause of many tropical diseases and their successful control. It is becoming increasingly apparent that understanding the genesis of Western diseases will require not only the knowledge and expertise of physicians from numerous specialities, but also food scientists, biochemists, food chemists, surface chemists and many others. A review of existing knowledge is an important first procedure in stimulating interdisciplinary research and discussion; *Western Diseases: their emergence and prevention* has taken this very important first step. The book amply demonstrates global interest in this subject, as well as the multifaceted approach that will be needed to fully understand and control these diseases.

It is also necessary to recognize the implications of these diseases for emerging nations. We should not be concerned with the genesis and control of these diseases only from the selfish viewpoint of the Western world. It seems that westernization is an inevitable consequence for developing areas. In this process we need to consider carefully whether Western influence in Africa, Asia, Central and South America and the Far East is unnecessarily imposing our diseases on other populations who are presently relatively free of them.

We also need to consider whether Western diets are contributing to the production of atherosclerosis, diabetes, hypertension and obesity. In the United States Senator George McGovern's Senate Select Committee on Nutrition and Human Needs have recommended *Dietary Goals for the United States* (1977). They recommended that the current US diet be altered: the proportion of energy derived from complex carbohydrates (starch foods) should be doubled and it should be derived from whole grains, the proportion of energy derived from sugar and fat should be considerably reduced, likewise salt. This book supports these recommendations.

This book, *Western Diseases: their emergence and prevention*, should help us to understand the consequences of our current mode of life.

Reference

Select Committee on Nutrition and Human Needs, United States Senate (1977). *Dietary Goals for the United States*, second edition. Washington, US Government Printing Office

Preface

This book attempts to discuss the commoner 'diseases of civilization'. The editors have been associated with the teaching of medicine in East Africa for a total of half a century (H. T. 1929–1958; D. B. 1948–1966). In retirement both have revisited East Africa; and one of us (D. B.) has travelled widely, visiting hospitals in all five continents. We taught medicine and surgery to students who, like ourselves, would treat African, Asian and European patients. It was relatively easy to explain the different incidence of infective diseases in these three communities, but it proved impossible to account for the glaring differences in the incidence of many non-infective diseases.

This problem was reviewed by one of us (H. T.) in *Non-infective Disease in Africa* as long ago as 1960. Cleave and Campbell's *Diabetes, Coronary Thrombosis and the Saccharine Disease* (1966) recently proved an enormous stimulus to both of us and led to our editing *Refined Carbohydrate Foods and Disease* (1975). Its sub-title, *Some Implications of Dietary Fibre*, emphasized the probable protective role of fibre against certain diseases of the large bowel and possibly also against some metabolic disorders such as diabetes mellitus and gallstones. In all of these diseases it was emphasized that a deficiency of dietary fibre was only one of many aetiological factors. For instance in diverticular disease low fibre diets were considered to be the major factor, but age, sex, genetic and other factors doubtless also operate.

The term 'diseases of civilization' is not appropriate: available evidence suggests that some of the diseases were present but uncommon in the ancient civilizations of Egypt, Greece, Rome, India and China. These diseases are those which are characteristic of modern affluent Western technological communities. This is probably the best definition of a 'Western disease'. Western adults live longer than in former centuries due to the conquest of most infections and the achievements of surgery. Western man frequently dies eventually of one of the disorders placed in the provisional list of Western diseases given at the end of this Preface. Available evidence suggests that several of these diseases have become commoner in the Western world in the past one hundred years. The lower reported incidence of many Western diseases in developing countries, especially in underprivileged socioeconomic groups, is not explained in our opinion by the lower proportion of older persons or by under-reporting, although both of these factors operate to produce low hospital diagnosis figures. Moreover some of these Western diseases, like appendicitis, are commoner in young adults and children, but appendicitis still remains uncommon among Africans in many parts of Africa, including urban areas with modern hospitals.

In recent years several doctors with long years of experience of teaching in the medical schools of southern Africa have coined the term 'Western diseases' for disorders the incidence of which increases in the black population as their diet and lifestyle become westernized, and a fair number of cases are found nowadays in African upper socioeconomic groups. These doctors therefore have written about the 'emergence' of these disorders in South African black populations: our experiences of the 'emergence' of certain Western diseases in Kenyans and Ugandans are the basis of the first two chapters. The title Western diseases is preferred to that of the diseases of civilization, for it proved obnoxious to teach African and Asian medical students that their communities had a low incidence of these diseases because they were uncivilized.

The term Western diseases has been restricted by common usage to disorders of uncertain aetiology. This restriction of the term perpetuates an artificial division of the diseases brought, often indirectly, by technological change, especially modern changes that followed the Industrial Revolution of the last century. This limitation of the term Western diseases is followed, but with regret, in this book owing to consideration of space. Motor car accidents, industrial hazards and pollution, cigarettes and the consumption of alcoholic spirits and of new drugs, are barely discussed, even if they are truly Western diseases as defined in this Preface.

The Western diseases are essentially the 'man-made diseases' and man is almost the only creature who profoundly alters his own environment. Eventually we will suggest that the increased incidence of these diseases reflects technological change, however simple. This technological change is usually modern, but not always so. Ancient technology made possible the preparation and transport of salt, it conferred the great benefits of increased food supply and it inaugurated the grinding of cereals, the crushing of sugar cane and the preparation of vegetable oils. Modern technology has altered radically the production and preparation of food, it has abolished hunger in many nations, it has also created affluence and has permitted the decrease of physical exertion. It has increased considerably the length of life and allowed the diseases of ageing to increase. It has changed in a profound manner the whole Western lifestyle, bringing many benefits but also introducing new risks, and increasing old risks, of certain diseases.

The incidence and variety of diseases in a community reflects always the interplay of many environmental factors on the genetic pool of the community. The appearance of disease in an individual reflects the influence of environmental factors in an individual phenotype who inherited his genes from the community pool. In relatively stable populations the community genetic pool alters only very slowly during very long periods of evolutionary time; in comparison the environment may alter very quickly. If environmental factors change *rapidly* then the pattern of environment-related diseases also changes rapidly. This book surveys in broad outline some changes in the pattern of non-infective disease that have occurred and are occurring in the modern world. In some respects it is almost a pioneer venture and pioneers make many mistakes. Future research will reveal several mistakes in this book; better data will accumulate, but something will survive and grow and perhaps contribute to a new world outlook in medicine.

Thirty-four contributors from five continents have written their own chapters, giving their experience of the changing pattern of non-infective disease as westernization occurs in certain communities. Contributors were sent a provisional list of Western diseases, listed at the end of this Preface. Some of our own experience in Kenyans and Ugandans is recorded in Part I. Part II considers evidence that environmental factors operate in the formation of cholesterol gallstones and renal stone, also in multiple sclerosis, rheumatoid arthritis and certain varieties of cancer. It must *not* be assumed that any, or all, of these disorders are *proved* to be Western diseases; contributors were asked to review evidence that environmental factors influence the incidence of these diseases. Part III examines the scanty data concerning the Western diseases among hunter-gatherer groups who are probably similar in many respects to those from whom the genetic pool of man was inherited. Part IV considers the incidence of Western diseases among peasant agriculturalists, Part V among migrants and Part VI in the people of the Far East. With considerable hesitation Part VII reports preliminary studies which suggest that some of the Western diseases—essential hypertension, angina and diabetes mellitus type II, formerly called maturity-onset diabetes —may regress if patients revert to the diet, and even the physical activity, of early peasant agricultural groups, who have a low incidence of these diseases. The editors have visited on several occasions all the medical centres reporting these surprising results. Part VIII summarizes the data and criticisms of the contributors' reports on any aspect of the overall hypothesis of the Western diseases.

Provisional list of Western diseases

Metabolic and cardiovascular: essential hypertension, obesity, diabetes mellitus (type II), cholesterol gallstones, cerebrovascular disease, peripheral vascular disease, coronary heart disease; varicose veins, deep vein thrombosis and pulmonary embolism.

Colonic: constipation, appendicitis, diverticular disease, haemorrhoids; cancer and polyp of large bowel.

Other diseases: dental caries, renal stone, hyperuricaemia and gout, thyrotoxicosis, pernicious anaemia, subacute combined degeneration, also other forms of cancer such as breast and lung.

Evidence is increasing that the following may prove to be Western diseases: irritable bowel syndrome, ulcerative colitis, Crohn's disease, hiatus hernia, pelvic phleboliths and certain autoimmune diseases (Chapter 27). The editors consider these are Western diseases but supporting publications are few.

The editors thank those who have made this investigation possible (H. T. the Pharmaceutical Division of Reckitt and Colman), also the publishers for helpful cooperation and Mrs. Priscilla Tippett for years of much helpful secretarial assistance.

While this book was being printed the editors heard, with deep regret, of the death of Professor Kelly West. His study of diabetes and other diseases in North American Indians (Chapter 9) is a worthy memorial.

Hugh Trowell
Denis Burkitt

References

Burkitt, D. P. and Trowell, H. C. (1975). *Refined Carbohydrate Foods and Disease. Some Implications of Dietary Fibre.* Academic Press, London

Cleave, T. L. and Campbell, G. D. (1966). *Diabetes, Coronary Thrombosis and the Saccharine Disease.* John Wright, Bristol

Trowell, H. C. (1960). *Non-infective Disease in Africa.* Edward Arnold, London

Contents

Part I

Emergence of Western diseases in
sub-Saharal Africans

1

Hypertension, obesity, diabetes mellitus and coronary heart disease

Hugh Trowell

High blood pressure emerges

'Consider the rise of blood pressure with age that is characteristic of most of our populations. I believe this rise is pathological'. (Peart, 1978)

'Prognostically ideal blood pressure seems to be "as low as possible" and in this sense the concept of "a case of hypertension" becomes inappropriate'. (Rose and Barker, 1979)

Blood pressure rises with age in most persons and in most populations. Professor W. S. Peart, Chairman of the Medical Research Council Working Party on Mild-to-Moderate Hypertension, has stated that this is pathological: if so most elderly persons suffer from it. Professor G. Rose, Professor of Epidemiology of the London School of Hygiene and Tropical Medicine, and Dr. D. J. P. Barker, Reader in Clinical Epidemiology of the University of Southampton, agree that ideal blood pressure does not rise with age. They illustrated this point by stating that '. . . in a man of 50 a systolic pressure of 150 mmHg is common (that is it is "statistically normal") and it is clinically normal, in the sense of being symptomless; but his risk of fatal heart attack is about twice that of his contemporary with a low blood pressure'.

This chapter discusses the emergence of a disease called 'blood pressure rising with age' in the Africans of Kenya and Uganda; they are called Kenyans and Ugandans. It will also discuss the disease called essential hypertension which is invariably preceded by blood pressure rising with age.

Communities with lifelong low blood pressure

Epstein and Eckhoff (1967) in their survey of the epidemiology of hypertension cited some 13 small, and usually isolated, ethnic groups in whom blood pressure did not rise with age. Shaper (1972) added other groups, as did Page (1976; 1979). New groups continue to be discovered, such as the Mzigua tribe in Tanzania (Vaughan, 1978), so that at least 30 ethnic groups, usually small in numbers, have been identified.

3

No reports have been traced concerning any large defined community, who changed slowly over the years from lifelong low blood pressure to blood pressure rising with age, until this was reported for Kenyans and Ugandans during the 50 years 1929–78 (Trowell, 1978a; 1980). I was in Kenya from 1929 to 1935, and in Uganda from 1935 to 1958, and revisited these countries in 1963 and 1970.

The crucial evidence concerns the lifelong low blood pressure during the years 1928–40 in Kenyans and Ugandans. These populations certainly have blood pressure rising with age and much essential hypertension nowadays: this is therefore discussed, but only briefly, at the end of this section. This evidence, based largely on the experience of the staffs of the medical schools of Kenya and Uganda, is unique: it is unlikely to be repeated in the future in any other large community. It involved the earliest blood pressure survey of age groups in an unacculturated mixture of several African tribes, coupled with the earliest comprehensive analysis of the African diet, supplemented by clinical reports and autopsy data spread over the next 50 years. No other survey of unacculturated ethnic groups with lifelong low blood pressure has been based on clinical and necropsy studies or an analysis of the diet, or been furnished with records extending over a period of 50 years.

Kenya and Uganda lifelong low blood pressure 1929–40

Kenya, Uganda and Tanzania were among the last African countries to be westernized, for in the days of only sea communications they were more remote from Europe than North, West or South Africa. Intertribal warfare, slave-raiding and roaming nomadic warriors like the Masai had previously been barriers to trade. No railways or permanent roads ran inland from the Indian ocean until the turn of the century. Metal currency came into common use in the Kenya highlands only in the 1920s; then Africans began to open shops. Throughout the Kenya highlands and the whole of Uganda there are few surface deposits of salt (page 11).

The sunny equatorial climate of Kenya, modified by altitude, encouraged thousands of British settlers to open farms in the 1920s. Scores of British doctors devoted their lives to medicine and surgery either in government service, or in missionary hospitals, or in private practice. Never before did, and probably never again will, so many resident doctors observe three million men, women and children, as in Kenya in the 1920s, emerge from preindustrial tribal life and undergo rapid westernization. A comparable number lived in Uganda wherein African kingdoms had welcomed some elements of westernization at least three decades earlier than occurred in Kenya. Disease patterns shifted earlier in Uganda than in Kenya. Doctors in all East African territories began to record their observations in the *Kenya Medical Journal*, founded in 1924, long before comparable medical journals emerged in West and Central Africa. Annual conferences of doctors in Kenya reflected their number; for instance 56 doctors attended the 1926 conference in Nairobi; in 1927 the Kenya Medical Association had 100 members with British qualifications.

Formal training of Kenyan hospital assistants (bush doctors) started in 1931 at Nairobi. I was responsible for their training from 1933 to 1935, then transferred to teach medicine at Mulago hospital and Makerere University in Kampala, Uganda, until 1958. It became incumbent on all teachers of medicine to collect data concerning the prevalance of the common diseases in Africans. From 1930 until 1935 doctors in Kenya were unanimous that they had never seen essential hypertension in an African and no case was reported either in Kenya and Uganda until 1941.

Necropsy studies of Kenyans 1927 until 1937

This conviction concerning the absence or rarity of essential hypertension stemmed largely from the necropsy studies of Vint (1936–37), who was Government pathologist from 1927 until 1953. He had been the first doctor in East Africa to devote himself exclusively to necropsies on Kenyans, Indians and Europeans, and was the medicolegal expert for the whole of the Kenya Colony. This involved receiving reports and specimens from doctors throughout the country. Necropsies were performed on the majority of patients dying in the Nairobi Native Civil Hospital and upon all prisoners and any African found dead in Nairobi township. African patients at the Nairobi Native Civil Hospital were drawn from *all* African highland tribes, among whom Kikuyu then, as nowadays, predominated.

Most African patients in Nairobi were young male adults, few were children, and only a minority were over 40 years of age; roughly 5 per cent has sufficient white hair and aged features to qualify, on medical certification, for exemption of taxation, as they were deemed to be over 60 years old. Vint in 1936–37 reported the results of his first thousand Kenyan necropsies. This article provided the basis of estimates concerning the prevalence of disease in Kenya Africans. Since Vint was at that time conducting research into brain structure, this organ was always examined. All the principal organs were weighed as a routine.

Among this thousand African necropsies there had been 56 cardiovascular deaths but no manifestation of essential hypertension or ischaemic heart disease, both of which were common in European and Indian persons. Eighty-nine Africans displayed advanced atherosclerosis of the aorta but the coronary arteries had been spared; 33 Africans had died of nephritis, usually chronic, and sections had confirmed the diagnosis. There had been 3 deaths from diabetes mellitus, but no case of appendicitis; the gallbladder was always opened but only one stone had been found, and this had been in a child. After some more years of experience Vint, in an undated personal communication to Akinkugbe (1972), stated categorically concerning Kenyans 'The writer has not seen a single case of essential hypertension, nor do the medical records of the (Kenya) Colony show evidence of the occurrence'.

Clinical studies 1923-34

Several clinical workers in Kenya confirmed the rarity of essential hypertension in Africans. For instance Jex-Blake (1934), who had retired early from the staff of a London teaching hospital in 1923, emigrated to Kenya to become the senior medical consultant in Nairobi, a position which he held for the next 30 years. After he had been in consultant practice for 11 years he reviewed his study of 200 patients with essential hypertension at the monthly BMA Nairobi meeting. All patients had been European or Asian; he had never seen or heard of a single case of essential hypertension in a Kenyan. He was aware of the results accruing in the necropsy studies of Vint (1936–37) and of the blood pressure survey of Donnison (1929), shortly to be discussed. In the light of these facts and his own observations he stated that among Kenyans 'essential hypertension must be exceeding rare'. I was among the 13 BMA members who attended the meeting and commented on the rarity of this disease in Kenyans. This discussion and the whole lecture was published in the *East African Medical Journal*, together with an Editorial article. Almost all the 150 doctors then practising in Kenya, Uganda and Tanganyika received a copy of this journal, but no one wrote challenging this statement until ten years later when Williams (1944) reported the first East African hospital cases. Previous erroneous generalizations of disease in Africans had stated that cancer was rare; this provoked in the next issues of the Kenya journal several case reports of hospital patients with cancer. The alleged rarity of peptic ulcer in Africans, mooted in the late 1930s in the same journal, soon elicited several case reports from many East African doctors. But no one reported essential hypertension in an African for several more years after the editorial article had summarized evidence of its rarity.

Blood pressure surveys in 1928 and 1941

The first blood pressure survey of Kenyans was conducted by Donnison (1929). He examined 1000 African men from a mixture of four Kavirondo Bantu and Nilotic tribes living near the Uganda border (Table 1.1). Ages ranged from 15 to 70 years and were assessed by tribal elders; 97 men were estimated to have been over 60 years. Women proved too nervous to volunteer for examination. This was the first large age group blood pressure survey in Africa. Blood pressure levels in men remained low, not rising with age, but after 40 years levels actually fell to average 105/60 mmHg in the 97 men aged more than 60 years. (Is this the biological norm for a community eating low sodium diets, as reported subsequently?)

Eight years later, because no doctor had challenged the findings of Donnison (1929), Jex-Blake (1934) and Vint (1936–37), Donnison (1937) wrote his book *Civilization and Disease*. This was the first modern book on this subject to be based on clinical and necropsy studies in Kenya and the Colonial Office yearly medical reports on hospital inpatient diagnoses in all British colonies. The diseases of civilization were considered to be essential hypertension, obesity, angina, ischaemic heart disease, cerebrovascular

Table 1.1 Blood pressure surveys of Kenyans and Ugandans

Year	Country	Tribes	Persons	Age groups years	BP change with age — men	BP change with age — women	Hypertension	Investigator
1928	Kenya	Kisii, Luo Suba, Kuria	1000[1]	15–70	fell	—[1]	nil	Donnison (1929)
1941	Uganda	Tesot Karamoja	456	21–50+	nil	nil	few	Williams (1941–1942)
1958 and 1961	Kenya	Kikuyu	529	20–80	systolic rose; diastolic fell[2]	systolic rose; diastolic fell[2]	nil	Williams (1969)
1963	Uganda	Ganda migrants	600 300	10–65+ 10–65+	rose[3] almost nil	rose[3] almost nil	present[2] nil	Shaper and Saxton (1969)

[1] Men only; in other surveys men and women almost equal in numbers
[2] In older age groups
[3] Equal in incidence to US white subjects

disease, diabetes, dental caries, appendicitis, gallstones, varicose veins, pernicious anaemia, renal calculus, thyrotoxicosis and toxaemia of pregnancy. In his opinion the psychosomatic stresses of civilized life caused essential hypertension and contributed to the aetiology of all diseases of civilization. Beyond a favourable review in the *East African Medical Journal* no comment has been traced concerning this book in any other African country. But by the late 1930s many doctors, especially those in West Africa and South Africa, had reported much hypertension in Africans, but acculturation had occurred many decades previously among Africans in these countries. The book spoke to dull ears, for many doubted its data: no one considered that essential hypertension could *emerge* as a disease in communities previously having lifelong low blood pressure.

The first blood pressure survey of Ugandans was conducted by Williams (1941–42) (Table 1.1). In this connection it is misleading to speak of Ugandans and Kenyans. A large mixture of small Bantu-speaking tribes had been further fragmented by invading Nilotic tribes from the Sudan and Hamitic tribes intruding from Abyssinia during several previous centuries. Intertribal warfare and slave-raiding, both accompanied by the capture of women and children, had occurred. The Uganda–Kenya boundaries altered from time to time; this had divided still further a hotchpotch of mixed tribal groups. Those examined by Donnison (1929) lay on the Kenya side of this 'border'; a similar mixture of tribes were examined by Williams (1941–42); they lived on the Ugandan side of the 'border'; both had been 'Ugandan' tribes a few years previously, before the 'border' was altered. He examined 456 men and women aged 21–50 years or more. Their blood pressure levels did not rise with age; however, they did not fall during middle-age as noted by Donnison (1929). It was therefore stated that '. . . essential hypertension among Africans in Africa is uncommon and its serious complications are quite rare'. Dr. A. W. Williams had been nine years in different districts of Uganda when he made this statement; within a few years he became Professor of Medicine at Makerere University Medical School in Kampala, Uganda, and this became the major centre of cardiovascular research in tropical Africa.

High blood pressure emerges in Uganda and Kenya after 1940

Blood pressure surveys 1941 until 1969

Williams (1941–42) actually found a few borderline hypertensive patients in his survey; 13 Ugandans had a diastolic blood pressure (IV phase) exceeding 90 mmHg (Table 1.1). Being desirous of establishing the presence of essential hypertension in East Africans it was decided that all patients in the 100 medical beds of Mulago hospital, Kampala, Uganda, who had systolic blood pressure >170 and/or diastolic blood pressure (IV phase) >95 mmHg should be referred to him. In this way 23 cases of essential hypertension were found during the next four years, most of whom were salaried, prosperous

Ganda men (Williams, 1944). Another 43 cases of hypertension were ascribed to renal disease; this was then, and for several subsequent years, the commoner cause of hypertension in this hospital. Cerebrovascular disease and angina were still considered to be very rare and malignant hypertension was not reported in an East African until 1953.

In 1958 and 1961 Williams (1969) (Table 1.1) conducted blood pressure surveys of Kikuyu men and women aged 20–80 years in the rural communities of Kiambu and Fort Hall in the Kenya highlands. Systolic blood pressure rose in older age groups in men and women, more in women than in men; diastolic blood pressure did not rise with age in either sex, but fell in most of the oldest age groups.

In 1963 Shaper and Saxton (1969) conducted a large blood pressure survey of 900 persons living in a rural community near Kampala, the capital of Uganda (Table 1.1). Two-thirds were local Ganda, a tribe that had been much acculturated from the beginning of the century. Both Ganda men and women had blood pressure rising steeply with age; they had similar levels and the same prevalence of hypertension as American white men and women. Ganda men and women were considerably lighter in body weight than American white subjects. One-third of the Uganda rural community were migrant labourers of many different tribes; they had been acculturated for fewer years and less in degree than the Ganda. These labourer groups had almost no rise of systolic or diastolic blood pressure with age. Dietary data in this survey were scanty and salt intakes were not assessed. Finally it was concluded that body weight had not influenced blood pressure levels in these two groups but that unspecified environmental factors must have operated to produce the different patterns of blood pressure changes with age.

Cerebrovascular disease 1940–70

Cerebrovascular disease (CVD) is the first arterial disease of clinical significance to emerge in Africans following acculturation (Walker, 1975). CVD was a rare disease in Ugandans in the 1940s. At Mulago hospital, Kampala, Muwazi and Trowell (1944) reported that '. . . we doubt if we have ever seen a case' of CVD due to essential hypertension: not a single case had been diagnosed in 269 consecutive neurological inpatients. Davies (1948b) reviewed the reports of 3000 Ugandan necropsies, those of the preceding 15 years at Mulago hospital; only 4 had died of cerebral haemorrhage, another 6 from essential hypertensive heart disease and one from coronary thrombosis.

Some 12 years later the second review of 700 consecutive Ugandan neurological admissions to Mulago hospital reported that 11 per cent had hypertensive CVD (Hutton, 1956). After the lapse of another 14 years the third review of 600 consecutive Ugandan neurological admissions to the same hospital reported that 34 per cent had hypertensive CVD (Billinghurst, 1970). Hypertension was considered to be the commonest cause of death in this series of neurological inpatients; it was specially common in elderly Ganda men.

Only a small proportion of these elderly Uganda patients die in hospital because relatives ask that an old man with an incurable disease be taken home to die. In young persons admitted to many tropical Africa hospitals the most important cause of severe and fatal hypertension is chronic renal disease, especially glomerulonephritis; these cases therefore often predominate in the necropsy records (Shaper, 1972).

Cardiovascular disease in East Africa and in South Africa in the 1970s

As already pointed out (page 4), it is not necessary to produce detailed evidence that essential hypertension has become a very common disease in recent years in the East Africans of Kenya, Uganda and Tanzania. Vaughan (1977) stated in a recent review that in the East African hospitals of these three countries essential hypertension accounted for 'something like 40 to 60 per cent' of the cardiovascular disease hospital diagnoses. During the years 1960–80 many articles had been published in the *East African Medical Journal* reporting the frequency of essential hypertension and recording some of its manifestations. For instance Awan *et al.* (1974) stated that essential hypertension was the commonest cause of congestive heart failure in the Kenyatta National hospital, Nairobi, and caused much hypertensive retinopathy. This university hospital had replaced the old Native Civil hospital wherein only 40 years before neither Jex-Blake (1934) nor I could find one case among the living nor Vint (1936–37) one case among the dead.

Even in Nairobi no one has produced figures that equal those found among South African Bantu. Doctors in that country have produced evidence that essential hypertension is '. . . an emerging disease among (South African) urbanized Blacks' and the second commonest cause of death in urbanized Bantu (Seedat *et al.* 1978). Many urban Bantu adults add sodium 300 mmol (salt 18 g) to their daily food (Seedat and Reddy, 1974). South African Bantu have been acculturated for a longer period of time and to a greater degree than Kenyans and Ugandans.

Salt in Kenya and Uganda diets

The Kikuyu diet during 1930 was typical of that eaten by other East African agricultural peasants living in an area of similar rainfall and altitude and was comparable to that of the subjects of the blood pressure surveys of Donnison (1929). The (British) Medical Research Council analysed fully the Kikuyu 1930 diet (Orr and Gilks, 1931). This was the first comprehensive analysis of an African diet before acculturation had much effect. It had been suspected that the meat-eating Masai had better nutrition than the Kikuyu who took little meat and milk. Neither tribe added shop salt to their food. It was, however, mere chance that this dietary survey coincided with the clinical and necropsy studies of blood pressure already mentioned.

The basis of the Kikuyu diet was home-grown lightly processed maize, millet, sweet potatoes, beans and plantains, a small amount of meat occasionally, negligible amounts of milk and almost no bought sugar or tea. An adult man ate on average 9·5 MJ/day (2250 kcal/d), derived from protein 19 per cent, fat 9 per cent, unrefined starch carbohydrate 72 per cent. Food was usually plentiful; there were two crops a year, land was almost always available for cultivation. Apart from a failure of one of the two yearly rainy seasons, there was seldom any shortage of food.

The MRC report also stated that '. . . a common practice throughout the Kikuyu Reserve is the preparation of a salt substitute by the burning of swamp plants . . . this custom (of adding the substitute) appears to be confined to the females and young children; men get little' (Orr and Gilks, 1931). Kikuyu men had a daily average intake of sodium 20 mmol (salt 1·3 g/d), Kikuyu women daily average intake of sodium was 65 mmol (salt 4·1 g/d). The report also noted that salt manufactured at Magadi in Masai territory was beginning to be sold in the Kikuyu Reserve and was already used in the Nairobi Native Civil hospital diets, from which adults had a daily average intake of sodium 225 mmol (salt 15 g/d), for salt ½ oz (14 g) had been added to the cereal food.

Large inland areas of Kenya and Uganda have no surface deposits of salt or salty earths; most tribes lived many hundreds of miles from the few dried-up saline lakes that lie scattered along one of the two arms of the Rift valley. The only large deposit of soda lay at Magadi, far towards the south, almost on the border between Kenya and Tanzania; manufacture of table salt started there in the 1920s. Previously Masai had roamed over the intervening grassy plains so that other tribes had little access to the Magadi soda deposits.

In the first years of the *Kenya Medical Journal* (1924–30) several articles commented on the absence of added salt in Kenyan diets; it was therefore advocated that the practice of South Africa should be followed; therein mine labourer daily diets had salt ½ oz (14 g) added (Wilson, 1925–26). Early administrators in Kenya and Uganda commented on the absence of salt in the diet of the Kavironda Bantu, examined by Donnison (1929) in his blood pressure survey: this tribe had therefore burnt water plants to provide a salt substitute (Johnston, 1902a).

In Uganda salt had always been difficult to obtain; it could be produced towards the distant Congo border from the saline deposits at Katwe or Kibero; these lay in the western arm of the Rift valley lakes. The porters who prepared the coarse salt could not be paid in currency; they received salt by way of wages, then carried it 200 miles eastward to the Ganda kingdom, wherein 'salt was a great luxury' (Roscoe, 1911). This salt did not travel furthest east across the Nile into eastern Uganda or across the Kenya border to the Kavirondo Bantu.

Salt intakes were certainly very low in almost all areas of inland Kenya and Uganda in the early decades of the twentieth century. Salt intakes started to rise in many areas in the 1920s and 1930s, first in urban areas and more among acculturated ethnic groups such as the Ganda in Uganda, and later in the Kikuyu in Kenya. This occurred when Magadi shop salt became available, and metal currency, transport and shops increased and dietary habits were changed in institutions wherein diets were supervised by Europeans, who were accustomed to high salt diets.

Sodium intake and lifelong low blood pressure

The relationship of lifelong low blood pressure in a community to a low sodium intake is becoming progressively clarified. Western man consumes daily sodium 100–300 mmol (salt 6–18 g) (Meneely and Battarbee, 1976a). On the other hand primeval herbivorous food-gatherer man, before he learned to kill large animals, or add salt to his food, ate daily sodium 10 mmol (salt 0·6 g/d). This still constitutes the assessed adult sodium requirement of man (Meneely and Battarbee, 1976a). Inherited physiological mechanisms were firmly encoded during the million or more years of food-gathering. Hunter-food-gatherer man, even if he derived half his energy from flesh foods, ate daily sodium 16 mmol (salt 1 g/d). Recently a food-gatherer group in Tanzania, the Hadza, were examined; blood pressure did not rise with age either in men or in women; they had just become peasant agriculturalists but added no salt to their food although they lived on the shores of a dried-up saline Rift valley lake (Barnicot *et al.*, 1972). They drank brackish water but even among them sodium intake would not have exceeded 65 mmol/d (salt 4 g/d) and was probably far less.

Ethnic groups who do not add common salt to their food have lifelong low blood pressure; *no exception to this generalization has been traced*. This is true of African Bushmen and Pygmies, Brazilian Indians, Australian Aborigines, Eskimos, Polynesians and Melanesians, also Kenya highland Africans (Table 1.1). Cattle-keeping Kenya Samburu and Masai, who take much sodium-rich milk, meat and blood, may have daily average sodium intakes rising to 50–70 mmol (salt 3–4 g/d) when energy intakes are high; these populations also have lifelong low blood pressure. However, when young Samburu nomads were drafted into the army and began to eat salted food the daily average sodium intake rose to 240 mmol (salt 15 g/d), then blood pressure levels rose significantly in the third year of military service (Shaper *et al.*, 1969). Like many Western men they were eating 24 times the sodium requirements of man.

Tobian (1979) has stated that communities eating an adult daily average sodium intake of less than 60 mmol (salt 4 g) have lifelong low blood pressure, but he cited only three ethnic groups, Polynesians, Melanesians and Samburu. Gliebermann (1973) produced evidence of comparable low intakes and lifelong low blood pressure in other groups.

Genetically controlled salt sensitivity varies considerably in animals and in man. It is suggested by way of an hypothesis of lifelong low blood pressure in man that almost all men can tolerate daily sodium intakes of 45–60 mmol (salt 3–4 g). Above this level of sodium intake an increasing proportion of salt-sensitive subjects develop blood pressure rising with age. Above yet another level of increased daily intake, say sodium 90–120 mmol (salt about 6–8 g) almost all salt-sensitive subjects develop blood pressure levels rising with age and a fair proportion develop essential hypertension, especially if they are overweight. Above this level of sodium intake (sodium about 100 mmol, salt 6 g/d) the development of essential hypertension depends much more on genetic salt sensitivity than on levels of sodium intake. This would explain why no correlation has been found in several groups of persons between sodium intakes in hypertensives and 'normotensives'.

Accessory aetiological factors

Obesity certainly raises blood pressure levels in persons eating high sodium diets, but there is no evidence that obesity in populations eating low sodium diets produces essential hypertension. Negative energy balance reduces blood pressure levels, but no one can survive indefinitely who remains in negative energy balance. Thus low energy diets cannot provide a permanent cure.

The psychological and socioeconomic stresses that accompany acculturation of peasants have been postulated to cause high blood pressure. On the other hand psychiatrists who have observed primeval peasant communities report that stress is common even in the least acculturated: they mourn frequent deaths even in the prime of life, fear evil spirits, dread charms, have much burning of their huts by personal enemies, and the murder rate is high (Carothers, 1953). Stress is there, but the pattern is different. Page (1979) found no correlation between the degree of acculturation and blood pressure levels in 8 Solomon island groups. He reported close correlation with sodium intakes in these islanders and outlined his studies of Gashgai nomads of Iran: they had remained quite unacculturated, but added much salt to their food, they also developed much hypertension.

Page (1979) therefore considered that low blood pressure populations '. . . had not yet been assimilated into the dominant Western civilization'. This will be only a matter of time, but for these unacculturated groups high blood pressure can be regarded as a Western disease. A comparable dietary change occurred in all other ethnic groups, usually many millennia ago, and strokes were commonly reported in middle-aged persons of many civilizations. Simple tools had made possible the preparation, transport and sale of salt: these were the mechanical harbingers of Western technology.

Essential hypertension treated by low sodium diet

Morgan *et al.* (1978) treated men with mild hypertension by advising a diet containing sodium 65–95 mmol/d (salt 4–6 g/d); they reported that 55 per cent slowly achieved normal diastolic blood pressure in spite of the fact that many of the patients did not appear to be eating sodium less than 95 mmol/d (salt 6 g/d), assessed by urinary excretion. Magnani *et al.* (1976) reported that 37 hypertensive patients treated by a diet containing daily sodium 48 mmol (salt 3 g) had as effective a reduction of blood pressure as a control group of 44 patients given hypotensive drugs, both groups treated for 15–21 months, but gave no details of the diet or of methods to check compliance.

Later in this book two medical centres report that the majority of their essential hypertension patients achieved normotension within a few weeks while eating a diet containing daily sodium less than 60 mmol (salt 4 g/d)

(Chapters 23 and 24). Many patients, previously treated with hypotensive drugs, were able to dispense with these drugs, others were able to receive a reduced dosage. The moderate reduction of energy in both diets probably accelerated the fall of blood pressure, but by itself would seldom convert essential hypertension to normotension. Other features, present in both therapeutic diets, require investigation. Both had a high potassium : sodium ratio and it has been postulated that this is protective (Meneely and Battarbee, 1976b). The protective action of polyunsaturated fats (Iacono *et al.*, 1975), and of cereal fibre (Wright *et al.*, 1979), features of one or other of the diets, await investigation.

Obesity emerges

Obesity in East Africans was rare in 1929 when I started medical work in Kenya. The late Sir Julian Huxley, a biologist of international repute, toured Kenya, Uganda and Tanganyika for 16 weeks in 1930; he recorded with amazement 'almost the only fat woman I saw in Africa' worked in the Nairobi brewery; he considered that beer might be fattening (Huxley, 1931). The theme of certain foods being fattening will recur in this chapter. At the present time the towns of East Africa contain many fat upper class Africans; their leaders seen on television are often grossly obese.

Slome *et al.* (1960) have recorded lifelong low body weight, falling after 30 years of age, among rural Zulu men and women of South Africa. Weight averaged 59 kg (130 lb) for rural Zulu men at 30 years, and rural Zulu women averaged 55 kg (120 lb) at that age; on the other hand urban Zulu men were 4·5 kg (10 lb) heavier at 30 years, and urban Zulu women had body weight rising until 50 years of age when it averaged 23 kg (50 lb) *more* than rural Zulu women. Comparable figures of lifelong low body weight, falling in middle-age, were recorded in Kenya Kikuyu rural men and women in 1929 (Orr and Gilks, 1931).

My interest was therefore aroused concerning the history of obesity. Obesity had apparently emerged as a *common* disorder in English upper social classes in the late eighteenth century (Trowell, 1975a). The glycosuria of diabetes was first reported in England, and in Europe, about the same time (page 24). Obesity and type II diabetes mellitus (page 24) are related diseases: in any community, they emerge, and prevalences increase, about the same period of time and always in upper social groups.

Hunter-gatherers

'The evidence is overwhelming that in some or many ways the control mechanism (of body weight) tends to break down in the affluent society'

(Margen, 1969). Garrow (1978) has summarized the modern literature on obesity and energy balance thus: 'Primitive man may have had an automatic pilot which regulated the amount of energy he spent in gathering food and the amount of primitive food he consumed to provide tolerable regulation of energy balance during his short life-span. Modern supermarket man has no such automatic faculty.'

An adult man, whether hunter-gatherer or supermarket man, consuming on average 1 per cent more energy per day than he expended would accumulate extra fat 1 kg/year: aged 30 years such a person might weigh nearly 30 kg (66 lb) more than someone who had been in long-term energy balance. Strong evolutionary pressures were at work in hunter-gatherers: if the man consistently ate too little he would become weak and unable to hunt; if he consistently ate too much, even by only 1 per cent, excessive weight would prevent him from catching his prey and his wife from gathering her quota of plant foods. Also a fat man and a fat woman would not easily escape animal and human predators.

Hunter-gatherers obtain most of their food from plant sources. Data from 58 contemporary hunting and gathering groups (Lee, 1968) reported that a plentiful and nutritionally adequate diet had been obtained in 2–3 hours' work a day, even less in certain circumstances (Sahlins, 1972). Animal foods supplied 25–35 per cent of the food; this was obtained by the men from hunting. Plant foods supplied 65–75 per cent of the food; this was gathered by women who stayed near the camp and also fed the children. If the diet of prehistoric hunter-gatherers resembled that of contemporary groups its approximate composition of energy was high protein 15–20 per cent, low fat 15–30 per cent, high unrefined starch (complex carbohydrates) 50–70 per cent, high fibre, no added milk, sugar, salt or alcohol. Those who have investigated hunter-gatherers state that it was the most successful and persistent adaptation man has ever achieved and that 'the biology of our species was created in that long gathering and hunting period' (Washburn and Lancaster, 1968). If the biology of the human species is adapted to the food and physical activity of hunter-gatherers and new diseases appear either in peasant agriculturalists or in modern man, these disorders should be regarded as possible maladaptations to a new environment. *This is the crux of this book.*

Modern methods of age assessment of contemporary hunter-gatherers show that life expectancy at birth is 22–29 years (Lozoff and Brittenham, 1977). Many therefore live until 30–39 years; they are old enough to display middle-aged obesity but this does not occur. Seven per cent of ! Kung African Bushmen were over 65 years of age, but all were slim (Truswell, 1977). The ancient misconception of the universal shortness of life in hunter-gatherers will not explain the absence of obesity at all ages among them. Obesity emerges as a new disease, rare in peasant agriculturalists, but common in modern society. Attention will therefore be directed towards two provoking suggestions of Garrow (1978): hunter-gatherers ate 'primitive food' and remained slim; modern man eats 'supermarket food' and often gets fat.

First agricultural revolution and peasant agriculturalists

The first Agricultural Revolution of the tenth millennium BC changed profoundly the sources of food supply, for men started to grow and store cereals; they ceased to be plant food-gatherers. The sources of mechanical energy however remained unchanged: these were human physical energy aided by domesticated animals (Cipolla, 1978). The common man was a peasant who grew and stored almost all his own food; he had little cash with which to buy other expensive foods, such as meat, milk, fat and oils. A few persons in the upper socioeconomic classes were able to purchase a more luxurious diet; some of these even became obese. These conditions prevail even today in many rural developing communities of Africa, Asia, South America and Oceania.

The composition of the diet of peasant agriculturalists even nowadays has changed only slightly from that of the hunter-gatherers. The protein content decreased moderately from about 15–30 per cent energy in hunter-gatherer diets to about 10–15 per cent in peasant agriculturalist diets. In terms of energy the starch foods (complex carbohydrates) increased slightly from about 50–70 per cent in most hunter-gatherer diets to about 60–75 per cent among peasant agriculturalists. Among the latter the starch foods remained lightly processed and they retained almost all of their original fibre, minerals and vitamins. Fat probably decreased from about 15–30 per cent energy in hunter-gatherer diets (unless they ate fat-storing polar animals) to about 10–15 per cent energy in the peasant diets.

Malnutrition among peasant agriculturalists reflects their poverty and lowly methods of food production and storage. If population density grows then infections increase and children suffer from protein-calorie malnutrition. Some undernutrition occurs fairly frequently at all ages, especially in poor social groups and at times of food shortage; severe famine may occur due to drought or some failure of the crops. It is extremely difficult to determine the prevalence of undernutrition among peasant agriculturalists even at the present time. Successive FAO Committees on Calorie Requirements have reduced their estimates of desirable energy intakes (FAO/WHO, 1973); previously inflated recommendations had exaggerated the reported prevalence of undernutrition in developing countries.

Poor developing peasant communities that are forced to rely unduly on a few cheap staple foods may develop specific vitamin and mineral deficiencies such as anaemia, xerophthalmia, beri-beri and pellagra, even goitre if soil and water contain little iodine. On the other hand metabolic and degenerative conditions, such as obesity, type II diabetes (page 22) and cardiovascular disease are far less common in developing rural peasant communities than in the Western developed communities. Table 1.2 offers an estimate of a British nutritionist (Miller, 1979) concerning the prevalence of malnutrition in developing communities and developed industrial Western communities at the present time. These figures are an informed guess, called a 'guestimate', but are based wherever possible by FAO/WHO surveys.

Although food shortages certainly occur in developing peasant rural communities, depending largely on population density and soil fertility, competent scientific observers have reported that where the population was not dense, the soil was fertile and two crops a year occurred, as in tropical countries, such as Uganda (Johnston, 1902b) and the Kenya Highlands (Orr and Gilks, 1931), body weight remained low throughout adult life. Their diet, resembling in its composition that of hunter-gatherers, and consumed *ad libitum*, protects against obesity. Obesity occurs almost exclusively in a few wealthy upper class peasants who purchase foods which are characteristic of more advanced technology.

Table 1.2   An estimate of the prevalence of malnutrition in the world in 1979[1]

	Developing communities (%)	Developed communities (%)
Obesity	3[2]	25
Heart disease[3]	2	30
Dental caries	10[4]	99
Undernutrition[5]	25	3
Anaemia[6]	30	5
Xerophthalmia	1	0
Total population (millions)	1750	1110

Source: Miller (1979), who commented:

[1] All figures are 'guestimates', but are based on modern surveys
[2] Increasing in urban areas
[3] Largely coronary heart disease in which malnutrition is one of many factors
[4] An Asian rate was cited, but it is impossible to quantify prevalence
[5] Almost certainly an overestimate
[6] Iron and folate deficiencies

Pastoralists

This summary of the diet and diseases of hunter-gatherers and peasant agriculturalists is based largely on a scheme presented by Truswell (1979) in the seventh edition of *Human Nutrition and Dietetics*. Another ethnic group, mentioned therein, are the pastoralists. They plant no crops, but follow their flocks of animals in arid grasslands; their diet is largely milk, meat and blood. Small amounts of plant foods and cereals are often obtained by trade with agricultural groups. Little is known about the nutrition of pastoralists, but serum cholesterol levels remain low in spite of high intakes of animal fat and cholesterol; fibre intakes remain low but some is taken in sour milk and in agricultural foods obtained by trading. Obesity remains rare, but may occur in women fattened for marriage, or for prestige after marriage, by large quantities of milk. The women may have little work to do in pastoral societies. Pastoralists appear well adapted to their traditional if unusual diet, one that has been consumed probably for several millennia.

Industrial Revolution and second Agricultural Revolution

The second Agricultural Revolution started in Europe towards the end of the eighteenth century (Cipolla, 1978). It was the first manifestation of modern technology as applied to agriculture. The Industrial Revolution occurred a century later in urban factories. The Agricultural Revolution employed methods of crop rotation and fertilizers, it improved both farm machinery and animal husbandry. It enabled the upper classes to become more wealthy, for trade prospered. It increased and altered the food supply. Animal products increased in the diet; no longer were many beasts slaughtered in the autumn; meat, butter and milk could be consumed throughout the year by those who could afford it. Overseas trade brought increased supplies of coffee, tea and chocolate (often drunk) and sugar intakes began to increase, likewise alcoholic beverages.

The English National Portrait Gallery, wherein portraits date back to the fourteenth century, clearly portrays that gross obesity, previously very rare even in the nobility, suddenly became extremely common in the upper social classes towards the end of the seventeenth century and even more so in the eighteenth century. Portraits even of young men and women usually portrayed protruding tummies and large double chins (Trowell, 1975a).

The Industrial Revolution soon followed in the nineteenth century and spread rapidly throughout Europe, North America and the urban areas of other continents. Machinery on the farms, mills and factories in the town, also improved methods of transport, all began to use for the first time new powerful sources of energy, and these were plentiful: coal, coal gas, petrol and electricity. The production of goods and wealth rose more rapidly than ever before. This permitted major changes in the production, storage, and processing of all foods. The milling of cereals permitted the production of more refined products so that white wheat flour contained less fibre and vitamins. Machines made possible the production of margarine and vegetable oils so that consumption of fats rose considerably; butter and milk consumption also increased. Sugar imports rose. Salt, sugar and fat were incorporated increasingly into many foods, snacks and drinks; these measures increased palatability and encouraged increased consumption of energy foods.

At the same time the consumption of all starch foods, chiefly bread and potatoes, fell dramatically, so that intakes of their associated fibre decreased for two reasons, less starch food and less fibre in this food. On the other hand, the consumption of vegetables and fruit steadily increased. Physical exertion decreased considerably as the machines replaced human exertion. The mounting production of goods created affluence; this spread slowly but eventually to all social classes in the industrial countries of the Western world. People began to be able to purchase almost all foods that they desired. Alcoholic drinks often increased. New habits such as cigarette smoking increased, but not before the twentieth century. Apart from the regular meals people began to use snacks and drinks for comfort feeding, thereby finding solace from the stress of living as a sensitive educated person in modern urban society. The advertisement of food and drink, and their subtle palatability, encouraged increased consumption.

In the present century and even before this date overweight seems to have increased in Britain and the United States with successive surveys (Garrow, 1978). This is exemplified by a report from the United States of men aged 30–34 years and 5 foot 8 inches (1·67 m) in height: in 1863 they averaged 148 lb (66 kg), but weight rose steadily so that in 1963 they averaged 170 lb (77 kg) (Van Itallie, 1978).

Modern dietary change

The development of the Industrial Revolution has permitted and encouraged the diets of Western countries to change considerably during the past 100 years 1880–1980. The changes in the Welsh rural diet from 1870 to 1977 (Hughes and Jones, 1979) are one example (Table 1.3). Antar *et al.* (1964), and others, have reported comparable changes in the United States diet during the same period of time. The 1870 Welsh rural diet resembled in many respects the 1970 diets in rural developing peasant communities of Africa, Asia and South America (Fig. 1.1). During the past hundred years the total protein content of the Welsh rural diet has not changed. In terms of energy percentages fats and oils have increased from 25 to 42, and the proportion of polyunsaturated fatty acids compared to total fat has decreased considerably; sugar has increased from 4 to 17, and cholesterol from 139 mg/d to 517 mg/d. On the other hand the percentage of starch foods has decreased considerably from 60 to 30. Cereal foods have become more refined so that, although vegetables and fruit have increased, dietary fibre average intakes have decreased from 65 g/d to 21 g/d. Other rural diets in Britain may not have changed quite as much as that of rural Wales.

Table 1.3   Dietary changes in rural Wales 1870–1977

	1870	1977
	energy %	
Protein	11	11
Fats, total	25	42
PUFA[1]	19	9
Sugar	4	17
Starch[2]	60	30
Dietary fibre (g/d)	65	21
Cholesterol (mg/d)	139	517

[1] Polyunsaturated fatty acids present in total fats
[2] Bread 903 g/d, potatoes 490 g/d, oatmeal 50 g/d

Source: Hughes and Jones (1979)

The Industrial Revolution has spread to developing countries during the present century. The composition of the traditional rural peasant diet is being slowly transformed until it begins to resemble the composition of modern Western diets. The degree of dietary change correlates with the degree of westernization, and with affluence. This is illustrated in Fig. 1.1, the data being derived from the FAO/WHO (1973) appraisal of food consumption in 85 countries of the world correlated with income, assessed as the gross domestic product per head per year, recorded in US dollars and shown in a logarithmic scale along the ordinate; the percentage of energy provided by various nutrients is shown along the abscissa. The main change occurs in the character of the energy foods: these are predominantly high fibre starch foods in poor developing countries (75 per cent) but are fibre-free fats and sugar (60 per cent) in affluent developed countries.

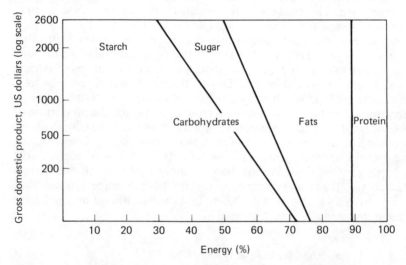

Fig. 1.1   Energy derived from starch and sugar carbohydrates, fats and protein in 85 countries recorded as percentages of energy in relation to income recorded as US dollars per head per year in 1962 in a logarithmetic scale (FAO/WHO, 1973)

Urban slums

Population pressure has forced many rural peasants to migrate in recent years to the modern towns of Asia, South America and Africa. Shanty towns grow to a fantastic size and unemployment may be common in these vast urban slums. An enormous social problem has arisen, compounded by violence and alcoholism. Overcrowding into insanitary conditions promotes an increase of infection and a high infant mortality rate.

The diet usually deteriorates; undernutrition may occur at all ages and protein-calorie malnutrition is rife among young children. Only the cheapest foods are eaten in a diet that is a mixture of the common traditional foods and low-priced Western food products. Refined cereals tend to replace less processed foodstuffs, so that cereal fibre intakes may drop to one-fifth, as occurred in urban South African Bantu (Lubbe, 1971). Sugar being cheap and tasty increases considerably, also fats if wages permit, but these rarely rise to Western levels.

Obesity then often becomes common, especially in women. It is regarded as a sign of health, prestige and beauty. This has been described in former years among the US black women, and nowadays in South African Bantu (Slome *et al.*, 1960) and in the urban shopkeepers of Asian towns. The prevalence of diabetes mellitus type II (page 25) increases. Salt is added to render the food more tasty, so that intakes may be high, and hypertension and strokes increase. Ischaemic heart disease, however, remains uncommon even in the presence of either diabetes or hypertension.

Aetiology of obesity

It is postulated that the essential cause of the high prevalence of obesity in the modern world has been the change in the character of the energy foods. Over half of the energy in the diet of hunter-gatherers and peasant agriculturalists came from high fibre starch foods; these diets even when consumed *ad libitum* accompanied lifelong low body weight. At least two-thirds of the energy in modern Western diets comes from fibre-free fat and sugar, also low fibre cereal products (Fig. 1.1). Doubtless many other psychological and social factors operate to increase the prevalence and severity of obesity in susceptible genotypes and others are completely protected by their inheritance.

This hypothesis has by no means been proved. Most physicians, however, advise obese patients to change their dietary pattern by decreasing fibre-free fat and sugar, both of which also increase palatability, also to change to high fibre starch foods (complex carbohydrates) and to increase fibre-containing vegetables and fruit (Craddock, 1978). Natural dietary fibre decreases absorbed energy by about 2 per cent (Southgate and Durnin, 1970); most of this unabsorbed energy is passed in the bulky stools. Heaton (1973) has summarized numerous reasons which explain how fibre-depleted energy foods (fat, sugar and refined cereals) might encourage obesity, but experimental proof is still scanty. Van Itallie (1978) concluded his review by stating 'The hypothesis that dietary fibre can protect against obesity therefore deserves further testing.' It seems likely that meals are terminated as a result of satiety signals arising from the gastrointestinal tract, principally from the small intestine. Dietary fibre, being unabsorbed, provides bulk in both the small and large intestine.

In the modern world psychological and social factors operate in the creation of many attitudes concerning feeding so that comfort-feeding, nibbling and drinking become firmly established habits. In the modern world many lose weight and remain slim only if they are very strongly motivated and receive sound medical advice (Garrow, 1978). It is extremely difficult to modify the food habits of a lifetime. Alcoholic drinks also encourage obesity.

Diabetes mellitus emerges

'Environmental factors sometimes account for differences as great as tenfold in the incidence of diabetes.' (West, 1979)

Diabetes rare in Kenya in 1930s

In 1933 the medical staff of the Nairobi African Hospital, Kenya, met to examine a patient having a disease not seen in an African by most doctors attending the meeting. I had not encountered diabetes mellitus since starting work at the 150-bed hospital some three years previously. During those years the non-fasting urines of all patients admitted to the separate African, Indian and European hospitals of Nairobi were sent for examination to the Medical Research Laboratory. The rarity of glycosuria in Africans, but not in other ethnic groups, over a period of several years received special mention in the annual reports (Harvey, 1951). In 1933 the patient was a fat African nurse-maid (ayah) living with her British employer. This coincidence supported the hypothesis that diabetes was a disease of civlization, rare among the relaxed Africans, but common among Europeans and Indians who were subjected to the psychosomatic stresses of civilized life. Four years later Donnison (1937), a colleague of mine in the Kenya Medical Service, wrote *Civilization and Disease*, in which he elaborated this hypothesis.

In East Africa in the 1930s obesity was rarely seen in Africans (page 14). Nowadays there are many obese Africans in all urban areas of East Africa and a large diabetes clinic at all town hospitals. This led me to examine the history of diabetes mellitus to see if the disease had been rare in other countries and subsequently had become common and whether this had paralleled the emergence of obesity as a common disorder (Trowell, 1975a).

No description of diabetes mellitus in ancient Greece and Rome

Medical historians are of two varieties. Most describe the discoveries of single individuals, on the other hand a few historians examine critically the growth of knowledge concerning specific diseases. The former group consider that diabetes mellitus was first described by Aretaeus, a physician in Alexandria in the second century AD. He was certainly the first to use the Greek term 'diabetes', often translated as 'siphon'. All historians state that he wrote that diabetes was 'fortunately rather rare'. Galen, the greatest medical authority in the Roman empire, lived in the second century AD; he borrowed the new term from Aretaeus and he recorded only two cases of diabetes during his many years of medical work in Rome and other cities. On the other hand another medical historian, Henschen (1966), considered that the medical literature of the ancient Mediterranean countries had always described diabetes insipidus, never diabetes mellitus, for 'none of these writers says a word about (urinary) sugar . . . (and) in the Hippocratic collection there is no account of the disease'. Aretaeus and Galen described clearly diabetes insipidus thus: 'he cannot be stopped drinking . . . thirst unquenchable . . . never stop making urine'. This passed through the body as through a siphon; hence the name of the disease. This is not a description of diabetes mellitus: it fits diabetes insipidus.

Avicenna (AD 980–1037), a famous Arab physician in Iran, clearly described diabetes mellitus and the 'residue of honey' in the urine. He did not mention how many diabetic patients he had encountered.

Not recorded by urinoscopy during the Middle Ages

Greek and Roman physicians in ancient times, and the physicians of the Middle Ages, attached great importance to a careful inspection of the patient's urine. This custom of urinoscopy was followed in England during the years of the Renaissance until it declined in the seventeenth century. Many medical manuals were published therefore during the Middle Ages and the reign of the Tudors concerning the colour and physical characteristics of the urine (Copeman, 1960). In spite of all this study of the urine during a period of 2000 years (BC 400 to AD 1600), no European physician is known to have described the characteristic features of the urine of diabetes mellitus: large in volume, watery, pale in colour, having an aromatic smell. Many a flask of the patient's urine must have lain for hours awaiting its inspection by the visiting physician, but no one noticed the simple fact, commented on repeatedly by sweepers in tropical hospitals, that ants and other insects swarm into a flask of sugary urine which, if spilled onto the floor, dogs lick up. All these points were vividly described by Indian physicians 2000 years ago.

Sugary urine recorded in India and China

The history of diabetes mellitus in India and China is completely different from that of the ancient world of Greece and Rome and of Europe prior to the seventeenth century. *Madhumeh* (honey urine) was graphically described as a *common* disease by more than one Indian physician, notably Charaka (*c* AD 150). About 2000 years ago it was written 'the urine is seen to be limp and sweet as honey . . . sticky . . . attraction of ants by the urine'. Tulloch (1962a) cited these words from two ancient Indian physicians. In his consideration of the history of the disease he did not even mention the dubious descriptions of the Greek and Roman authors, but then he, like the Indian physicians, and the present author, had worked in the tropics.

The sweet urine of diabetes mellitus was clearly described in China in the seventh century AD (Gwei-Djen and Needham, 1967).

Emergence of diabetes mellitus in seventeenth-century England

Willis in 1673 was the first doctor in modern Europe to describe, however briefly, that diabetic urine tasted 'wonderfully sweet as if imbued with honey or sugar'. A century later Dodson in 1776 proved by fermentation that a sugar-like substance was present in the urine in diabetes mellitus. Small wonder that soon afterwards Frank in 1794 was able to distinguish the difference between diabetes mellitus and diabetes insipidus, and became the discoverer of the latter disease (Singer and Underwood, 1962). As discussed previously (page 18), there is a good deal of evidence that obesity, present in a few aristocrats of ancient Egypt, Greece and Rome, was uncommon in the English aristocracy until it appeared among them as a common disorder in the eighteenth century. Obesity and diabetes mellitus (type II) usually emerge together about the same time in any community that is becoming affluent, wherein the wealthy are able to consume more fat, oil, sugar, meat, wine and beer, also refined cereals, such as white bread and white rice. Little is known concerning the ancient date when, in India and China, rice began to be hulled to produce brown rice, then milled to produce unpolished, low fibre white rice, finally polished to produce polished white rice. Boiled white rice contains far less dietary fibre than white wheat bread. Perhaps this explains why diabetes mellitus emerged as a common disease at an early date in India and China.

Designated a Western disease

Tulloch (1962a) reviewed diabetes in the tropics. He showed that its prevalence rates probably differ considerably from one tropical community to another, but his data were limited to hospital admissions and clinic attendances. Standardized diabetes prevalence surveys in the various ethnic groups of South Africa, including rural and urban Bantu, led Jackson (1971), who conducted many of these surveys, to review the world epidemiology of this disease. He concluded that 'certainly the incidence of diabetes is likely to increase with urbanization, or as the complexity of civilization takes hold of any racial group'. When more surveys in South Africa confirmed this prophecy, Jackson (1978) stated 'certainly changes in life style, associated with urbanization and the adoption of "Western civilization", have produced manifold increases in the incidence of diabetes'.

Diabetes mellitus common in urban Kenyans in 1970s

Diabetes prevalence surveys have not been conducted in East Africa. Hospital admissions, usually for some complication of diabetes such as coma, have increased considerably. Only two African diabetes patients per year were treated in *all* Kenya hospitals during the years 1926–30 (Trowell, 1960); that was the period during which I arrived in Kenya and heard that it was a rare disease. Seventeen African diabetes patients were admitted to the Kenyatta National Hospital, Nairobi, during 1955 (Tulloch, 1962b), but 132 patients during 1975 (Mngola *et al.*, 1977). Increased medical facilities and a larger population partially explain the rising number of patients, but probably there has been an increased prevalence of diabetes mellitus in Kenyans comparable to that which has occurred in South African Bantu. Sophisticated prevalence surveys in South Africa have reported increased incidence of diabetes associated with westernization of the diets. Available evidence suggests that diabetes mellitus emerged slowly in East Africans in the 1920s and 1930s, specially in urban communities.

Varieties of diabetes and their treatment

Diabetes mellitus (DM) is a collection of heterogenous syndromes. The National Institutes of Health of the United States has recently classified these into four main varieties (National Diabetes Data Group, 1979). Type I, insulin-dependent DM, was formerly termed juvenile DM but it may occur at any age; insulin is essential and patients are prone to ketosis. It should be added that type I DM is a very rare condition in the *young children* of many tropical communities (Tulloch, 1962c), also rare in Japanese children (page 345). Type II, non-insulin-dependent DM, usually but not always occurs in the obese; this was formerly termed maturity-onset DM, but it occurs -occasionally in children. In both type I and type II DM genetic and environmental factors operate. A large change in the incidence or prevalence of any variety of DM in a defined population is due to changed environmental factors.

Impaired glucose tolerance (IGT) has also been defined by the US group, already mentioned, in terms of an abnormal oral glucose tolerance test. This variety (IGT) was called formerly borderline or subclinical diabetes. IGT is very common in ageing Western populations, especially in those who are obese. It is said to be less common in ageing primeval populations (page 438). Since an arbitrary line separates IGT from DM much uncertainty remains concerning whether IGT is a pathological condition or is due to normal ageing. One study (O'Sullivan, 1979) reported that IGT had deteriorated slowly in certain selected US women, some of whom eventually developed DM. Most persons, however, who have IGT do not develop DM. Possibly IGT will come to be regarded as a risk factor of DM type II.

A hypothesis has been proposed that fibre-depleted starch foods (complex carbohydrates) are diabetogenic in susceptible phenotypes (Trowell, 1975b); also that a high intake of high fibre starch food is a protective factor and might prove beneficial in the treatment of diabetes (Trowell, 1978b). It is suggested therefore that type I and type II DM should be treated by a diet the composition of which resembles that of peasant agriculturalists who rarely develop either disease. This diet is low fat, low sucrose, high unrefined starch, high fibre. It has been called a high carbohydrate, high fibre diet (HCF diet) in the

United States. Anderson (Chapter 22) reports the regression of type II DM and decreased insulin requirements in type I diabetes in patients treated by HCF diets. Blood lipids also decrease during treatment. It is also suggested that persons having impaired glucose tolerance (IGT) should eat increased amounts of fibre-rich starch foods (complex carbohydrates).

The United States Senate Select Committee on Nutrition and Human Needs (1977) has recommended that the whole US population should double the consumption of complex carbohydrates (starch foods) and increase whole grain products, thereby increasing the dietary fibre intakes (page viii). This recommendation was based largely on evidence produced concerning coronary heart disease, obesity and dietary fibre: the question of diabetes received less consideration by this committee.

The epidemiology of diabetes mellitus in Africa and other tropical countries is complicated by the presence of malnutrition diabetes (McMillan and Geevarghese, 1979). This can be classified as secondary diabetes. It is associated with chronic pancreatitis caused probably by the ingestion of cyanide-containing food such as cassava. Another variety of secondary diabetes in Africa is associated with excessive deposits of iron in pancreas and liver caused probably by high intakes of iron from iron cooking pots and alcoholic beverages (West, 1978). Secondary diabetes is usually progressive and marked improvement by a change of diet cannot be expected.

Coronary heart disease emerges

All available evidence suggests that coronary heart disease (CHD) is the last major cardiovascular Western disease to emerge; the last gastro-intestinal disease to emerge is diverticular disease. The emergence of CHD in East Africans is most clearly documented. First, there was the stage of reported absence: Vint (1936–37) reported no CHD in the first thousand Kenyan autopsies. Second, there was the first report of CHD, made by a pathologist (Davies, 1948a, b); one Ganda woman among 2994 autopsies, dating from 1931 to 1946 at Makerere University Medical School, Uganda, had clear signs of myocardial infarction. Third, there was the first clinical report of CHD, a typical case in a middle-aged Ugandan High Court Judge who ate a partially westernized diet (Trowell and Singh, 1956). There has been usually a competition to report first cases of any Western disease in an East African: Ojiambo (1968) in Kenya and Nhonoli (1968) in Tanzania, reported first cases of CHD in these countries.

CHD risk factors and protective factors

CHD remains, even nowadays, an uncommon disease in South African blacks. Among the million Bantu of Johannesburg CHD death rates are only about 1–2 per cent of those in South African whites of similar age and sex (Chapter 18). It has proved difficult to explain the rarity of CHD in South African blacks in terms of recognized risk factors. Possibly these risk factors have not operated since childhood, but whatever the explanation, CHD is emerging very slowly in South African blacks. Seftel (1978) analysed five of the CHD 'risk factors in the Western way of death', as he termed it, both during childhood and adult life. He listed these Western risk factors in order of priority: affluence, little physical exercise, high fat, high cholesterol diets, and hyperlipidaemia. All these operated he considered less in blacks than in whites, and the former smoked only about half as many cigarettes as the latter.

Walker (1973), however, has pointed out that among the urban blacks in regular employment in Johannesburg, 45 per cent of those aged 30–39 years have serum cholesterol levels greater than 5·8 mmol/l (220 mg/dl) compared with 55 per cent in South African whites and Indians of similar age and sex, but there is far less CHD in blacks than in the other two communities. Hypertension is both common and severe in South African blacks but these hypertensive persons rarely develop CHD (Seedat and Pillay, 1976). Diabetes mellitus type II is fairly common in South African urban blacks but CHD and large-vessel atheromatous disease is rare among them (Seftel and Walker, 1966).

These remarkable anomalies might be explained either by protective ethnic genetic factors, but these have not been demonstrated in CHD, or by unrecognized environmental protective factors. A hypothesis was therefore proposed that a high consumption of starchy carbohydrate foods containing their full complement of dietary fibre appears to protect against CHD (Trowell, 1976). A high consumption of starch foods (complex carbohydrates) is usually accompanied by a low intake of fat, the latter being atherogenic. The low intake of fat, however, need not occur if energy intakes are high to provide for much physical activity. This occurred in South African urban blacks whose average daily intake was 17 MJ (4000 kcal/d), derived from starch 500 g, fat 125 g, of which animal fat was 105 g/d, and protein 126 g/d (Lubbe, 1971). The lightly refined maize (corn) meal eaten by urban blacks still contains a fair amount of dietary fibre: can this be a protective factor?

A few recent reports from Britain lend some support to this suggestion. Foster *et al* (1978) reported a higher prevalence (57 per cent) of diverticular disease among English myocardial infarct patients than among matched controls (25 per cent). Cereal fibre protects against diverticular disease. In a 10-year survey of CHD and diet in English men Morris *et al* (1977) reported that only 5 men in the high cereal fibre intake group developed CHD compared to 25 men in the low cereal fibre intake group, although serum cholesterol levels were similar in the two groups. Prospective studies are required and mechanisms identified before this hypothesis can be regarded as established.

In Chapter 23 (Diehl and Mannerberg) and Chapter 24 (Dodson and Humphreys) report the regression of angina and CHD risk factors of hyperlipidaemia, by increased exercise and a diet resembling that of peasant agriculturalists. More clinical trials, however, are required to establish the efficacy of these therapeutic measures. But if peasant agriculturalists rarely get CHD, why not try the effect of eating a similar diet?

References

Akinkugbe, O. O. (1972). *High Blood Pressure in the African*, 18. Churchill-Livingstone, Edinburgh

Antar, M. A., Ohlson, M. A. and Hodges, R. E. (1964). Changes in the retail market food supplies in the United States in the last seventy years in relation to the incidence of coronary heart disease, with special reference to dietary carbohydrates and essential fatty acids. *American Journal of Clinical Nutrition,* **14,** 169–179

Awan, A. W., Ojiambo, H. P., Ogada, T. and Gitau, W. (1974). Hypertensive retinopathy at Kenyatta National Hospital. *East African Medical Journal,* **51,** 304–320

Barnicot, N. A., Bennett, F. J., Woodburn, J. C., Pilkington, T. R. E. and the late Antonis, A. (1972). Blood pressure and serum cholesterol in the Hadza of Tanzania. *Human Biology,* **44,** 87–116

Billinghurst, J. R. (1970). The pattern of adult neurological admissions to Mulago Hospital, Kamrala, June 1966–May 1968. *East African Medical Journal,* **47,** 653–663

Carothers, J. C. (1953). *The African Mind in Health and Disease:* a study of ethno-psychiatry. World Health Organization, Geneva

Cipolla, C. M. (1978). *The Economic History of World Population*, seventh edition, 17. Penguin, Harmondsworth

Copeman, W. S. C. (1960). *Doctors and Disease in Tudor Times*, 118. Dawson, London

Craddock, D. (1978). *Obesity and its Management*, 13. Churchill-Livingstone, London

Davies, J. N. P. (1948a). Causes of sudden death in Africans. *East African Medical Journal,* **25,** 322–330

Davies, J. N. P. (1948b). Pathology of Central African natives. IX: Cardiovascular diseases. *East African Medical Journal,* **25,** 454–467

Donnison, C. P. (1929). Blood pressure in the African native. *Lancet,* **i,** 6–7

Donnison, C. P. (1937). *Civilization and Diseases*. Baillière, Tindall and Cox, London

Epstein, F. H. and Eckhoff, R. D. (1967). The epidemiology of high blood pressure—geographical distributions and etiological factors. In: *The Epidemiology of Hypertension*, 155–160. Editors J. Stamler, R. Stamler and T. N. Pullman. Grune and Stratton, New York

Food and Agriculture Organization/World Health Organization (1973). *Protein and Energy Requirements*, Technical Report Series No. 522, 20. WHO, Geneva

Foster, K. J., Holdstock, G., Whorwell, P. J., Guyer, P. and Wright, P. (1978). Prevalence of diverticular disease of the colon in patients with ischaemic heart disease. *Gut,* **19,** 1054–1056

Garrow, J. S. (1978). *Energy Balance and Obesity in Man*, second edition, 144. Elsevier, Amsterdam

Gliebermann, L. (1973). Blood pressure and dietary salt in human populations. *Ecology of Food and Nutrition,* **2,** 143–156

Gwei-Djen, L. and Needham, J. (1967). Records of disease in Ancient China. In: *Diseases in Antiquity*, 235. Editors D. Brothwell and A. T. Sandison. Thomas, Springfield

Harvey, D. (1951). *Records of the Medical Research Laboratory, Nairobi*, No. 9, cited by Trowell, H. C. (1960). *Non-Infective Disease in Africa*, 310. Edward Arnold, London

Heaton, K. W. (1973). Food fibre as an obstacle to energy intake. *Lancet*, **ii**, 1418–1421

Henschen, F. (1966). *The History of Diseases*, 195. Longmans, London

Hughes, R. E. and Jones, E. (1979). A Welsh diet for Britain? (Letter). *British Medical Journal*, **2**, 1145

Hutton, P. W. (1956). Neurological disease in Uganda. *East African Medical Journal*, **33**, 209–223

Huxley, J. (1931). *Africa View*, 162. Chatto and Windus, London

Iacono, J. M., Marshall, M. W., Dougherty, R. M. and Wheeler, M. A. (1975). Reduction in blood pressure associated with high polyunsaturated fat diets that reduce blood cholesterol in man. *Preventive Medicine*, **4**, 426–443

Jackson, W. P. U. (1971). Diabetes mellitus in different countries and different races. Prevalence and major features. *Acta Diabetologia Latina*, **7**, 361–401

Jackson, W. P. U. (1978). The genetics of diabetes mellitus. *South African Medical Journal*, **53**, 481–490

Jex-Blake, A. J. (1934). High blood pressure. *East African Medical Journal*, **10**, 286–300

Johnston, H. (1902a). *The Uganda Protectorate*, vol. 2, 745. Hutchinson, London

Johnston, H. (1902b). *Ibid.*, 98

Lee, R. B. (1968). What hunters do for a living, or, How to make out on scarce resources. In: *Man the Hunter*, 30–48. Editors R. B. Lee and I. DeVore. Aldine, Chicago

Lozoff, B. and Brittenham, G. M. (1977). Field methods of health and disease in pre-agricultural societies. In: *Health and Disease in Tribal Societies*. Ciba Foundation Symposium, 49 (new series), 49–67. Elsevier, Amsterdam

Lubbe, A. M. (1971). A comparative study of rural and urban Venda males. Dietary assessment. *South African Medical Journal*, **45**, 1289–1297

Magnani, B., Ambrosioni, E., Agosta, R. and Racco, F. (1976). Comparison of the effects of pharmacological therapy and a low-sodium diet on mild hypertension. *Clinical Science and Molecular Medicine*, **51**, 625S–626S

Margen, S. (1969). Energy balance with increasing weight. In: *Obesity*, 78. Editor N. Wilson. Davis, Philadelphia

McMillan, D. E. and Geevarghese, P. J. (1979). Dietary cyanide and tropical malnutrition diabetes. *Diabetes Care*, **2**, 202–208

Meneely, G. R. and Battarbee, H. D. (1976a). Sodium and potassium. In: *Nutrition Reviews' Present Knowledge in Nutrition*, fourth edition, 259–279. Nutrition Foundation, New York

Meneely, G. R. and Battarbee, H. D. (1976b). High sodium–low potassium environment and hypertension. *American Journal of Cardiology*, **38**, 768–785

Miller, D. S. (1979). Prevalence of nutritional problems in the world. *Proceedings of the Nutrition Society*, **38**, 197–205

Mngola, E., Radia, R. G. and Shah, M. V. (1977). Retrospective study of diabetic ketosis coma seen at Kenyatta National Hospital in Africans in 1975. *East African Medical Journal*, **54**, 593–594

Morgan, T., Adam, W., Gillies, A., Wilson, M., Morgan, G. and Carney, S. (1978). Hypertension treated by salt restriction. *Lancet*, **i**, 227–230

Morris, J. N., Marr, J. W. and Clayton, D. G. (1977). Diet and heart: a postscript. *British Medical Journal*, **2**, 1307–1314

Muwazi, E. M. K. and Trowell, H. C. (1944). Neurological disease among African natives of Uganda: a review of 269 cases. *East African Medical Journal*, **21**, 3–19

National Diabetes Data Group (1979). Classification and diagnosis of diabetes mellitus and other categories of glucose intolerance. *Diabetes*, **28**, 1039–1057

Nhonoli, A. M. (1968). Heart disease in Dar-es-Salaam. *East African Medical Journal*, **45**, 118–121

Ojiambo, H. (1968). Ischaemic heart disease in a Kenyan African. Case report and brief review of the literature. *East African Medical Journal*, **45**, 133–135

Orr, J. B. and Gilks, J. L. (1931). *Studies of Nutrition. The Physique and Health of Two African Tribes*. Medical Research Council Special Report Series, No. 155. His Majesty's Stationery Office, London

O'Sullivan, J. B. (1979). Prevalence and course of diabetes modified by fasting blood glucose levels: implications for diagnostic criteria. *Diabetes Care*, **2**, 85–90

Page, L. B. (1976). Epidemiological evidence on the etiology of human hypertension and its possible prevention. *American Heart Journal*, **91**, 527–534

Page, L. B. (1979). Salt and hypertension: epidemiology and mechanisms. In: *Hypertension. Determinants, Complications and Intervention*. The Fifth Hahnemann International Symposium on Hypertension, 1–11. Editors G. Onesti and C. R. Klimt. Grune and Stratton, New York

Peart, W. S. (1978). Mild hypertension. In: *Royal College of Physicians of London Advanced Medicine*, **14**, 87–93. Editor D. J. Weatherall. Pitman Medical, London

Roscoe, J. (1911). *The Baganda*, 438. London, Macmillan

Rose, G. and Barker, D. J. P. (1979). *Epidemiology for the Uninitiated*, 5. British Medical Association, London

Sahlins, M. (1972). *Stone Age Economics*. Aldine, Chicago

Seedat, Y. K. and Pillay, N. (1976). Rarity of myocardial infarction in African hypertensive patients (Letter). *Lancet*, **ii**, 46–47

Seedat, Y. K. and Reedy, J. (1974). A study of 1,000 South African non-white hypertensive patients. *South African Medical Journal*, **48**, 816–820

Seedat, Y. K., Seedat, M. A. and Nkomo, M. N. (1978). The prevalence of hypertension in the urban Zulu. *South African Medical Journal*, **53,** 923–927

Seftel, H. C. (1978). The rarity of coronary heart disease in South African Blacks. *South African Medical Journal*, **53,** 99–104

Seftel, H. C. and Walker, A. R. P. (1966). Vascular disease in South African Bantu diabetics. Clinical notes. *Diabetologia*, **2,** 286–290

Shaper, A. G. (1972). Cardio-vascular disease in the tropics. III. Blood pressure and hypertension. *British Medical Journal*, **3,** 805–807

Shaper, A. G., Leonard, P. J., Jones, K. W. and Jones, M. (1969). Environmental effects on the body build, blood pressure and blood chemistry of nomadic warriors serving in the army in Kenya. *East African Medical Journal*, **46,** 282–289

Shaper, A. G. and Saxton, G. A. (1969). Blood pressure and body build in a rural community in Uganda. *East African Medical Journal*, **46,** 228–245

Singer, C. and Underwood, E. A. (1962). *A Short History of Medicine*, second edition, 544. Clarendon Press, Oxford

Slome, G., Gampel, B., Abramson, J. H. and Scotch, N. (1960). Weight, height and skin fold thickness of Zulu adults in Durban. *South African Medical Journal*, **34,** 505–509

Southgate, D. A. and Durnin, J. V. (1970). Calorie conversion factors. An experimental reassessment of the factors used in the calculation of the energy value of human diets. *British Journal of Nutrition*, **24,** 517–535

Tobian, L. (1979). Interrelationships of sodium and hypertension. In: *Hypertension. Determinants, Complications and Intervention*. The Fifth Hahnemann International Symposium on Hypertension, 13–32. Editors G. Onesti and C. R. Klimt. Grune and Stratton, New York

Trowell, H. C. (1960). *Non-infective Disease in Africa*, 306. Edward Arnold, London

Trowell, H. (1975a). Obesity in the Western world. *Plant Foods for Man*, **1,** 157–165

Trowell, H. C. (1975b). Dietary-fiber hypothesis of the etiology of diabetes mellitus. *Diabetes*, **24,** 762–765

Trowell, H. (1976). Definition of dietary fiber and hypotheses that it is a protective factor in certain diseases. *American Journal of Clinical Nutrition*, **29,** 417–427

Trowell, H. (1978a). Hypertension and salt (Letter). *Lancet*, **i,** 204

Trowell, H. (1978b). Diabetes mellitus and dietary fiber of starchy foods. *American Journal of Clinical Nutrition*, **31,** S53–S57

Trowell, H. C. (1980). From normotension to hypertension in Kenyans and Ugandans 1928–78. *East African Medical Journal*, **57,** 167–173

Trowell, H. C. and Singh, S. A. (1956). A case of coronary heart disease in an African. *East African Medical Journal*, **33,** 391–394

Truswell, A. S. (1977). Diet and nutrition of hunter-gatherers. In: *Health and Disease in Tribal Societies*, Ciba Foundation Symposium 49 (new series), 213–226. Elsevier, Amsterdam

Truswell, A. S. (1979). Historical and geographic perspectives. In: *Human Nutrition and Dietetics*, seventh edition, 1–5. Editors S. Davidson, R. Passmore, J. F. Brock and A. S. Truswell. Churchill-Livingstone, Edinburgh

Tulloch, J. A. (1962a). *Diabetes Mellitus in the Tropics*, 2. Livingstone, Edinburgh

Tulloch, J. A. (1962b). *Ibid.*, 42

Tulloch, J. A. (1962c). *Ibid.*, 64

United States Senate Select Committee on Nutrition and Human Needs (1977). *Dietary Goals for the United States*, 12–13. US Government Printing Office, Washington

Van Itallie, T. B. (1978). Dietary fiber and obesity. *American Journal of Clinical Nutrition*, **31**, 543–552

Vaughan, J. P. (1977). A brief review of cardiovascular disease in Africa. *Transactions of the Royal Society of Tropical Medicine and Hygiene*, **71**, 226–231

Vaughan, J. P. (1978). A cardiovascular survey in rural Tanzania. *East African Medical Journal*, **55**, 380–388

Vint, F. W. (1936–37). Postmortem findings in the natives of Kenya. *East African Medical Journal*, **13**, 332–340

Walker, A. R. P. (1973). Studies bearing on coronary heart disease in South African populations. *South African Medical Journal*, **47**, 85–90

Walker, A. R. P. (1975). The epidemiological emergence of ischemic arterial diseases. *American Heart Journal*, **89**, 133–136

Washburn, S. L. and Lancaster, C. S. (1968). In: *Man the Hunter*, 303. Editors R. B. Lee and I. DeVore. Aldine, Chicago

West, K. W. (1978). *Epidemiology of Diabetes and its Vascular Lesions*, 334–336. Elsevier, New York

West, K. W. (1979). Introduction: Proceedings of the Kroc Foundation international conference on epidemiology of diabetes and its macro-vascular complications. *Diabetes Care*, **2**, 63–64

Williams, A. W. (1941–42). The blood pressure of Africans. *East African Medical Journal*, **18**, 109–117

Williams, A. W. (1944). Hypertensive heart disease in the native population of Uganda. *East African Medical Journal*, **21**, 328–335, 368–378

Williams, A. W. (1969). Blood pressure differences in Kikuyu and Samburu communities in Kenya. *East African Medical Journal*, **46**, 262–272

Wilson, C. J. (1925–26). Native diet: a lesson from Rhodesia. *Kenya Medical Journal*, **2**, 337–342

Wright, A., Burstyn, P. G. and Gibney, M. J. (1979). Dietary fibre and blood pressure. *British Medical Journal*, **2**, 1541–1543

2

Surgical diseases of the large bowel and other related diseases

Denis Burkitt

Emergence of Western diseases in sub-Saharal Africa

More information is available as to the emergence of characteristically Western diseases in sub-Saharal Africa than in most other parts of the world. Moreover the marked influence of Western culture, and of dietary customs in particular, in South African urban communities has resulted in new patterns of disease that are in contrast to those in rural communities still largely dependent on subsistence farming. Since authors of other chapters will describe the situation with regard to the emergence of these diseases in particular countries or population groups, the situation in sub-Saharal Africa as a whole will be used to illustrate the pattern of emergence of these diseases.

In this chapter diseases which are usually considered to belong to the province of the surgeon, with the exception of gallstones which are dealt with in Chapter 3, will be considered. They will be examined in the order in which they initially emerge or increase in prevalence in developing countries following impact with Western culture and technology.

These diseases include appendicitis, haemorrhoids, varicose veins, large bowel tumours, hiatus hernia, deep vein thrombosis, pelvic phleboliths and diverticular disease of the colon. It is significant that the order in which these diseases normally appear with increasing age in Western countries is the same as that in which they appear with passage of time in developing countries following impact with Western culture. This observation suggests that they may be in part the result of varying periods of exposure to similar environmental factors.

Doctors from 60 hospitals in 13 countries in sub-Saharal Africa replied to questionnaires asking for their impressions based on personal experience of the order of emergence of these diseases. All but four were convinced that a rise in the prevalence of appendicitis and haemorrhoids preceded that of varicose veins, and doctors in all five hospitals questioned in India were of the same opinion. All who replied to the questionnaire agreed that hiatus hernia, large bowel cancer and diverticular disease were among the latest of the characteristically Western diseases to increase in prevalence in developing countries (Burkitt, 1977).

Appendicitis

This is the first of the so-called Western diseases of primarily surgical interest to emerge in developing countries. In assessing the prevalence of this disease it is important to distinguish between acute appendicitis, which is probably always an obstructive phenomenon initially, and so-called chronic appendicitis, which is now considered a diagnosis of dubious validity. Whenever possible it is also important to distinguish between appendicectomy rates and the incidence of acute appendicitis verified by pathological reports.

Prevalence in rural Africa

All papers published prior to 1940 indicated the rarity of appendicitis in sub-Saharal Africa (Burkitt, 1975a).

Sir Albert Cook, the founder of Mengo Mission Hospital in Kampala, Uganda, in 1897 wrote in his memoirs in 1945 'Appendicitis is astonishingly rare in natives. Dr. Stones' [a colleague of his] 'recently searched among the carefully kept records of the hospital and among 47 211 in-patients found only 6 cases. This does not apply to Europeans and Indians in Uganda who frequently need apprendicectomy' (Cook, 1945). It is still possible to find hospitals in Africa in which doctors have worked for over 10 years without encountering a case of appendicitis.

There was no case of appendicities amongst 1000 consecutive Kenyan autopsies performed in Nairobi by Vint (1937).

In an attempt to ascertain the prevalence of acute appendicitis in mainly rural communities in sub-Saharal Africa, over 100 hospitals serving such communities were circulated monthly with a simple questionnaire asking for particulars on any patients seen with appendicitis and some other characteristically Western diseases. Of 96 rural hospitals reporting from 15 countries in Africa 74, that is 71 per cent, saw less than one case in a year. Only three saw over four cases, and on questioning it became evident that two of these hospitals were reporting patients who were not suffering from appendicitis, and one was including appendices that only contained worms. Eight of 14 hospitals serving mainly rural communities in the Indian subcontinent saw no case of appendicitis during a year when they were submitting monthly returns. Only one reported over three cases. The patients reported were almost invariably those whose contact with Western culture had led to the inclusion of Western-type foods in their diet.

Increasing prevalences in urban communities

During the past 25 years the number of patients with acute appendicitis admitted annually to large urban hospitals throughout sub-Saharal Africa has risen in most instances from less than 5 to over 50 a year. For example, in 1952 only two cases of appendicitis were admitted annually to the large university teaching hospital in Kampala, Uganda (Burkitt, 1952).

L. Oluminde (personal communication, 1976) has pointed out that whereas appendicectomies accounted for 18 per cent of abdominal emergencies admitted to the Lagos Teaching Hospital in the period 1957–61, they accounted for no less than 43 per cent by 1974. In summarizing he stated that '. . . acute appendicitis, which 50 years ago was extremely rare in Africa, was the most common cause of acute abdomen encountered'. A similar experience has been reported from Ghana (Badoe, 1967). Whereas in the 1940s and '50s only 5–10 cases were admitted annually to Korle Bu Teaching Hospital in Accra, in twelve months of 1959–60 some 70 appendicectomies were performed, all for acute appendicitis; during twelve months of 1965–66 another 130 appendicectomies had been performed. During this period a further 65 patients were treated conservatively and another 14 had their abscesses drained. Even following this increase the prevalence of appendicitis in Ghana was still much lower than in Britain. It was estimated that in the former it was 2·2 per 10 000 of the population per year and in the latter 30·9 per 10 000.

It must be noted that even in South African townships in which food of Africans has been influenced towards Western dietary customs more than elsewhere in the continent, the prevalence of appendicitis remains considerably lower than it is in white communities (Walker *et al.*, 1979).

Kakande *et al.* (1978) reviewed medical records at Mulago Hospital, Kampala, for the six years 1970–75 inclusive of all patients admitted and subsequently diagnosed as appendicitis. Of the 241 cases admitted, 86 (36 per cent) were diagnosed finally as acute appendicitis, an average of 6 cases of acute appendicitis per year. He comments that of the 67 appendicitis patients whose occupation was known 26 (39 per cent) were students, and that the majority of all the patients were urban or semi-urban dwellers, whereas the majority of the population of Buganda were rural.

Osman (1974) traced the increase in prevalence of appendicitis in the Sudan by comparing the relative number of cases admitted with those of diseases, such as hernia, which did not change with alterations of lifestyle. There was a steady increase in the prevalence of appendicitis from 1928 to 1931, then four times as many inguinal hernias as cases of appendicitis were admitted, but in recent years the ratio had been reversed. Osman emphasized that whereas appendicitis was still rare in tribal situations it had become increasingly common among more westernized Sudanese.

When appendicitis first emerges in a country most patients are adults. This pattern is beginning to change in Nigeria: Taiwo *et al.* (1977) reported 46 cases of appendicitis in children between the ages of 1 and 13 years in the 8-year period 1963–71. In view of the fact that over 13 000 children were admitted to the Paediatric Hospital during this period the condition was still relatively rare there in comparison with European countries.

The relationship between the prevalence of appendicitis and diet was demonstrated by the observations that in at least two situations during the 1939–45 war appendicitis began to appear for the first time amongst African troops after they were supplied with British army rations when they were attached to British regiments (Burkitt, 1975a).

Pathological features and postulated pathogenesis

The pathological changes in acute appendicitis are almost invariably generalized within, and confined to, the part of the appendix that is distal to a more or less well-defined line of demarcation between normal and diseased tissue. This suggests that the initial lesion is an obstruction, beyond which pressures build up and deprive the mucosa of its blood supply. This in turn paves the way for bacterial invasion and subsequent inflammation. This is the only concept of the pathogenesis of appendicitis that is consistent with the pathological, clinical and epidemiological features of the disease. For instance, the first clinical manifestation of acute appendicitis is intermittent *central* abdominal pain due to obstruction.

If it is agreed that appendicitis is usually, if not always, the result of lumen obstruction, what causes the obstruction? The most commonly demonstrated cause is the impaction of a faecolith, an unusually desiccated and consequently hard particle of faecal material. This has been observed, however, only in about 10 per cent of cases of acute appendicitis (Horton, 1977; Johnson, 1978). It has been postulated that in other cases the obstruction may be caused by exaggerated muscle contraction occasioned by the presence of solid faecal particles in the lumen, which are more difficult to expel than are the semi-fluid contents which are normal in this part of the gut. The situation may be analogous to that in the sigmoid colon in which excessive contracture of circular muscle can occlude the whole lumen of the colon and then generate pressures sufficient to force diverticula of mucosa through the muscle wall (Painter, 1975). Evidence is accumulating which suggests that appendicitis occurs frequently only in populations in which solid faecal particles are commonly present in the lumen of the appendix, and it may be that herein lies a clue to the causation of the disease. Factors which contribute to the presence of firm small faecal masses within the large bowel are probably similar to those which contribute to the presence of solid faecal material in the appendix. This is due to excessive absorption of water from the gut in the absence of sufficient fibre to retain it.

Haemorrhoids

It is difficult to estimate with an accuracy the prevalence of haemorrhoids in a community. The diagnosis is imprecise and liable to include other anal conditions. Even the previously accepted nature of the disease has recently been challenged, for Thomson (1975) has provided convincing evidence that the concept of haemorrhoids being varicosities of anal veins, analogous to the varicose veins in the legs, is no longer tenable. It appears that they should be viewed rather as a prolapse of vascular submucosal anal cushions, which in their natural position and size are normal, and not pathological structures encircling the anal canal. These anal cushions have the function of maintaining faecal continence.

The frequency of complications of a disease is usually related to its overall prevalence and these are sometimes more readily recognized than is the uncomplicated disease. An attempt was therefore made to assess the frequency of haemorrhoids in sub-Saharal African populations by enquiring for particulars of any patients seen with either bleeding or prolapsed piles. Monthly returns from 77 mainly rural hospitals in sub-Saharal Africa indicated on average that less than 3 patients with bleeding or prolapsed haemorrhoids were diagnosed annually in each hospital (Burkitt, 1975b). This suggests a very much lower prevalence of the disorder than that observed in Western countries.

With a disease occurring as often as haemorrhoids the word 'common' is entirely relative. It might be used if this disorder was present in 5–10 per cent of adults in a community; this would be a very high prevalence in the case of many other diseases. This figure, say for haemorrhoids in sub-Saharal Africans, would, however, denote relative rarity in comparison with the situation in North America where this disorder has been estimated to affect, to some extent, one in two of the entire population over the age of 50 years.

Postulated causation

Previously held concepts of the causation of haemorrhoids, such as man's erect posture, or absence of valves in the portal system, are no longer tenable in view of the epidemiological features of the disease.

Thomson (1975) has related the condition to constipation. The abdominal straining, that is necessitated to assist the evacuation of small firm faecal masses, engorges the submucosal anal cushions. Then the oft-repeated shearing stress, occasioned by the passage of hard faecal masses through the anal canal, forces the anal cushions down the canal, rupturing their attachments to the sphincters. Both the straining and the undue firmness of the faecal matter are the result of low fibre diets.

Varicose veins

The prevalence of varicose veins in different communities has been much easier to estimate than that of haemorrhoids. The universal experience of doctors in third world countries has for long indicated that this disorder is much less common in such situations than it is in Western communities. This has now been substantiated by specific population surveys. Once again the word common is relative and even a prevalence of 10 per cent in people over the age of 30 years in third world countries is far below that in North America. Confusion has also occurred in that merely unduly prominent veins have been included under the term varicose.

In a survey of a total community in North America 19 per cent of men and 44 per cent of women over the age of 30, 23 per cent of men and 54 per cent of women over the age of 40, and 42 per cent of men and 64 per cent of women over the age of 50 had varicose veins (Coon and Collier, 1959).

In a survey in Egypt 6 per cent of factory women had varicose veins (Mekkey *et al.*, 1969).

In an African hospital varicose veins were present late in pregnancy in 9·7 per cent, 3·2 per cent and 1·5 per cent of Indian, African and Arab women respectively (Burkitt *et al.*, 1976). Both in Africa and in India this disorder appears to be more prevalent in men than in women.

Daynes and Beighton (1973) found a frequency of 7·7 per cent in South African women and Skaug (in Burkitt *et al.*, 1976) observed varicose veins in only 2 of 174 (1·1 per cent) adult men and in 3 of 163 (1·8 per cent) women living in a tribal Tanzanian situation.

Postulated pathogenesis

Previously incriminated factors in the causation of varicose veins such as man's erect posture, constrictive clothing, pregnancy and even heredity are no longer tenable as primary causative factors in the light of the epidemiology of the disease.

It has been postulated that a major causative factor is the raised pressure transmitted to the major venous channels in the abdomen, and thence to the leg veins, during abdominal straining. These bouts of raised pressure result in venous dilatation with consequent incompetence of the valves; this is a progressive and sequential process from above downwards (Burkitt, 1976).

Hiatus hernia

This disorder is almost certainly rare among Africans in all parts of sub-Saharal Africa. The most comprehensive study which has been done is that of Bassey *et al*. (1977) who deliberately searched for evidence of hiatus hernia in a prospective radiological study of the upper gastrointestinal tract in over 1000 adult Nigerians and was able to detect it in only 4.

In Nairobi, Kenya, Whittaker (1966) found only one case in 1319 barium meal examinations in Africans. In Kampala, Uganda, Moore (1967) found 25 in 786 barium meal examinations, almost all of the small stenosing type. In Dar-es-Salaam, Tanzania, Grech (1965) found only one in 733 barium meal examinations in Africans. Archampong *et al.* (1978) reported the frequency of 20 per cent in Ghana, over 40 times higher than that reported by Bassey *et al.* (1977) in Lagos. Diagnostic criteria, or the age structure of the two populations, adopted in the two reports must have differed, as such a discrepancy between two African communities living in almost identical circumstances would be inconceivable. Higher figures, though lower than those for Europeans, have been reported in Bantu urban communities in South Africa. M. Moshal (personal communication, 1977) found that the lower oesophageal sphincter commonly straddled the diaphragm in urban South African Bantu, as it does in North Americans, whereas Bassey *et al.* (1977) found it to be almost invariably below the diaphragm in Nigerians.

Postulated pathogenesis

It has been postulated that hiatus hernia is the result of raised intra-abdominal pressures caused by straining at stool or in other ways (Burkitt, 1975c). This is the only hypothesis postulated that is consistent with epidemiological evidence.

If a ball with a hole in its wall and containing water is squeezed, the water is expressed through the hole. The abdominal cavity can be considered as a ball, the hole representing the hiatus in the diaphragm through which the oesophagus passes. Abdominal straining when sitting on a toilet seat has been shown to raise subdiaphragmatic pressures to 19·0 kPa (195 cmH₂O), whereas the intrathoracic pressures rise to only 6·6 kPa (67 cmH₂O). The disparity between the supra- and infradiaphragmatic pressures is 12·4 kPa (128 cmH₂O). When squatting, the traditional position for defaecating, intra-abdominal and intrathoracic pressures were found to be only 13·0 and 5·3 kPa (132 and 54 cmH₂O), a difference of only 8·7 kPa (88 cmH₂O) respectively (Fedail *et al.*, 1979). It would thus appear that both fibre-depleted diets and raised toilet seats may contribute to the causation of hiatus hernia.

Deep vein thrombosis (DVT) and pelvic phleboliths

Venous thrombosis is much less common in third world communities than it is in Western countries, and resultant pulmonary embolism is particularly rare in the former. This occurs in spite of the fact that similar surgery is performed without the use of anticoagulants even in elderly patients. Pelvic phleboliths have been shown to be calcified clots in pelvic veins, and their geographical distribution appears to be similar, if not identical, to that of DVT. The prevalence of phleboliths is easy to assess by examining pelvic radiographs.

The relative frequency of phleboliths was estimated by examining pelvic radiographs of 155 Tanzanians and comparing them with those of 155 age- and sex-matched Britons. Phleboliths were observed in 19 per cent of the former and 66 per cent of the latter (Burkitt *et al.*, 1977).

Kloppers and Fehrsen (1977) compared 727 black and 823 white South Africans of comparable age and sex, and found phleboliths in 13·5 per cent of the former and in 44·7 per cent of the latter. J. Ward and J. Reinhardt (personal communication, 1979) in a prospective radiological study of black and white Americans of comparable age and sex found the prevalence of phleboliths almost identical in the two populations.

Tumours of the large intestine

Cancer

Incidence rates of malignant tumours of the large bowel, and of the colon in particular, are more directly related to the extent of economic development than are those of any other form of cancer. All published figures from sub-Saharal Africa show low rates for Africans, yet black and white North Americans are comparably affected today.

Over most of sub-Saharal Africa colorectal cancer appears to represent a fairly constant figure of approximately 2 per cent of all malignant tumours (Burkitt, 1971). It would appear that these tumours can result from factors independent of contact with Western culture; also that the rise in prevalence above this minimum is the result of other factors introduced into the environment.

Tumours of the large bowel are among the last of characteristically Western diseases to increase in prevalence following impact with Western technology.

Postulated causation

It is now generally accepted that dietary factors are dominant in the pathogenesis of large bowel cancer.

Opinions differ as to the mechanisms involved, but the weight of informed opinion considers that diets rich in fat, and in animal fat in particular, predispose to cancer development, and that dietary fibre, and cereal fibre in particular, exert a protective influence. Hill (1974) incriminates derivatives of bacterial action on primary bile acids; Bruce, *et al.* (1979) have presented evidence that the effective carcinogen may be a nitrosamine compound, and Cruse *et al.* (1979) have argued that cholesterol itself may act as a promoter of cancer. Walker and Burkitt (1976) have presented evidence to suggest that whatever factors are responsible for the causation of colorectal cancer, dietary fibre, by diluting and hastening the evacuation of carcinogens, reduces their potency and can thus be viewed as protective.

Polyps

The contrast between the prevalence of large bowel polyps as found in sub-Saharal Africa and in Western countries is much greater than that between prevalence of cancer in these communities. Whereas intestinal polyps can be found in some 20 per cent of necropsies in North America (Arminski and McLean, 1964), their rarity in sub-Saharal Africa can be illustrated by the fact that even in Johannesburg, the largest urban community in southern Africa, only 6 polyps were found amongst all necropsies and surgical biopsy material over a period of 14 years in a Bantu 2000-bed hospital (Bremner and Ackerman, 1970). Templeton (1973) found only one adenomatous polyp in 40 000 surgical biopsies in Kampala, Uganda, over a 5-year period. The rarity of adenomatous polyps of the bowel even in Asia suggests that their prevalence does not significantly increase until after large bowel malignant tumours become more common.

Epidemiological evidence suggests that cancer and polyps of the bowel share common causative factors. In Western countries the majority of cancers are believed to arise in pre-existing polyps (Hill *et al.*, 1978).

Diverticular disease of the colon

This is probably the last of the characteristically Western diseases of the large bowel to emerge in developing countries. Until recently it has been almost unknown throughout sub-Saharal Africa, being rarely seen even in large populations such as Johannesburg and Durban in South Africa and Lagos and Ibadan in Nigeria. Recently Calder (1979) and Archampong *et al.* (1978) have, however, reported this disease in the hospitals of the capitals of Kenya (15 cases in 2 years) and Nigeria (16 cases in 3 years). This still probably represents a low incidence of the disease, since both investigators appear to have searched for cases among the 200 to 350 barium enemata examinations performed during the period under review. The occurrence of diverticular disease is believed to depend on a long period of exposure to low fibre diets, while appendicitis occurs even in young persons eating low fibre diets. In no country in the world has diverticular disease ever been observed to emerge as a common disorder until about 20–40 years after appendicitis became common.

Postulated pathogenesis

It is now generally accepted that diverticula are protrusions of mucosa forced through the muscle wall of the colon as a result of raised intraluminal pressures. These are occasioned by the increased efforts required to propel along the colon faecal content which is reduced in volume and increased in viscosity as a result of excessive water loss. This in turn is a result of the low fibre content of the diet (Painter, 1975).

References

Archampong, E. Q., Christian, F. and Badoe, E. A. (1978). Diverticular disease in an indigenous African community. *Annals of the Royal College of Surgeons of England*, **60**, 464–470

Arminski, T. C. and McLean, D. W. (1964). Incidence and distribution of adenomatous polyps of the colon and rectum based on 1,000 autopsy examinations. *Diseases of the Colon and Rectum*, **7**, 249–261

Badoe, E. A. (1967). Acute appendicitis in Accra. *Ghana Medical Journal*, **6**, 69–75

Bassey, O. O., Eyo, E. E. and Akinhanmi, L. A. (1977). Incidence of hiatus hernia and gastro-oesophageal reflux in 1030 prospective barium meal examinations in adult Nigerians. *Thorax*, **32**, 356–359

Bremner, C. G. and Ackerman, L. V. (1970). Polyps and carcinoma of the large bowel. *Cancer*, **26**, 991–999

Bruce, W. R., Varghese, A. J., Wang, S. and Dion, P. (1979). The endogenous production of nitroso compounds in the colon and cancer at that site. *Proceedings of the Princess Takamtsu Conference*, Tokyo, Japan

Burkitt, D. P. (1952). Acute abdomens—British and Baganda compared. *East African Medical Journal*, **29**, 190–194

Burkitt, D. P. (1971). Epidemiology of cancer of the colon and rectum. *Cancer*, **28**, 3–13

Burkitt, D. P. (1975a). Appendicitis. In: *Refined Carbohydrate Foods and Disease*, 87–97. Editors D. P. Burkitt and H. C. Trowell. Academic Press, London

Burkitt, D. P. (1975b). Haemorrhoids, varicose veins and deep vein thrombosis; epidemiological features and suggestive causative factors. *Canadian Journal of Surgery*, **18**, 483–488

Burkitt, D. P. (1975c). Hiatus hernia. In: *Refined Carbohydrate Foods and Disease*, 161–169. Editors D. P. Burkitt and H. C. Trowell. Academic Press, London

Burkitt, D. P. (1976). Varicose veins. Facts and Fantasy. *Archives of Surgery*, **III**, 1327–1332

Burkitt, D. P. (1977). Relationship between diseases and their etiological significance. *American Journal of Clinical Nutrition*, **30**, 262–267

Burkitt, D. P., Latto, C., Janvrin, S. B. and Mayou, B. (1977). Pelvic phleboliths. Epidemiology and postulated etiology. *New England Journal of Medicine*, **296**, 1387–1389

Burkitt, D. P., Townsend, A. J., Patel, K. and Skaug, K. (1976). Varicose veins in developing countries. *Lancet*, **ii**, 202–203

Calder, J. F. (1979). Diverticular disease of the colon in Africans. *British Medical Journal*, **1**, 1465–1466

Cook, A. R. (1945). *Uganda Memories*, 49. Uganda Society, Kampala

Coon, W. W. and Collier, F. A. (1959). Some epidemiological considerations of thrombo-embolism. *Surgery, Gynaecology and Obstetrics*, **109**, 487–501

Cruse, P., Lewin, M. and Clark, C. G. (1979). Dietary cholesterol is co-carcinogenic for human colon cancer. *Lancet*, **i**, 752–755

Daynes, G. and Beighton, P. (1973). Prevalence of varicose veins in Africans. *British Medical Journal*, **3**, 354

Fedail, S. S., Harvey, R. F. and Burns-Cox, C. J. (1979). Abdominal and thoracic pressures during defaecation. *British Medical Journal*, **1**, 91

Grech, P. (1965). Radiological analysis of lesions of the upper intestinal tract during a four-year period in Africans in Tanganyika. *East African Medical Journal*, **42**, 106–116

Hill, M. (1974). Bacteria and the etiology of colonic cancer. *Cancer*, **34**, 815–818

Hill, M. J., Morson, B. C. and Bussey, H. J. R. (1978). Aetiology of adenoma–carcinoma sequence in large bowel. *Lancet*, **i**, 245–247

Horton, L. W. L. (1977). Pathogenesis of acute appendicitis. *British Medical Journal*, **3**, 1672

Johnson, J. R. (1978). Pathogenesis of acute appendicitis. *British Medical Journal*, **1**, 305

Kakande, J., Kavuma, J. and Kayondo, J. (1978). Appendicitis in Mulago Hospital, Kampala. *East African Medical Journal*, **55**, 172–176

Kloppers, P. J. and Fehrsen, G. S. (1977). Phleboliths, western diseases in developing peoples; in search of a marker. *South African Medical Journal*, **51**, 745–746

Mekkey, S., Schilling, R. S. F. and Walford, J. (1969). Varicose veins in women cotton workers. An epidemiological study in England and Egypt. *British Medical Journal*, **2**, 591–595

Moore, E. W. (1967). Radiological experience of upper intestinal tract disease in Kampala, Uganda. *East African Medical Journal*, **44**, 513–517

Osman, A. A. (1974). Epidemiological study of appendicitis in Khartoum. *International Surgery*, **59**, No. 4, 218–221

Painter, N. S. (1975). *Diverticular Disease of the Colon*, 110–121. William Heinemann, London

Taiwo, O. I., Itayemi, S. O. and Seriki, O. (1977). Acute appendicitis in Nigerian children. *Tropical and Geographical Medicine*, **29**, 35–46

Templeton, A. C. (editor) (1973). *Tumours in a Tropical Country*, 52–70. Heinemann Medical Books, London

Thomson, W. H. F. (1975). The nature of haemorrhoids. *British Journal of Surgery*, **62**, 542–552

Vint, F. W. (1937). Post-mortem findings in the natives of Kenya. *East African Medical Journal*, **13**, 332–340

Walker, A. R. P. and Burkitt, D. P. (1976). Colonic cancer—hypotheses of causation, dietary prophylaxis and future research. *American Journal of Digestive Diseases*, **21**, 910–917

Walker, A. R. P., Walker, B. F. and Segal, I. (1979). Faecal pH value and its modification by dietary means in South African black and white school-children. *South African Medical Journal*, **55**, 495–498

Whittaker, L. R. (1966). A review of a series of radiological examinations of the upper alimentary tract in African patients. *East African Medical Journal*, **43**, 336–340

Part II

Environmental factors of certain diseases

3

Gallstones

Kenneth Heaton

In Western civilization biliary calculi nearly always arise within the gall-bladder, but in the Far East pigment-rich calculi often arise within the ducts, probably due to parasitic infestation and infection of the ducts. Such bile duct stones become less common as westernization proceeds, and they will not be considered further.

Gallbladder calculi are traditionally classified by simple visual inspection into cholesterol, pigment and mixed stones. However, modern methods of analysis show that nearly all stones contain a mixture of crystalline and amorphous substances deposited on an amorphous organic matrix (Sutor, 1979). In a survey of 578 gallstones, mainly from England, 43 per cent consisted of cholesterol, with or without small beads of calcium palmitate, 13 per cent were composed of calcium salts (carbonate, phosphate, palmitate and bilirubinate), 42 per cent contained both cholesterol and calcium salts, and the remaining 2 per cent were amorphous or of unidentified material (Sutor, 1979). Calcium-rich stones correspond roughly with the clinician's pigment stones. Their aetiology is poorly understood. They occur as often in men as in women and are usually found in elderly people (Soloway *et al.*, 1977). Their incidence is increased in haemolytic states and also, for unknown reasons, in cirrhosis of the liver. Otherwise, environmental factors have not been identified. It is possible that pigment stones have aetiological factors in common with cholesterol-rich stones since, in hamsters, there is little or no difference between diets which induce the two types of stone (Soloway *et al.*, 1977).

The rest of this chapter is concerned with the common cholesterol-rich gallstone and the supersaturated bile which underlies it. Much progress has been made in recent years in understanding the pathogenesis of super-saturated bile.

Metabolic basis of cholesterol gallstones

The essential biochemical abnormality is the secretion by the liver of bile which contains an excess of cholesterol in relation to the two substances, bile acids and lecithin, which solubilize cholesterol by incorporating it into detergent micelles. Hepatic bile, that is, bile freshly secreted into the canaliculi, is supersaturated when the rate of cholesterol secretion is excessive or the rate of bile acid and lecithin secretion is inadequate. The bile in which gallstones form is the bile which is diverted into the gallbladder as digestion ceases, to be retained and concentrated there until the next meal is taken. In this process, much or most of the bile acid pool is removed from the entero-hepatic circulation and sequestered in the gallbladder. Hence, the main determinant of the bile acid and, secondarily, lecithin content of the relaxed gallbladder is the size of the bile acid pool. In non-obese gallstone patients the bile acid pool is reduced from the normal mean of about 6 mmol to 3–4 mmol and, consequently, their gallbladder bile is supersaturated in the face of relatively normal cholesterol secretion. The cause of the small pool is not established but is widely ascribed to suppression of bile acid synthesis by the liver. Certainly, the rate-limiting enzyme in bile acid synthesis (cholesterol 7α-hydroxylase) is less active in the gallstone patient's liver than in that of controls. It is not known whether this difference is congenital or acquired. However, there is much evidence that bile acid synthesis decreases in animals fed semisynthetic diets rich in fibre-free sucrose or glucose (Heaton, 1972).

Cholesterol secretion into bile is excessive in many gallstone patients, especially those who are obese. It is also excessive in many obese people without gallstones, but they seem to cope with this by having normal or large bile acid pools. Cholesterol secretion depends, at least in part, on the rate of cholesterol synthesis, and the enzyme which controls the rate of cholesterol synthesis (HMGCoA-reductase) is overactive in the livers of gallstone patients. Again, little is known about the factors affecting this enzyme, but it is probably increased in obesity and may be stimulated by insulin.

Thus the two metabolic abnormalities of gallstone patients—excessive secretion of cholesterol and a small bile acid pool—are probably both due to altered enzymatic activity in the liver, leading to enhanced synthesis of cholesterol and suppressed synthesis of bile acids respectively. Epidemiology strongly suggests that one or both of these biochemical perversions is caused by environmental factors.

Epidemiology

Geographical variations

Accurate information on the prevalence of gallstones in different communities is lacking since the disease is non-fatal and usually asymptomatic. The best available figures are from autopsy series, although these are always from urban areas and from a selected population. It is difficult to compare the data from different series because their age and sex composition varies, and prevalence increases with age and is two or more times greater in women than in men. For a mixed population a single figure cannot meaningfully be used to express prevalence. The prevalence in elderly women, which is the maximum possible, is a rough indicator of the gallstone-proneness of a

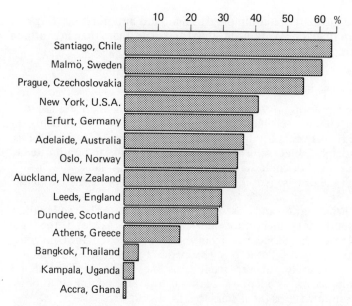

Fig. 3.1 Prevalence of gallstones in women aged 70–79 years in 14 different countries. The data are taken from autopsy surveys published since 1951

population. As shown in Fig. 3.1, the gallstone-proneness of westernized countries varies between 30 and 60 per cent, the highest published figures being from Chile, Sweden and Czechoslovakia (Marinovic *et al.*, 1972; Cleland, 1953; Rodewald, 1957; Newman and Northup, 1959; Torvik and Høivik, 1960; Watkinson, 1967; Douss and Castleden, 1973; Záhoř *et al.*, 1974; Bateson and Bouchier, 1975). For third world countries, data are necessarily more scanty, but the following figures seem reliable: Thailand, 4·4 per cent; Uganda, 3 per cent (probably pigment stones); and Ghana, 0 per cent (Edington, 1957; Stitnimankarn, 1960; Owor, 1964). An intermediate place is occupied by Greece. Thus, there are good grounds for the belief that gallstones are common or very common in all westernized countries but are rare or uncommon in developing countries.

Systematic postal questioning of doctors in outlying hospitals in Africa, India, Arabia and New Guinea has confirmed that patients with gallstones are rarely seen in the rural areas of these countries (less than 0·1 per cent of surgical admissions) (Burkitt and Tunstall, 1975). On the other hand, in the urbanized blacks of Johannesburg, gallstones are quite common, being found in 12 per cent of elderly females (Becker and Chatgidakis, 1952). An urban–rural difference has also been reported from Japan, cholesterol-rich stones being found much more commonly in the cities than in the country (Yagi, 1960; Maki, 1961).

Prevalence may vary in different regions of a country. There is some evidence that gallstones are commoner in Scotland and northern England than in southern England (Watkinson, 1967) and in northern than in southern India (Malhotra, 1968).

Changes in gallstone incidence

Changes on emigration are poorly documented. When an Italian was admitted to hospital in the 1960s the probability of the admission being for gallstones was 1·5 per cent in Italy itself but 4·8 per cent in Melbourne (Hills, 1971). In Philadelphia, blacks are at least as likely as whites to be admitted to hospital for treatment of cholesterol-rich gallstones (Trotman and Soloway, 1973), although the disease is still rare in West Africa, where the US blacks originated.

Changes on urbanization and westernization are suggested by the Japanese and Johannesburg data mentioned above. Between 1949 and 1964 the autopsy prevalence of gallstones rose from 2·5 to 6·1 per cent in the University of Tokyo Department of Pathology (Kameda, 1967). It is said that the Canadian Eskimo rarely suffered from gallstones when he lived in his traditional, nomadic way, but the disease is now very common amongst Eskimos living in townships (Schaefer, 1971).

Since World War Two there has been a world-wide increase in the number of patients undergoing surgery for gallstones. This has been documented in England, France, Sweden, Canada, Greece and South Africa (Heaton, 1973; Plant *et al.,* 1973; Kalos *et al.,* 1977). The magnitude of the increase has been between 2·5 and 6. Readier diagnosis may explain part of this change. However, it is unlikely to explain the finding in several studies that there has been a disproportionate increase in younger people and also in men—the least susceptible groups in the population. When a disease spreads to involve less susceptible people it suggests that the pathogenic factors have intensified.

Epidemiology of supersaturated gallbladder bile

In high incidence countries like the USA and Sweden, unselected members of the population have bile which is nearly saturated or supersaturated with cholesterol, but in rural Africans and Japanese bile is almost always highly unsaturated (Redinger and Small, 1972; Heaton *et al.,* 1977). Within a westernized population, bile becomes more saturated with cholesterol with increasing age (Valdivieso *et al.,* 1978).

Conclusions from epidemiology

Incomplete as they are, the epidemiological data do suggest that gallstones are essentially a disease of civilization and especially of modern western culture. This of itself leaves open many possible explanations, but the only theories which command any credence today are nutritional ones. Evidence for these comes from disease associations, animal models and dietary experiments.

Related diseases and metabolic disturbances

Many within-patient associations have been suggested but few are supported by satisfactory statistics. Even the well-known Saint's triad of gallstones, diverticular disease and hiatus hernia is unsupported by statistical evidence as being more than a coincidence (Kaye and Kern, 1971). Gallstones and diverticular disease are not especially prone to occur in the same patient at autopsy (Eide and Stalsberg, 1979) and adequate studies in living subjects have not been reported. However, patients with hiatus hernia have twice the expected prevalence of gallstones and their gallbladder bile is unexpectedly rich in cholesterol (Capron *et al.*, 1978). Since there is no obvious mechanism whereby one disease could cause the other, these findings suggest there is a common point in their pathogenetic pathways or a common aetiology. Obesity is common with both diseases but not invariably present and, in any case, the hiatus hernia patients studied by Capron *et al.* (1978) were matched with controls of similar body weight. It has been proposed that hiatal herniation results from straining at stool and so from low residue diets (Burkitt and James, 1973), but direct evidence is lacking.

The other well-documented associations of gallstones are obesity, diabetes and hypertriglyceridaemia. The connection between these four diseases is very close. If a person has any one of them he (or more likely she) is at increased risk of having all the other three (for references see Heaton, 1973; 1975). Furthermore, a woman with gallstones has on average gained more weight since maturity than one without, even if she is not frankly obese; her fasting blood sugar is higher and her fasting triglycerides are higher (Heaton, 1973; 1979). Conversely, people who are obese, or hypertriglyceridaemic, or have maturity-onset diabetes, not only have an increased risk of gallstones but also a strong tendency to secrete bile which is supersaturated with cholesterol (Bennion and Grundy, 1975; Angelin, 1977; Haber and Heaton, 1979). Even in apparently healthy women, with plasma lipids in the normal range for Britain, supersaturated gallbladder bile is more likely to be found if plasma triglycerides are at the upper end of the normal range (Thornton *et al.*, 1979).

The common factor in these four metabolic abnormalities seems to be overnutrition or surplus energy intake. A lowered calorie intake is the most effective treatment for maturity-onset diabetes and hypertriglyceridaemia as well as obesity. It also results in a lower output of cholesterol into the bile and less saturated gallbladder bile, at any rate once the subject is stable at his lower weight (Bennion and Grundy, 1975; Shaffer and Small, 1977).

The association between gallstones and coronary heart disease is controversial but on balance the evidence does favour its existence (Heaton, 1973). There is no relationship between serum cholesterol on the one hand and gallstones or the cholesterol saturation of gallbladder bile on the other, but it has recently been found that there is quite a good inverse correlation between bile saturation and the plasma level of high density lipoprotein, especially if this is expressed as a per cent of total cholesterol (Fig. 3.2). This suggests that the risk of gallstones and the risk of coronary heart disease are linked, but the nature of the link is unknown.

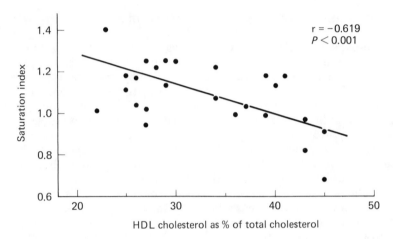

Fig. 3.2   Relationship between the cholesterol saturation of gallbladder bile aspirated from the duodenum and the plasma concentration of high density lipoprotein (HDL) cholesterol, expressed as a percentage of total plasma cholesterol, in 25 healthy non-obese women aged 40–44 years (Thornton *et al.*, 1979)

Two other disorders, pacreatis and ileal resection, are often associated with gallstones but the relationships are probably due to cause and effect so they are not relevant to the present discussion.

Iatrogenic gallstones are being increasingly recognized. Oestrogen therapy, including the contraceptive pill, and regimens aimed at lowering the serum cholesterol, including clofibrate and the low cholesterol, high poly-unsaturated fat diet, all increase the risk of gallstones and render bile more saturated with cholesterol. However, these therapies were all introduced after gallstones had already become common.

Case-control studies

Sarles has reported four studies performed in France over 21 years in which the habitual diet of gallstone patients was compared with that of matched controls (Sarles *et al.*, 1970; 1978). In every study the mean energy (calorie) intake was higher in the patients, though insignificantly so in the last study. In the one study where individual foods were reported patients ate less vegetables and fruit and more white bread. In other words, their carbo-hydrate intake was more refined. Patients also admitted to more psychological stresses (Sarles *et al.*, 1969); perhaps this contributed to their greater food intake.

Two studies in Australia did not show higher energy intakes in gallstone patients than controls (Wheeler *et al.*, 1970; Burnett, 1971), but these studies were not so well designed as the French ones.

Diet-induced gallstones in animals

Wild animals very rarely form gallstones. However, cholesterol-rich gall-stones have been induced by giving an artificial diet in hamsters, mice, prairie dogs, rabbits and squirrel monkeys, and they have been recorded in baboons eating a relatively natural diet. The experimental diets have varied greatly in their composition (Table 3.1). Often cholesterol has been added, but not always (and in the original hamster model of Dam it was absent). The only feature which all these diets have in common is that they are semisynthetic or semipurified. In effect this means that the carbohydrate component of lithogenic diets is always a refined or fibre-depleted material, usually glucose or sucrose but sometimes corn starch. The only published exception to this rule is the gerbil which will form cholesterol-rich gallstones on ordinary, unpurified chow, but this is achieved only by feeding so much cholesterol that the liver becomes stuffed and swollen with it (Bergman and van der Linden, 1971).

Table 3.1   Diets used to produce cholesterol-rich gallstones in animals

Animal	Special features of diet	Carbohydrate in diet	Reference
Hamster	Best if fat-free	72% glucose or sucrose	Dam (1971) Hikasa *et al.* (1969)
Mouse	31% fat Added cholesterol and cholic acid	51% glucose	Tepperman *et al.* (1964)
Prairie dog	41% fat Added cholesterol 2·6% cellulose	34% sucrose 14% corn starch	Brenneman *et al.* (1972)
Rabbit	15% olive oil 15% cellulose	7% sucrose $6\frac{1}{2}$% glucose 6% corn starch	Borgman and Haselden (1968)
Squirrel monkey	25% butter Added cholesterol	44% sucrose	Osuga and Portman (1971)

The idea that it is lack of fibre which explains the lithogenicity of these diets is supported by two observations. In the hamster, the diet loses its effect if it is supplemented with bulking agents such as agar and carboxy-methyl-cellulose, or if the animal is allowed to eat the straw laid on the floor of its cage (Hikasa *et al.*, 1969). In the rabbit, stones dissolve rapidly if ordinary fibre-rich chow is fed. The lithogenic rabbit diet contains cellulose but this is purified crystalline cellulose (Alphacel) which is not to be equated with natural cell-wall material.

Effect of dietary modification on bile composition in man

Fat

Altering the amount or type of fat in the diet has no consistent effect in short-term experiments (Dam *et al.*, 1967; Sarles *et al.*, 1970). No long-term studies have been reported. However, a low saturated fat, low cholesterol diet was associated with increased gallstones at autopsy in California veterans (Sturdevant *et al.*, 1973).

Cholesterol

Results have been conflicting. In one study, eating 5–10 eggs a day failed to increase the bile cholesterol content of young volunteers after six weeks; in fact, it tended to decrease it (Dam *et al.*, 1971). In another, adding 750 mg cholesterol (equivalent to three eggs) daily to a liquid formula diet raised the cholesterol content of healthy men's duodenal bile from 8·1 to 10·9 moles per cent (DenBesten *et al.*, 1973). The relevance of studies with liquid formula diets is hard to assess and the subjects in this study already had unusually saturated bile on the formula diet alone.

Dietary fibre

Addition of wheat bran to a normal Western diet has been studied by three groups. In Bristol, Pomare *et al.* (1976) fed bran in the maximum tolerated dose, usually 20–40 g/d, to women with radiolucent gallstones and after six weeks their bile was significantly less saturated with cholesterol. The change was modest and in most subjects bile was still supersaturated. In healthy young men, bran 30 g/d made no difference at all, but their bile was un-saturated initially (Wicks *et al.*, 1978). Similar findings were reported from Adelaide (Watts *et al.*, 1978); raw bran 30 g/d reduced bile saturation in women with supersaturated bile but had no effect in men with already unsaturated bile. From Edmonton, McDougall *et al.* (1978) reported that cooked bran 50 g/d caused such a sharp drop in saturation index that in most patients bile became unsaturated.

The mode of action of bran is uncertain. In all three studies there was a fall in the biliary content of deoxycholate, a bacterially degraded bile salt absorbed from the colon. Feeding deoxycholate has been reported to increase the cholesterol saturation of bile (Low-Beer and Pomare, 1975), while removing it by giving the antimicrobial drug metronidazole had the opposite effect (Low-Beer and Nutter, 1978). It is possible, therefore, that bran acts by removing deoxycholate from bile. This could happen as a result of reduced bacterial activity or interference with absorption from the colon. The finding that the fall in biliary deoxycholate takes four weeks or more to develop led Wicks *et al.* (1978) to suggest that it is the formation rather than absorption of deoxycholate which is affected.

In a seemingly discordant study, Meyer *et al.* (1979) reported no improvement in the bile of four grossly obese women given bran for six weeks. However, a huge dose of bran was used and the subjects developed bile acid malabsorption which is not a physiological effect.

So far all studies with bran have been of relatively short duration, maximum two months, and no studies have been reported with other fibre supplements.

Refined carbohydrate

The refined carbohydrates—chiefly sugar and white flour—are foods which have been artificially depleted of fibre. Their effect on bile is being explored in Bristol. Preliminary results are available on 13 subjects with gallstones or supersaturated bile who have been studied after seven weeks on an *ad lib.* diet rich in refined carbohydrates and after seven weeks on an *ad lib.* diet devoid of these foods. In all but one subject, bile was less saturated on the unrefined diet, mean saturation index $1\cdot20 \pm 0\cdot42$ *vs* $1\cdot50 \pm 0\cdot37$ (Thornton, Emmett and Heaton, unpublished data). In all subjects calorie intake was also lower on the unrefined diet and all but two lost weight. However, the average weight loss was only $1\cdot6$ kg, which is unlikely to account for the improved bile composition. Dietary fibre intake was higher on the unrefined diet.

Summary and conclusions

Cholesterol-rich gallstones are a disease of civilization, especially of modern Western civilization. The disease seems to have increased everywhere in the last three decades and to be involving younger people. Gallstones and the secretion of bile supersaturated with cholesterol are closely associated with obesity, maturity-onset diabetes and raised plasma triglycerides. This points to overnutrition as a key factor. Overnutrition leads to excess secretion of cholesterol into bile. A particular role for refined or fibre-depleted carbo-hydrate is suggested by three observations: diets which induce cholesterol gallstones in animals are generally rich in refined carbohydrate; replacing refined with unrefined carbohydrate in the diet of gallstone patients renders their bile less saturated with cholesterol; and adding bran to the diet has the same beneficial effect. Other environmental factors are drugs and diets which lower the serum cholesterol and therapy with oestrogens.

References

Angelin, B. (1977). Cholesterol and bile acid metabolism in normo- and hyperlipoproteinaemia. *Acta Medica Scandinavica*, Suppl. 610, 1–40

Bateson, M. C. and Bouchier, I. A. D. (1975). Prevalence of gallstones in Dundee: a necropsy study. *British Medical Journal*, **4**, 427–430

Becker, J. P. and Chatgidakis, C. B. (1952). Carcinoma of the gallbladder and cholelithiasis on the Witwatersrand. *South African Journal of Clinical Science*, **3**, 13–22

Bennion, L. J. and Grundy, S. M. (1975). Effects of obesity and caloric intake on biliary lipid metabolism in man. *Journal of Clinical Investigation*, **56**, 996–1011

Bergman, F. and van der Linden, W. (1971). Reaction of the Mongolian gerbil to a cholesterol-cholic acid-containing gallstone inducing diet. *Acta Pathologica et Microbiologica Scandinavica*, **79**, 476–486

Borgman, R. F. and Haselden, F. H. (1968). Cholelithiasis in rabbits: effects of diet upon formation and dissolution of gallstones. *American Journal of Veterinary Research*, **29**, 1287–1292

Brenneman, D. E., Connor, W. E., Forker, E. L. and DenBesten, L. (1972). The formation of abnormal bile and cholesterol gallstones from dietary cholesterol in the prairie dog. *Journal of Clinical Investigation*, **51**, 1495–1503

Burkitt, D. P. and James, P. A. (1973). Low-residue diets and hiatus hernia. *Lancet*, **ii**, 128–130

Burkitt, D. P. and Tunstall, M. (1975). Gallstones: geographical and chronological features. *Journal of Tropical Medicine and Hygiene*, **78**, 140–144

Burnett, W. (1971). The epidemiology of gallstones. *Tijdschrift voor Gastroenterologie*, **14**, 79–89

Capron, J-P., Payenneville, H., Dumont, M., Dupas, J-L. and Lorriaux, A. (1978). Evidence for an association between cholelithiasis and hiatus hernia. *Lancet*, **ii**, 329–331

Cleland, J. B. (1953). Gallstones in seven thousand post-mortem examinations. *Medical Journal of Australia*, **2**, 488–489

Dam, H. (1971). Determinants of cholesterol cholelithiasis in man and animals. *American Journal of Medicine*, **51**, 596–613

Dam, H., Kruse, I., Jensen, M. K. and Kallehauge, H. E. (1967). Studies on human bile. II. Influence of two different fats on the composition of human bile. *Scandinavian Journal of Clinical and Laboratory Investigation*, **19**, 367–378

Dam, H., Prange, I., Jensen, M. K., Kallehauge, H. E. and Fenger, H. J. (1971). Studies on human bile. IV. Influence of ingestion of cholesterol in the form of eggs on the composition of bile in healthy subjects. *Zeitschrift für die Ernährungswissenschaft*, **10**, 178–187

DenBesten, L., Connor, W. E. and Bell, S. (1973). The effect of dietary cholesterol on the composition of human bile. *Surgery*, **73**, 266–273

Douss, T. W. and Castleden, W. M. (1973). Gallstones and carcinoma of the large bowel. *New Zealand Medical Journal*, **77**, 162–165

Edington, G. M. (1957). Observations on hepatic disease in the Gold Coast: with special reference to cirrhosis. *Transactions of the Royal Society for Tropical Medicine and Hygiene*, **51**, 48–55

Eide, T. J. and Stalsberg, H. (1979). Diverticular disease of the large intestine in Northern Norway. *Gut*, **20**, 609–615

Haber, G. B. and Heaton, K. W. (1979). Lipid composition of bile in diabetics and obesity-matched controls. *Gut*, **20**, 518–522

Heaton, K. W. (1972). *Bile Salts in Health and Disease*, 184–195. Churchill-Livingstone, Edinburgh

Heaton, K. W. (1973). The epidemiology of gallstones and suggested aetiology. *Clincis in Gastroenterology*, **2**, 67–83

Heaton, K. W. (1975). Gallstones and cholecystitis. In: *Refined Carbohydrate Foods and Disease. Some Implications of Dietary Fibre*, 173–194. Edited by D. P. Burkitt and H. C. Trowell. Academic Press, London

Heaton, K. W. (1979). Diet and gallstones. In: *Gallstones, Hepatology Research and Clinical Issues*, vol. 4, 371–389. Edited by M. M. Fisher, C. A. Goresky, E. A. Shaffer and S. M. Strasberg. Plenum, New York

Heaton, K. W., Wicks, A. C. B. and Yeates, J. (1977). Bile composition in relation to race and diet: studies in Rhodesian Africans and in British subjects. In: *Bile Acid Metabolism in Health and Disease*, 197–202. Edited by G. Paumgartner and A. Stiehl. MTP Press, Lancaster

Hikasa, Y., Matsuda, S., Nagase, M., Yoshinaga, M., Tobe, T., Maruyama, I., Shioda, R., Tanimura, H., Muraoka, R., Muroya, H. and Togo, M. (1969). Initiating factors of gallstones, especially cholesterol stones (III). *Archiv für Japanische Chirurgie*, **38**, 107–124

Hills, L. L. (1971). Cholelithiasis and immigration. *Medical Journal of Australia*, **2**, 94–95

Kalos, A., Delidou, A., Kordosis, T., Archimandritis, A., Gananis, A. and Angelopoulos, B. (1977). The incidence of gallstones in Greece: an autopsy study. *Acta Hepato-Gastroenterologica*, **24**, 20–23

Kameda, H. (1967). Gallstones, compositions, structural characteristics and geographical distribution. In: *Proceedings of 3rd World Congress of Gastroenterology, Tokyo, 1966*. Vol. 4, 117–124. Karger, Basel

Kaye, M. D. and Kern, F. (1971). Clinical relationships of gallstones. *Lancet*, **i**, 1228–1230

Low-Beer, T. S. and Nutter, S. (1978). Colonic bacterial activity, biliary cholesterol saturation, and pathogenesis of gallstones. *Lancet*, **ii**, 1063–1065

Low-Beer, T. S. and Pomare, E. W. (1975). Can colonic bacterial metabolites predispose to cholesterol gallstones? *British Medical Journal*, **1**, 438–440

Maki, T. (1961). Cholelithiasis in the Japanese. *Archives of Surgery*, **82**, 599–612

Malhotra, S. L. (1968). Epidemiological study of cholelithiasis among railroad workers in India with special reference to causation. *Gut*, **9**, 290–295

Marinovic, I., Guerra, C. and Larach, G. (1972). Incidencia de litiasis biliar en material de autopsias y analisis de composicion de los calculos. *Revista Medica Chile*, **100**, 1320–1327

McDougall, R. M., Yakymyshyn, L., Walker, K. and Thurston, O. G. (1978). The effect of wheat bran on serum lipoproteins and biliary lipids. *Canadian Journal of Surgery*, **21**, 433–435

Meyer, P. D., DenBesten, L. and Mason, E. E. (1979). The effects of a high-fiber diet on bile acid pool size, bile acid kinetics and biliary lipid secretory rates in the morbidly obese. *Surgery*, **85**, 311–316

Newman, H. F. and Northup, J. D. (1959). The autopsy incidence of gallstones. *International Abstracts of Surgery*, **109**, 1–13

Osuga, T. and Portman, O. W. (1971). Experimental formation of gallstones in the squirrel monkey. *Proceedings of the Society of Experimental Biology and Medicine,* **136,** 722–726

Owor, R. (1964). Gallstones in the autopsy population at Mulago Hospital, Kampala. *East African Medical Journal,* **41,** 251–253

Plant, J. C. D., Percy, I., Bates, T., Gastard, J. and Hita de Nercy, Y. (1973). Incidence of gallbladder disease in Canada, England and France. *Lancet,* **ii,** 249–251

Pomare, E. W., Heaton, K. W., Low-Beer, T. S. and Espiner, H. J. (1976). The effect of wheat bran upon bile salt metabolism and upon the lipid composition of bile in gallstone patients. *American Journal of Digestive Diseases,* **21,** 521–526

Redinger, R. N. and Small, D. M. (1972). Bile composition, bile salt metabolism and gallstones. *Archives of Internal Medicine,* **130,** 618–630

Rodewald, H. (1957). Zur Pathologie der Gallenblase II. Mitteilung über die Häufigkeit der Gallensteine. *Zentralblatt für Allgemeine Pathologie und Pathologische Anatomie,* **96,** 300–302

Sarles, H., Chabert, C., Pommeau, Y., Save, E., Mouret, H. and Gérolami, A. (1969). Diet and cholesterol gallstones. *American Journal of Digestive Diseases,* **14,** 531–537

Sarles, H., Gérolami, A. and Bord, A. (1978). Diet and cholesterol gallstones. A further study. *Digestion,* **17,** 128–134

Sarles, H., Hauto, J., Planche, N. E., Lafont, H. and Gérolami, A. (1970). Diet, cholesterol gallstones, and composition of the bile. *American Journal of Digestive Diseases,* **15,** 251–260

Schaefer, O. (1971). When the Eskimo comes to town. *Nutrition Today.* November/December, 8–16

Shaffer, E. A. and Small, D. M. (1977). Biliary lipid secretion in cholesterol gallstone disease. The effect of cholecystectomy and obesity. *Journal of Clinical Investigation,* **59,** 828–840

Soloway, R. D., Trotman, B. W. and Ostrow, J. D. (1977). Pigment gallstones. *Gastroenterology,* **72,** 167–182

Stitnimankarn, T. (1960). The necropsy incidence of gallstones in Thailand. *American Journal of the Medical Sciences,* **240,** 349–352

Sturdevant, R. A. L., Pearce, M. L. and Dayton, S. (1973). Increased prevalence of cholelithiasis in men ingesting a serum cholesterol lowering diet. *New England Journal of Medicine,* **288,** 24–27

Sutor, D. J. (1979). The composition of gallstones. In: *Gallstones. Hepatology Research and Clinical Issues,* Vol. 4, 19–29. Edited by M. M. Fisher, C. A. Goresky, E. A. Shaffer and S. M. Strasberg. Plenum, New York

Tepperman, J., Caldwell, F. T. and Tepperman, H. M. (1964). Induction of gallstones in mice by feeding a cholesterol-cholic acid containing diet. *American Journal of Physiology,* **206,** 628–634

Thornton, J. R., Heaton, K. W., MacFarlane, D. G. and Bolton, C. H. (1979). Bile saturation and plasma lipids: an association with high-density lipoprotein. *Gut,* **20A,** 931

Torvik, A. and Høivik, B. (1960). Gallstones in an autopsy series. Incidence, complications and correlations with carcinoma of the gallbladder. *Acta Chirurgica Scandinavica*, **120**, 168–174

Trotman, B. W. and Soloway, R. D. (1973). Influence of age, race or sex on pigment and cholesterol gallstone incidence. *Gastroenterology*, **65**, 573

Valdivieso, V., Palma, R., Wünkhaus, R., Antezana, C., Severin, C. and Contreras, A. (1978). Effect of aging on biliary lipid composition and bile acid metabolism in normal Chilean women. *Gastroenterology*, **74**, 871–874

Watkinson, G. (1967). The autopsy incidence of gallstones in England and Scotland. *Proceedings of 3rd World Congress of Gastroenterology, Tokyo, 1966*, Vol. 4, 157–162. Karger, Basel

Watts, J. McK., Jablonski, P. and Toouli, J. (1978). The effect of added bran to the diet on the saturation of bile in people without gallstones. *American Journal of Surgery*, **135**, 321–324

Wheeler, M., Hills, L. L. and Laby, B. (1970). Cholelithiasis: a clinical and dietary survey. *Gut*, **11**, 430–437

Wicks, A. C. B., Yeates, J. and Heaton, K. W. (1978). Bran and bile: time-course of changes in normal young men given a standard dose. *Scandinavian Journal of Gastroenterology*, **13**, 289–292

Yagi, T. (1960). Some observations on chemical components of gallstones in the Sendai district of Japan. *Tohoku Journal of Experimental Medicine*, **72**, 117–130

Záhoř, Z., Sternby, N. H., Kagan, A., Uemera, K., Vaněček, R. and Vichert, A. M. (1974). Frequency of cholelithiasis in Prague and Malmö. An autopsy study. *Scandinavian Journal of Gastroenterology*, **9**, 3–7.

4

Renal stone

Norman Blacklock

Stones of renal origin include those, such as cystine and uric acid, in which there is a specific metabolic abnormality; these account for approximately 15 per cent. Magnesium ammonium phosphate stones also occur in the upper urinary tract, are usually large and are often 'staghorn' in type. They are invariably associated with an infected urine and are found frequently in women and in the elderly of both sexes. Nearly 80 per cent of renal stones are calcium stones, either calcium oxalate, calcium phosphate or a mixture of both. If it is correct to assume that the proportion of metabolic and infected stones is approximately the same in all series throughout the world, then epidemiological studies are largely considering the phenomenon of the calcium stone in which calcium oxalate is the commonest constituent. Hyperparathyroidism can account for between 1 and 4 per cent of any calcium stone series.

Calcium stone formation

Physicochemical factors

Calculi are predominantly crystalline substances and their formation in the urinary tract is attributable to the precipitation of the solid phase from a supersaturated solution (Robertson et al., 1976). Urine is usually in the metastable zone of saturation between solubility and crystal formation limits. In this state, spontaneous formation of crystals is unlikely to occur but, if a nucleus of crystalline or organic material is present, then crystallization will take place on this. If the urine becomes oversaturated, spontaneous crystallization is likely. This may be modified by inhibitors in the urine and it has been suggested that lack of these inhibitory factors is another factor in calcium stone disease.

A feature of any series of calcium stone formers is the large proportion whose metabolism at the time of investigation shows no abnormality to indicate an increased risk of calcium oxalate crystallization in the urine.

Whilst the analysis of 24-hour urine collections shows that between 40 and 60 per cent of calcium stone formers excrete calcium at higher rates than normal, this is dependent on the ingestion of food, since excretion rates are normal in the majority of specimens collected after overnight fasting. Furthermore, Bulusu *et al.* (1970) and Robertson and Morgan (1972) observed that the extent of the hypercalciuria represented only a relatively small increase in mean calcium excretion, there being considerable overlap between normal and stone-forming subjects. Nordin *et al.* (1976) suggested from the data available that there was nothing to indicate a specific abnormality in calcium handling but observed that the risk of stone formation was increased six times with increase of urine calcium excretion from 300 mg to 600 mg daily.

The mechanism of this hypercalciuria is probably absorptive and intestinal absorption of ^{47}Calcium was found increased in approximately 70 per cent of solitary stone formers and in 90 per cent with multiple or recurrent calcium stones (Blacklock and Macleod, 1974). The stone risk increased six-fold with a rise in radiocalcium absorption from 0·5 ml to 1·2 ml per hour (Nordin *et al.*, 1976). This raised rate of absorption may be secondary to a renal phosphate 'leak', the resultant hypophosphataemia stimulating increased formation of 1,25-dihydroxycholecalciferol (1,25-DHCC) in the kidney.

Hyperuricosuria (high urate excretion) has been observed in calcium oxalate stone formers and in one series occurred in 26 per cent with or without hypercalciuria; it was more prevalent in those with recurrent calculi (Coe and Kavalach, 1974). The rate of urate excretion in the urine is influenced by the consumption of purine-containing foods—meat, fish, poultry—and varies with the endogenous production of urate and its handling by the kidney. Coe and Kavalach (1974) found the purine intake of calcium stone formers to be significantly greater than that of a group with no history of stone, the dietaries being otherwise similar. The stone formers consumed more meat, fish and poultry and less bread, grain and starch. There was some evidence suggesting increased production of endogenous urate in these circumstances. The hyperuricosuria therefore appeared to be related to diet, and they concluded that the substitution of bread, grain and starch for meat, fish and poultry might decrease it. Although uric acid or calcium urate may individually crystallize within the urine, the significance of raised urinary uric acid is the evidence that it can interfere with the action of an important acid mucopolysaccharide inhibitor of calcium oxalate crystallization (Robertson *et al.*, 1976).

To summarize these metabolic findings in calcium stone formers, the conclusion is that, whilst a minor metabolic abnormality is detectable in approximately 60 per cent, the extent of this is only such that the abnormal values in the various parameters lie mainly at the upper or lower levels of normal. From this point of view the disease has been aptly called 'idiopathic'. Further important observations are that the dietary structure can influence significantly these values and that the diet typical in the affluent westernized communities aggravates the extent of any abnormality (Andersen, 1972).

It is interesting to correlate these findings with the epidemiology of this condition.

Epidemiology

There has been considerable increase in the incidence of idiopathic renal stone in Europe, North America, Australasia and Japan within the present century (Grossman, 1938; Inada *et al.*, 1958; Andersen, 1969; Fig. 4.1). This has been progressive up to the present except for interruptions during the two world wars in countries in which dietary restrictions were severe (Schumann, 1963; Fig. 4.2). Whereas the disease formerly affected predominantly adults, it now occurs in children and has entirely displaced bladder stone as a childhood entity (Ghazali *et al.*, 1973). Renal stone varies in prevalence between 3 and 13 per cent in affluent industrialized communities (Blacklock, 1969; Ljunghall and Hedstrand, 1975; Scott *et al.*, 1977). The prevalence in the USA is around 12 per cent, and the direct medical cost of the disease has been estimated to be in excess of 47 million dollars per year (Finlayson, 1974).

Renal stone is rare among persons living in poor or primitive socio-economic circumstances and is very rare in African Bantu living under tribal conditions (Modlin, 1969). An apparently similar relative immunity of the Negro in the USA during the early decades of the present century (Reaser, 1935) was lost later with greater affluence and the adoption of the lifestyle of his white countrymen (Quinland, 1945). Other associations with affluence are the occurrence of the condition in south-east European immigrants

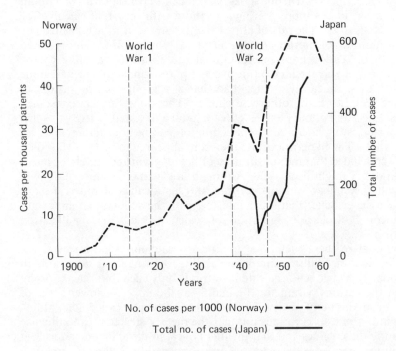

Fig. 4.1   Change in incidence of renal stone in Oslo City Hospital, Norway, 1900–60 (Andersen, 1969) and in Japan 1935–55 (Inada *et al.*, 1958)

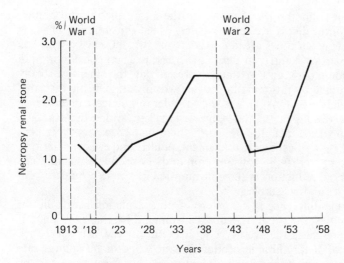

Fig. 4.2   Incidence of renal stone at necropsy in Leipzig, Germany 1913–58 (Schumann, 1963)

shortly after their arrival in industrial Germany (Boshamer, 1961) and the high prevalence of the condition in the more affluent Arabs of the Arabian peninsula.

Whilst a familial predisposition has been found implying genetic factors and there is the evidence for a familial idiopathic hypercalciuria (Coe, *et al.,* 1979), the spouses of some hypercalciuric stone formers were found also to have hypercalciuria (White *et al.,* 1969); this suggested the influence of a domestic factor which was most likely to be dietary. Ljunghall and Hedstrand (1975) also noted a greater incidence of stones in first degree relatives of stone formers than in a reference population of normal people.

To summarize, from being virtually unknown in historical times, renal stone has become significant as a common morbid condition in the affluent, westernized countries within the last 80 years whilst remaining rare in communities where the people live in primitive and poor conditions. If the predisposition to the minor metabolic abnormalities described in the previous section is present in the same proportion of the poor communities, as is most likely, their immunity must be dependent on the absence of a risk factor or factors common in the environment of the affluent communities. These are most likely to be associated with dietary structure.

Dietary factors

Dietary changes

Dietary changes from the historical past, when renal stone was uncommon, to the present are similar to the dietary differences which exist between the

poor and affluent communities of today. In the latter, the fat and animal
protein content of the diet is five times greater, whilst consumption of sugar
or sugar products is ten times greater (Anderson, 1972). Cleave (1974) has
described the progressive and considerable increase in sugar consumption in
the United Kingdom between 1850 and the present day, the otherwise steady
rise being interrupted by rationing in the two world wars. During the same
period of time Inada *et al*, (1958) noted the considerable increase in incidence
of renal stone in the Japanese, and Kagawa (1978) recorded the dramatic
change in the Japanese diet. In summary, there had been a 200 per cent
increase in sugar, 700 per cent increase in meat, poultry and egg consumption
and a 1500 per cent increase in consumption of diary products. There was a
concomitant overall reduction in the consumption of rice to a quarter, and
of barley, potatoes and vegetables.

Another notable difference is the extent of fibre depletion in the diet of
affluent communities; the tribal Africans consuming three times the amount
of dietary fibre present in the average UK diet (Burkitt and Trowell, 1975).
The importance of dietary fibre in producing satiety and modifying the rate
and overall absorption of nutrients and minerals has been described by
Haber *et al*. (1977). One of the implications of fibre depletion in the circumstances of nutrient surplus is that overnutrition is likely.

Sucrose

Hodgkinson and Heaton (1965), Lindeman *et al*. (1967) and others have
observed that both protein and glucose can increase the rate of urinary
calcium excretion and Lemann *et al*. (1969) noted that the glucose effect was
exaggerated in calcium stone formers. This suggested to Schwille *et al*. (1974)
that the basic metabolic fault might be a disorder of carbohydrate metabolism.
Recent studies have shown that either sucrose, or sucrose-containing products, when added as supplements to a standard diet, increase the frequency
and magnitude of diurnal peaks of urinary calcium concentration in a
majority of normal subjects. Urinary oxalate excretion and concentration
are increased concomitantly so that the formation product of calcium oxalate
is exceeded and there is the risk of spontaneous crystallization (Hargreave
et al., 1977; Thom *et al*., 1980). The mechanism of the effect of sucrose and
glucose on urinary calcium and oxalate excretion is not yet clear. It is likely,
however, to be mediated by the metabolic response to sucrose ingestion
which principally involves both insulin (Defronzo *et al*., 1975) and glucagon.

Whilst these changes in the pattern of excretion of calcium, oxalate and
other electrolytes have been observed to follow the ingestion of sucrose,
Kang *et al*. (1977) observed that the ingestion of sucrose by laboratory animals
resulted in a diffuse intercapillary glomerulosclerosis and that urinary excretion of N-acetyl-β-glucosaminadase, an indicator of renal tubular damage
(Dance and Price, 1970), was significantly greater throughout sucrose
feeding. The potential of ingested sucrose to produce damage in tubular cells
is of interest in view of the observations of Malek and Boyce (1973), Anderson
(1969) and others of microcalculi in histological studies of renal biopsies or

resection specimens from calcium stone formers. The location of these was both within the lumen of the tubule and in the tubule cells. They have been postulated to be the initial nidus on which subsequent crystallization takes place in stone formation. The aetiology of these lesions has so far been unexplained, but if sucrose ingestion is found in the human to induce increased rates of urinary excretion of N-acetyl-β-glucosaminadase, as occurs in certain laboratory animals, it is possible, if speculative, that excessive sucrose ingestion over a period, such as in childhood, may be a cause. Calcified deposits in the tubular cells form the basis of the fixed particle mechanism propounded by Finlayson and Reid (1978) as the essential prerequisite in the renal tubule for the development of urolithiasis.

Whilst the increased mean intestinal absorption of calcium observed in stone formers may be the result of increased plasma levels of 1,25-DHCC (Haussler *et al.*, 1976), sucrose has been found to induce significant increase in the rate of radiocalcium absorption (Macleod and Blacklock, 1979). This occurred both in normal subjects and in idiopathic calcium stone formers, but was proportionately less in the latter in view of their spontaneously higher rate of absorption. There is a greater spontaneous urinary excretion rate of oxalate in calcium oxalate stone formers, and Hagler and Hermann (1973) observed that they excreted much larger amounts of dietary oxalate than normal subjects. Although the mechanism of this is not clear there is the possibility that, with the more complete absorption of calcium in the upper intestine in stone formers, the lesser amount of residual calcium will precipitate and trap less dietary oxalate in the intestinal lumen, more oxalate remaining in solution and therefore available for absorption. If this is the mechanism involved, then any food constituent such as sucrose which will enhance calcium absorption from the intestine may be expected to increase the amount of dietary oxalate absorbed and therefore to increase urinary oxalate excretion. Thom *et al.* (1980) found that available carbohydrate and sucrose supplements to a standard diet increased the frequency and magnitude of peaks of urinary oxalate concentration in a majority of the normal subjects studied, these peaks coinciding with those of calcium concentration. The overall result of this supplementation of a standard diet was significantly to increase the number of occasions when the calcium oxalate formation product of the urine was exceeded, i.e. oversaturation, with the likelihood of inducing spontaneous crystallization.

To summarize, there is evidence that sucrose ingestion induces renal tubular cell damage in animals and that available carbohydrate and sucrose supplements change the urinary electrolyte profile of normal subjects so that there is increased risk of calcium oxalate crystallization. The latter effect is exaggerated in known calcium oxalate stone formers.

Animal protein

Another feature of the dietary structure of the affluent communities is the large amount of animal protein and with the confirmation of this in dietary information obtained from known stone formers, Robertson *et al.* (1979)

have studied the influence of increments of animal protein on the excretion rates of calcium, oxalate and uric acid. They found that these were all significantly increased, so that there was a greater likelihood of spontaneous calcium oxalate crystallization, both from the increase in the activity product of calcium oxalate to formation product levels, and from the interference with the effect of the acid mucopolysaccharide inhibitor of calcium oxalate crystallization by the increased urinary levels of uric acid.

Fibre

The properties of dietary fibre in the alimentary tract are both physical and physicochemical. On the physical side, the fibre absorbs water, increases stool bulk and in this way there is a shorter intestinal transit time. This on its own may have an influence on oxalate absorption. Additionally, however, cereal fibre can trap and diminish the extent of absorption of nutrients such as the sugars (Haber et al., 1977). Wheat bran has been observed to improve glucose tolerance and reduce plasma glucose in diabetics (Jeffreys, 1974). Kiehm et al. (1976) found that a high fibre, high carbohydrate diet diminished requirement of sulphonylureas or insulin in diabetic patients, whilst Miranda and Horwitz (1978) observed a lower mean serum glucagon with high fibre (20 g/d) diets. These effects of dietary fibre in modifying the metabolic response to energy-dense nutrients are of significance in calcium stone disease in view of the probable mediation of glucagon and insulin in renal function and urinary electrolyte secretion (Defronzo et al., 1975).

Macleod and Blacklock (1979) have found that wheat bran diminished [47]Calcium absorption from the intestine in a group of normal subjects by as much as 50 per cent, also that the increase in [47]Calcium absorption which had been induced by sugar was negated when wheat bran was given at the same time as the sugar and calcium carrier in the radiocalcium uptake test. This may be due either to the cereal fibre trapping the sugar or specifically absorbing the calcium or to a combination of both. The reduced plasma level of glucagon observed by Miranda and Horwitz (1978) with high fibre diets may also be involved.

The dietary hypothesis of the 'stone wave'

In suggesting that dietary constituents altered stone incidence within any population group, Andersen (1972) stipulated the need to demonstrate a biochemical pathway between dietary structure and urine composition favouring the formation of the type of stone prevalent within the group. The evidence of metabolic studies of idiopathic calcium stone formers has shown that, although there is abnormality in some, this is usually minor in degree and dependent on diet, disappearing in the fasting state. Stone formers therefore appear to be phenotypes whose minimal aberrations of metabolism are aggravated by overnutrition consequent upon a nutrient-rich and fibre-poor diet. Andersen's hypothesis appears largely to have been substantiated by the research work already described, since the dietary structure typical of the affluent, westernized countries has been shown to increase the likelihood of calcium oxalate crystallization in the urine at the same time as reducing the activity of acid mucopolysaccharide inhibitors of crystallization. It is therefore probable that this has been the trigger mechanism responsible for the great increase in renal stone during the present century—the 'stone wave'. McCance and Widdowson (1946) observed that the fibre-enriched, sugar- and animal protein-reduced wartime diet resulted in significant reduction in urinary calcium levels. The significance of this was not appreciated, however, by them at that time.

The implication of these observations is that idiopathic calcium urolithiasis, whatever the minor metabolic abnormalities present, can probably be diminished in incidence or prevented by a change to a dietary structure which is less energy dense than at present, containing less animal protein and sugar and more cereal and other sources of fibre. The progressive increase in incidence of renal stone might therefore be arrested and even reversed if appropriate change in dietary style is acceptable to a majority of people.

References

Andersen, D. A. (1969). Historical and geographical differences in the pattern of incidence of urinary stones considered in relation to aetiological factors. *Proceedings of the International Symposium on Renal Stone Research,* 7–32. Editors A. Hodgkinson and B. E. C. Nordin. Churchill, London

Andersen, D. A. (1972). Environmental factors in the aetiology of urolithiasis. *Proceedings of the International Symposium on Renal Stone Research,* 130–134. Editors D. L. Cifuentes, A. Rapado and A. Hodgkinson. Karger, Basle

Anderson, C. K. (1969). Renal histological changes in stone formers and non-stone formers. *Proceedings of the International Symposium on Renal Stone Research,* 133–136. Editors A. Hodgkinson and B. E. C. Nordin. Churchill, London

Blacklock, N. J. (1969). The pattern of urolithiasis in the Royal Navy. In: *Ibid.,* 33–48. Churchill, London

Blacklock, N. J. and MacLeod, M. A. (1974). Calcium-47 absorption in urolithiasis. *British Journal of Urology,* **46,** 377–384

Boshamer, K. (1961). *The Calculous Areas of the World. Handbook of Urology,* **10,** 34–50. Springer Verlag, Berlin

Bulusu, L., Hodgkinson, A., Nordin, B. E. C. and Peacock, M. (1970). Urinary excretion of calcium and creatinine in relation to age and body weight in normal subjects and patients with renal calculus. *Clinical Science,* **38,** 601–612

Burkitt, D. P. and Trowell, H. C. (1975). *Refined Carbohydrate Foods and Disease. Some Implications of Dietary Fibre.* Academic Press, London

Cleave, T. L. (1974). *The Saccharine Disease. Conditions Caused by the Taking of Refined Carbohydrates, such as Sugar and White Flour.* John Wright, Bristol

Coe, F. L. and Kavalach, A. G. (1974). Hypercalciuria and hyperuricosuria in patients with calcium nephrolithiasis. *New England Journal of Medicine*, **291**, 1344–1350

Coe, F. L., Parks, J. H. and Moore, E. S. (1979). Familial idiopathic hypercalciuria. *New England Journal of Medicine*, **300**, 337–340

Dance, N. and Price, R. G. (1970). The excretion of N-acetyl-β-glucosaminidase and β-galactosidase by patients with renal disease. *Clinica Chimica Acta*, **27**, 87–92

Defronzo, R. A., Cooke, C. R., Andres, R., Faloona, G. R. and Davies, P. J. (1975). The effect of insulin on renal handling of sodium, potassium, calcium and phosphate in man. *Journal of Clinical Investigation*, **55**, 845–855

Finlayson, B. (1974). Renal lithiasis in review. *Urological Clinics of North America*, **1**, 181–212

Finlayson, B. and Reid, F. (1978). The expectation of free and fixed particles in urinary stone disease. *Investigative Urology*, **15**, 442–448.

Ghazali, S., Barratt, T. M. and Williams, D. I. (1973). Childhood urolithiasis in Britain. *Archives of Diseases in Childhood*, **48**, 291–295

Grossman, W. (1938). Current urinary stone wave in central Europe. *British Journal of Urology*, **10**, 46–54

Haber, G. B., Heaton, K. W., Murphy, D. and Burroughs, L. F. (1977). Depletion and disruption of dietary fibre. *Lancet*, **ii**, 679–682

Hagler, L. and Hermann, R. H. (1973). Oxalate metabolism. I. *American Journal of Clinical Nutrition*, **26**, 758–765. II. 882–889. III. 1006–1010

Hargreave, T. B., Sali, A., MacKay, C. and Sullivan, M. (1977). Diurnal variation in urinary oxalate. *British Journal of Urology*, **49**, 597–600

Haussler, M. R., Baylink, D. J., Hughes, M. R., Brumbaugh, P. F., Wergedal, J. E., Shen, F. H., Nielsen, R., Counts, S. J., Bursac, K. M. and McCain, T. A. (1976). The assay of 1 alpha 25 dihydroxy-vitamin D_3: Physiologic and pathologic modulation of circulating hormone levels. *Clinical Endocrinology*, **5**, 151S–165S

Hodgkinson, A. and Heaton, F. W. (1965). The effect of food ingestion on the urinary excretion of calcium and magnesium. *Clinica Chimica Acta*, **11**, 354–362

Inada, T., Miyazaki, S., Omori, T., Nihira, H. and Hino, T. (1958). Statistical study on urolithiasis in Japan. *Urologia Internationalis, Basle*, **7**, 150–165

Jeffreys, D. B. (1974). The effect of dietary fibre on the response to orally administered glucose. *Proceedings of the Nutrition Society*, **33**, 11A–12A

Kagawa, Y. (1978). Impact of westernisation on the nutrition of Japanese: changes in physique, cancer, longevity and centenarians. *Preventive Medicine*, **7**, 205–217

Kang, S. S., Price, R. G., Bruckdorfer, K. R., Worcester, N. A. and Yudkin, J. (1977). Renal damage in rats caused by dietary sucrose. *Biochemical Society Transactions*, **5**, 235–236

Kiehm, T. G., Anderson, J. W. and Ward, K. (1976). Beneficial effects of a high carbohydrate, high fiber diet on hyperglycemic men. *American Journal of Clinical Nutrition*, **29**, 895–899

Lemann, J., Piering, W. F. and Lennon, E. J. (1969). Possible role of carbohydrate-induced calciuria in calcium oxalate kidney-stone formation. *New England Journal of Medicine*, **280**, 232–237

Lindeman, R. D., Adler, S., Yiengst, M. J. and Beard, E. S. (1967). Influence of various nutrients on urinary divalent cation excretion. *Journal of Laboratory Clinical Medicine*, **70**, 236–245

Ljunghall, S. and Hedstrand, H. (1965). Epidemiology of renal stone in a middle aged population. *Acta Medica Scandinavica*, **197**, 439–445

Macleod, M. A. and Blacklock, N. J. (1979). The influence of glucose and wheat bran on calcium absorption. *Journal of the Royal Naval Medical Service*, **65**, 143–146

Malek, R. S. and Boyce, W. H. (1973). Intranephronic calculosis; its significance and relationship to matrix in nephrolithiasis. *Journal of Urology*, **109**, 551–555

McCance, R. A. and Widdowson, E. M. (1946). *An Experimental Study of Rationing*, 41–42. MRC Special Report Series No. 254. His Majesty's Stationery Office, London

Miranda, P. M. and Horwitz, D. L. (1978). High-fiber diets in the treatment of diabetes mellitus. *Annals of Internal Medicine*, **88**, 482–486

Modlin, M. (1969). Renal calculus in the Republic of South Africa. *Proceedings of the Renal Stone Research Symposium, Leeds*, 49–58. Editors A. Hodgkinson and B. E. C. Nordin. Churchill, London

Nordin, B. E. C., Peacock, M. and Marshall, D. H. (1976). Calcium excretion and hypercalciuria. In: *Urolithiasis Research. Proceedings of Stone Symposium, Davos*, 101–115. Editors H. Fleisch, W. G. Robertson, L. H. Smith and W. Vahlensieck. Plenum, New York

Quinland, W. S. (1945). Urinary lithiasis. Review of 33 cases in Negroes. *Journal of Urology*, **53**, 791–804

Reaser, E. F. (1935). Racial incidence of urolithiasis. *Journal of Urology*, **34**, 148–155

Robertson, W. G. and Morgan, D. B. (1972). The distribution of urinary calcium excretions in normal persons and stone-formers. *Clinica Chimica Acta*, **37**, 503–508

Robertson, W. G., Peacock, M., Marshall, R. W., Marshall, D. H. and Nordin, B. E. C. (1976). Saturation-inhibition index as a measure of the risk of calcium oxalate stone formation in the urinary tract. *New England Journal of Medicine*, **294**, 249–252

Robertson, W. G., Peacock, M., Heyburn, P. J., Hanes, F., Rutherford, A., Clementson, E., Swaminathan, R. and Clark, P. B. (1979). Should recurrent calcium-containing stone-formers become vegetarians? *British Journal of Urology*, **51**, 427–431

Schumann, H. R. (1963). Die Haufigkeit der Urolithiasis in Sektions-gut des Pathologischer. Institutes St. George, Leipzig. *Zentralblatt fur Allgemeine Pathologie und Pathologische Anatomie*, **105**, 88–94

Schwille, P. O., Scholz, D., Hagemann, G. and Sigel, A. (1974). Metabolic and glucose load studies in uric acid, oxalic and hyperparathyroid stone formers. *Advances in Experimental Medicine and Biology*, **41**, 485–494

Scott, R., Freeland, R., Mowat, W., Gardiner, M., Hawthorne, V., Marshall, R. M. and Ives, J. G. J. (1977). The prevalence of calcified upper urinary tract stone disease in a random population—Cumbernauld Health Survey. *British Journal of Urology*, **49**, 589–595

Thom, J. A., Morris, J. E., Bishop, A. and Blacklock, N. J. (1980). Effect of dietary sucrose on urinary calcium oxalate activity product. *Proceedings of the International Urinary Stone Conference, 1979*. Editors G. Brockis and B. Finlayson. PSG Publishing (in press), Littleton, Massachusetts.

White, R. W., Cohen, R. D., Vince, F. P., Williams, G., Blandy, J. and Tresidder, G. C. (1969). Minerals in the urine of stone-formers and their spouses. *Renal Stone Research Symposium, Leeds*, 289–296. Editors A. Hodgkinson and B. E. C. Nordin. Churchill, London

5

Multiple sclerosis

Emer Shelley and Geoffrey Dean

Introduction

Multiple sclerosis (MS) is a chronic neurological disease of unknown cause. It is a demyelinating disease with loss of the myelin sheath which normally coats nerve axons, associated with an inflammatory cell infiltrate. In patients with a compatible history, and in whom there is no alternative explanation, the diagnosis of MS depends on the demonstration of objective signs of lesions at two or more distinct sites in the central nervous system (CNS). Women are affected slightly more frequently than men, and at a younger age. In countries where MS is common, the risk of developing the disease rises in adolescence, reaches a peak in the early thirties, and falls away in the sixth decade.

Studies of the epidemiology of MS have shown major differences in the incidence of the disease among people of the same genetic stock living in different environments. It is hoped that defining and comparing high and low risk areas will lead to discovery of the causative factor or factors of the disease.

Using information from many different studies it is possible to divide the world into high, medium and low risk zones, with prevalence rates of $\geqslant 40$, 20–39 and <20 per 100 000 population respectively. There are areas for which no data is available, and many border areas between zones of different risks have not yet been studied. Nevertheless the relationship between prevalence rates in an area, and latitude north or south of the equator is apparent. This relationship can be seen by looking at prevalence and mortality rates within an individual continent which spans a wide range of latitudes.

In North America, MS was found to be less common in New Orleans than further north. The incidence and prevalence of MS among the white population showed a three-fold increase between New Orleans (30 degrees N) and Boston (42 degrees N) and Winnipeg (50 degrees N). The rates for Negroes were also higher in Boston than in New Orleans (Westlund and Kurland, 1953). Other studies have looked at the prevalence of MS among US ex-servicemen being treated within the Veterans Administration. Prevalence, by place of birth was found to increase from south to north along the Pacific Coast, and on the Atlantic seaboard, as well as in the Mississippi Valley. A further study of army veterans by Kurtzke *et al.* (1975) showed that MS was less frequent in American blacks than in whites, and again found that in blacks, as in whites, the disease is less frequent in the south than in the north. Alaska, Mexico and South America seem to be areas of low MS risk.

In Europe the high risk zone extends from 45 to 65 degrees N latitude. There is a medium risk zone to the south and also to the north of the high risk zone. Iceland, the British Isles, northern France, Holland, Belgium, Germany and Poland lie within the high risk zone. Very high prevalence rates (> 1/1 000) have been reported from Orkney and Shetland, and in north-east Scotland. The Scandinavian countries also have a high risk except along the Atlantic coast of Norway and in the extreme north. If the prevalence of MS continued to increase with increasing distance from the equator, one would expect high prevalence in people living near the Arctic, for example in Laplanders and Eskimos. As far as is known, these groups do not have a high prevalence of MS. A low rate of MS was reported among the Eskimos in the area around Anchorage, Alaska, during the period 1950–63.

The situation in southern Europe is less clear. Intermediate or low rates have been reported from Italy, Sardinia, southern France and southern Switzerland. Immigrants to England from Italy had the same risk of being hospitalized with MS as the United Kingdom-born, immigrants from Spain had an intermediate risk, but no MS patients were found among the immigrants from Malta although the expected number was 9·7. The high prevalence of MS among Italian immigrants suggests that the prevalence in Italy as a whole is not greatly different to that in the United Kingdom (UK). Recent studies found a high rate in Enna city, Sicily (53 per 100 000) but a very low rate in the neighbouring islands of Malta (4 per 100 000). Further study of 'border' areas between places of different risk for MS could yield important information on the environmental and genetic factors responsible for the disease.

In the USSR an increase in frequency was reported as one moved northward from Baku (40 degrees N) to Archangel (66 degrees N). All of Asia is low risk. It is not yet known where the border zone lies between the high risk of the USSR and the low risk in Asia. Careful studies have confirmed that MS is rare in Japan and showed no gradient between Kumamoto (33 degrees N) and Sapporo (43 degrees N). Australia and New Zealand are medium risk zones and show a gradient of increasing frequency of MS with increasing distance from the equator. Reports from Queensland suggest that even when close to the equator, people of European stock retain a significant risk of developing MS.

Race

The frequency of MS is not constant throughout the world. The question arises as to whether the distribution of MS can be accounted for by the distribution of different racial groups. Many of the temperate regions where high MS rates have been reported are inhabited by Caucasians. Mongoloid and Negro groups in the same area have been reported to have lower rates of

MS than Caucasians. However, MS declines in frequency with latitude in both Caucasians and Negroes. It is likely that environmental factors account for many of the racial differences in the frequency of MS.

Migration

The relative importance of environmental as opposed to racial or genetic factors has been highlighted by studying the frequency of MS in groups of migrants, comparing the prevalence of MS in the migrants with the prevalence in their country of origin and in the country to which they emigrated.

South Africa is an area of low risk for MS. The disease is extremely uncommon among the Cape Coloured and the Indian people of South Africa, and no single case of MS has yet been found among South Africa's 17 million Bantu, though there are good Bantu hospitals with well-trained neurologists in the large cities. Immigrants from northern Europe had a three times greater risk of MS than immigrants from the Mediterranean countries, and white immigrants from other African states had a low risk. The risk of developing MS in an English-speaking white South African-born was between a third and a quarter, and in the Afrikaans-speaking white South African-born only one-eleventh the risk in the immigrants from the UK and north and central Europe (Dean and Kurtzke, 1971).

The South African findings were confirmed in Israel by Leibowitz *et al.* (1972) who found that immigrants from northern Europe had a high risk of developing MS but immigrants from Africa and Asia had only one-third of this risk.

Age of migration
Those who migrate from Europe to South Africa below the age of 15 years have a low risk of developing MS. The same was true for those who emigrated from Europe to Israel below the age of 15.

Migration from low to high risk areas
In a recent study of first hospital admissions for MS among immigrants in Greater London, there was a marked deficit of cases in immigrants from New Commonwealth Asia of Indian and Pakistani ethnic origin and among Africans and Indians from the New Commonwealth countries of Africa. Immigrants from the New Commonwealth America (the West Indies) had a higher risk of developing MS than Asians and Africans but still only one-seventh of that in the United Kingdom-born (Dean *et al.*, 1976). This suggests a very low incidence of MS in these people and that their risk was not increased by emigrating to an area of high risk. It will be of interest to study the incidence of MS among the UK-born children of immigrants from low risk parts of the world, to see if their risk of MS is that of their parents or if it increases towards the higher risk that occurs in England. Such a study would distinguish further between racial and environmental factors which lead to the development of MS. The low incidence of MS among the immigrants mentioned above contrasted with that of immigrants from other European

countries, Australia, Canada, New Zealand and the Middle East. This second group of immigrants had an incidence of MS which was only slightly less than that of the UK-born London residents.

In summary, those who migrate from a high risk zone to a low risk zone keep their high risk, unless they migrate below the age of 15. Conversely, emigrating to England from low risk parts of the world did not seem to increase the risk of developing MS.

Environmental factors

Epidemiological studies suggest that an environmental factor (or factors) plays some role in the causation of MS. Furthermore this environmental influence may be associated to some extent with latitude. Nevertheless, the distribution of MS does not accord well with the hypothesis that it is due to direct action of climate on the body, in the same sense that frostbite or cancer of the skin is directly related to climate. For instance, the coldness of winter is closely related to the distance from the ocean, but this is not correlated with the prevalence of MS.

In 1967, a theory was proposed which still best fits the epidemiological facts (Dean, 1967). It seems most likely that MS is normally an infection of infancy, probably a virus gastrointestinal infection. Those who escape early infection because of a high level of domestic hygiene may, if they are so predisposed, develop the adult form of the disease, that is, MS. According to this theory, the South African Bantu, Coloured and Asian living in primitive conditions in a warm country are almost invariably infected in early infancy. It is well established that South African infants have a very high morbidity and mortality from gastrointestinal infections. Poskanzer *et al.* (1963) suggested that one could compare MS with poliomyelitis. In the latter disease, the paralytic form occurred most commonly in those with a high level of social hygiene, who therefore were liable to miss an early non-paralytic form of the disease in infancy. Paralytic poliomyelitis in adult South Africans was much more common among the White than among the Coloured, Asian and Bantu, and in adults at least twice as common among immigrants from the UK and Europe as among the white South African-born.

Which virus?

The search for a virus which might play a role in causation of MS began in earnest with the recognition that some animal diseases were caused by 'slow viruses'. Studies of visna in sheep demonstrated virus growing in the brain during an incubation period of many months. The first recognized example of slowly progressive virus infection in man was subacute sclerosing panencephalitis (SSPE). The relationship between SSPE and measles virus was recognized in 1967. There is widespread infection in the brain with large amounts of virus antigen and a pronounced antibody response. Kuru and Creutzfeld–Jakob disease are two other progressive diseases which cause degeneration of the human brain and have since been associated with virus-like agents.

These associations between slowly progressive neurological disease and virus-like particles led to a study of the serology of MS. The presence of a slightly raised titre of measles antibody in a group of MS patients when compared with a group of normal controls was first described in 1962. This slightly raised titre of measles antibody has been found in many other studies. Other groups of MS patients have had increased titres of antibody to other viruses such as herpes virus and pox virus. However, these studies have all involved small numbers of patients. It is likely that in a study with a large group of patients and controls that only antibody to measles virus would be increased in MS when compared with controls (Frazer, 1977).

The need for caution in interpreting this association between raised measles antibody titres and the occurrence of MS has been stressed. Field used the following graphic analogy: 'For many years there has been a highly significant statistical correlation between the declining stork population in Sweden and the falling birth rate, but this does not mean that storks bring babies.' The only conclusion one can safely draw from this finding of raised antibody titres to measles virus in MS is that the measles antibody levels act as a marker of an abnormal immune response to viruses in patients with MS.

Evidence for a transmissible agent

In 1947 there was a report of the development of MS in 4 out of 7 scientists working on swayback in lambs. This 'outbreak' was reviewed in 1975 by Symonds who suggested that handling sheep's brains, in the presence of an asymptomatic virus infection, may have induced a hypersensitivity reaction resulting in demyelination. Another interesting report was that scrapie (a 'slow virus' neurological disease) was produced in Icelandic sheep, 16–21 months after intracerebral inoculation of brain from a patient who died of acute MS. This work has not been confirmed by others.

Perhaps the most exciting work in this area, which has been confirmed by a number of workers, has been the discovery of the 'granulocytopenic factor'. Carp *et al.* (1972) found that inoculation of mice with MS tissue produced a granulocytopenia (a reduction in the circulating white blood cells). Serum from these mice with granulocytopenia caused a fall in the cell levels in other mice. They suggested a possible filterable agent with a size of 25–50 nanometres.

Since then cell cultures of mouse fibroblasts have been inoculated with MS material. Subsequent subcultures showed a significant reduction in cell yield in the MS infected cultures. The cell-free lysate from the eighteenth passage produced a granulocytopenia when inoculated into mice. This evidence suggests that a transmissible agent plays some role in the aetiology of MS.

MS in the Faröe islands

No cases of MS were recorded on these islands between 1929 and 1943, and only 2 cases with onset between 1960 and 1974. However, from 1944 to 1960 there was an epidemic of MS, with 18 definite cases recorded on the islands (Kurtzke and Hyllested, 1975). It was suggested that a virus was introduced to the Faröe islands during the British occupation from 1940 to 1944. This virus might have spread among the indigenous population and then disappeared within a few years of introduction. This postulated 'slow virus' could have led to MS with an incubation period of 2–17 years.

Cook *et al.* (1978) have suggested that the infectious agent concerned in this outbreak might have been canine distemper virus, since a severe epidemic of distemper occurred in the canine population after the arrival of British troops in the early 1940s. Examination of earlier veterinary records showed that canine distemper had not been reported on the islands before 1939. There is now strict control on the import of dogs and there has been no canine distemper on the islands since 1956. This report is of particular interest since the viruses of canine distemper and of human measles are so alike antigenically that the measles virus has been used to vaccinate puppies against canine distemper. Canine distemper virus is a paramyxovirus which can produce a neurological demyelinating disease in dogs with many similarities to MS. Cook *et al.* (1978) stress that the only link to date between MS and canine distemper virus is a temporal one and that further research is required.

Diet

The myelin sheath is mainly composed of lipids. Many studies have looked at lipid metabolism in the CNS, and at the utilization of dietary lipids in MS. There is some epidemiological evidence of a possible correlation between the geographical distribution of MS and dietary fat. In 1953 Swank suggested that the high prevalence of MS in the more northern countries was due to a high fat intake. Sinclair suggested in 1956 that it was not simply a diet high in animal fats that led to an increased risk of MS in these northern countries, but a diet which was relatively deficient in polyunsaturated fatty acids (Mertin and Meade, 1977). Swank showed that the incidence and prevalence of MS was high in inland areas of Norway, in contrast to the low risk coastal areas. The coastal regions have a lower fat intake, with a higher proportion of polyunsaturated fatty acids. The higher incidence of MS in the cantons of Switzerland which are German speaking, compared with Italian- and French-speaking cantons, has also been attributed to the former's high fat consumption.

There is a change in the relative proportions of saturated and unsaturated fatty acids in the brain lipids of patients with MS. It has been suggested that an excess of saturated fatty acids might cause CNS membranes to become rigid. This alteration in structure could cause susceptibility to attack by a pathogenic agent and lead to destruction of myelin.

In MS patients, platelet stickiness is increased. Swank suggested that disordered fat transport in MS leads to intravascular aggregation of platelets and red blood cells (sludging). The resulting decrease in oxygen availability in brain tissue could cause perivascular demyelination. In human subjects, a diet low in saturated fatty acids and rich in polyunsaturated fatty acids caused a significant reduction in platelet aggregation in flowing blood (Hornstra *et al.*, 1973).

The above evidence has led to clinical trials of dietary therapy in the treatment of MS. Swank (1970) reported that oil supplements with a low animal fat intake for more than 20 years gave better relapse and survival rates when compared with rates reported in the literature. The trial did not include control subjects. Swank could conclude, however, that 'patients who consumed the least amount of fat and the largest amounts of fluid oils deteriorated less than those who consumed more fat and less oil'.

Millar *et al.* (1973) carried out a double-blind trial of linoleate supplementation in the diets of MS patients. They found that the rate of relapse per patient year was less for the treated group than for the control group, though the difference was not statistically significant. However, there was a significant reduction in the severity of relapses in the treated group. Millar *et al.* (1973) confirmed that platelet adhesiveness is greater in MS patients than in normal controls. Serial observations during linoleate supplementation showed no significant change in platelet stickiness. Serum linoleate is reduced in MS, and oral supplementation produced an increase in serum linoleate. Linoleate increased from 28·6 per cent (when expressed as a percentage of the total fatty acids) prior to the trial, to 36·3 per cent after 9–12 months' supplementation with linoleate. The numbers in this trial were small. While dietary therapy has never been adequately shown to have beneficial effects, many believe that further large-scale trials are justifiable.

Vitamin D

In 1929 Hess noted that 'a map of the incidence of rickets is the practical equivalent of a map of deficiency of sunlight'. However, there were some populations who did not get rickets in spite of their northern location. The Japanese, also the Eskimos of northern Greenland, had a very low incidence of rickets. These people also have a low risk of MS. The relationship between rickets and sunlight, vitamin D and fish oils is now proven. There has been speculation as to whether MS might also be linked in some way to vitamin D.

If vitamin D and MS were in some way associated, then variations in incidence of MS with sunshine and latitude and also differing racial susceptibility might be explained. Sunshine and vitamin D synthesis and therefore calcium metabolism are related to skin pigmentation. Alter and Harshe (1975) speculated that calcium levels, mediated by racially determined skin pigment, may influence the risk of MS and help account for racial differences in frequency. As was seen in South Africa, there is an inverse relationship between the degree of skin pigmentation and the racial risk of developing MS. Within the Caucasian race in the United States and in Europe, as pigmentation lessens from south to north, the incidence of MS increases.

It has been shown that the calcium ion can affect signs and symptoms in MS. The demyelinated fibre is very sensitive to changes in calcium ion concentration (Halliday and McDonald, 1977). The question of seasonal variation in 25-hydroxycholecalciferol (a vitamin D metabolite) is controversial. No seasonal variation in ionized calcium has been demonstrated. Further research is required into the ionized calcium levels in different racial groups and in patients with MS.

Dental caries

Craelius (1978) noted that casual comparison of the WHO map of dental caries throughout the world reveals a striking parallel with the incidence of MS. Furthermore, dental examination of MS patients found a high rate of caries among them, when compared with an age-matched group of epileptics. Craelius took 45 geographical areas throughout the world, and ranked the prevalence of MS with an index of dental health. He found a correlation coefficient of 0.78 ($P < 0.001$) and concluded that there is a close relationship between world-wide MS and dental disease rates. He noted that dental caries rates are low in tropical countries and increase with north and south latitude, except for Japan, and among the Eskimos in Alaska. The parallel between MS and dental caries remained when Craelius extended his study beyond geographic variation and looked at differences in MS and caries by race and sex.

Craelius recounted that dental surveys in the Isle of Lewis showed that caries increased from very low rates in 1938 to high rates in 1968. Dietary surveys were carried out in conjunction with the dental surveys. In the interval between the surveys there was a substitution of meat for fish, resulting in an increase in fat consumption, and a decreased intake of vitamin D and trace minerals. The incidence of MS on the Shetland islands has increased markedly since 1954 and they too have had a dietary change away from fish.

Cancer of the colon

Wolfgram (1975) took WHO mortality statistics and attempted to find diseases with similar geographic distribution to MS. He looked at mortality for 83 diseases in 36 countries. Only one disease, cancer of the colon, showed a positive correlation with MS. In addition to a low fibre diet, a diet high in fat and high in animal protein may be important in the aetiology of cancer of the colon (Hutt and Burkitt, 1977).

In summary, MS has a geographic distribution which suggests that it occurs more frequently in regions with a high intake of animal fats and a low intake of polyunsaturated fatty acids. Dietary supplementation with linoleate may improve the clinical course of MS. The disease may be associated with alterations in vitamin D and calcium metabolism. The distribution of MS is similar to other diseases which are associated with dietary factors, such as dental caries and carcinoma of the colon. Thus many distinct pieces of evidence point to a dietary factor (or factors) which increases susceptibility to MS, or to a factor which protects against the development of the disease.

Genetic factors

In addition to environmental factors one must also look at genetic factors which predispose to the development of an illness. MS occurs with increased frequency among close relatives of patients with MS. Millar and Allison (1954) reported a survey in Northern Ireland. Out of a total of 668 families, they found 44 families (6·6 per cent) in which two or more members were affected. The frequency of MS in the siblings of patients with MS was between five and fifteen times greater than the prevalence rate in the general population. This increased frequency of MS among relatives of patients has been observed in many other studies. It is difficult to assess the relative contribution of shared genetic and environmental factors. The low rate of concordance in monozygotic twins suggested that the familial clustering is due to common exposure to an environmental agent.

Histocompatibility types

Interest in genetic factors which may influence susceptibility to MS, was reawakened with the discovery of tissue antigens which are important in transplantation. The major histocompatibility complex in man is known as the Human Leucocyte Antigen (HLA) system. The genes which control the expression of antigens which are detected by lymphocytotoxic antibodies are designated A, B, and C. The gene determining mixed lymphocyte culture reaction is called D. It has been agreed to number the antigens, prefixed by the letter which denotes the determining gene (e.g. HLA–A3, HLA–B13). Antigens which have been less precisely defined have the letter w (for workshop) included, as in HLA–Bw37.

It is accepted that HLA types A3, B7 or Dw2 are found more frequently in patients with MS than in the general population. Dw2 is more strongly associated with MS than is B7 which in turn is more strongly associated than A3. The mechanism by which these genes cause increased susceptibility to MS is unknown. It may be that these genes are responsible for, or are closely related to, genes which are responsible for immune responses.

The association between MS and HLA types helps to explain the familial and geographic incidence of the disease. In some families the development of MS has been shown to segregate with histocompatibility type. There is some evidence that the prevalence of MS in a population parallels the prevalence of HLA–A3 and HLA–B7 in that population. These antigens are rare, as is MS, in those of Japanese and Indian origin. It is not yet known on a worldwide basis how closely HLA–A3 and HLA–B7 parallel the prevalence of MS.

Immunology and demyelination

The animal model for human MS is experimental allergic encephalomyelitis (EAE). Repeated injections of aqueous solutions of rabbit brain into monkeys produces a diffuse encephalomyelitis. EAE, however, is an acute monophasic condition. Recently a more chronic form of EAE, more closely resembling

MS, has been produced by injecting nervous tissue into juvenile guinea-pigs of a special inbred strain. The antigen responsible for producing EAE is a basic protein of the myelin sheath. Electron micrographs of EAE have shown macrophages sited between myelin folds and apparently stripping myelin off the axon. In the rat, susceptibility to EAE has been shown to be under the control of immune response genes, closely linked to the major histocompatibility locus. This is of special interest in view of the association between MS and certain histocompatibility types.

Vessels of very early MS lesions are surrounded by plasma cells, lympho-cytes, and microglia (the CNS macrophages). Histochemical studies of MS plaques have shown loss of myelin basic protein together with high levels of proteolytic enzymes. These enzymes most likely originate in the infiltrating inflammatory cells and cause destruction of the myelin sheath.

Hypothesis

Knowledge derived from epidemiology, virology, pathology, immunology and other disciplines must be coordinated in any hypothesis of the aetiology of MS. It seems likely that a transmissible agent, probably a virus, is involved in the initiation of the disease. Demyelination could be the end result of a non-specific immunological reaction to a variety of viruses. More probably it is caused by a specific virus. This virus could be widespread in tropical countries and cause a common disease of childhood or infancy. As one moves from the equator, with more temperate climates and better domestic hygiene, more individuals could reach adult age without encountering the virus.

Some races and some populations may be more vulnerable to attack by the hypothetical virus. Alternatively the virus may lie dormant within the CNS and its reactivation may be due to a factor or factors in those at high risk. HLA type has been shown to influence susceptibility. The world-wide HLA distribution may explain racial differences in prevalence of MS. Another factor which may help to explain racial and geographic variation is differing vitamin D and calcium metabolism with skin pigment and sunlight.

The similar world-wide distribution of MS, dental caries and carcinoma of the colon, suggests that dietary factors may play some role in the aetiology of MS. A diet low in polyunsaturated fatty acids and high in animal fat may cause myelin to be abnormally rigid and more easily destroyed during a viral infection. A diet high in animal fat may also cause sludging of red cells and platelet aggregation, leading to hypoxia within the CNS. This could also cause the myelin sheath to be vulnerable to destruction by a viral agent.

It is possible that abnormal structure or function of myelin may render it more likely to be injured, and thereby initiate an autoimmune type of con-tinuing destruction within the CNS. The HLA types which are associated with MS may promote this abnormal immune response or may act as a marker for another gene which is responsible for the immunological disorder.

It is probable that several factors in combination will be shown to be responsible for the causation of MS. It is also likely that the varying prevalence of the disease among the different peoples of the world will prove to be an important clue when the mystery of MS is finally solved.

References

Alter, M. and Harshe, M. (1975). Racial predilection in multiple sclerosis. *Journal of Neurology*, **210**, 1–20.

Carp, R. I., Licursi, P. C., Merz, P. A. and Merz, G. S. (1972). Decreased percentage of polymorphonuclear neutrophils in mouse peripheral blood after inoculation with material from multiple sclerosis patients. *Journal of Experimental Medicine*, **136**, 618–629

Cook, S. D., Dowling, P. C. and Russell, W. C. (1978). Multiple sclerosis and canine distemper. *Lancet*, **i**, 605–606

Craelius, W. (1978). Comparative epidemiology of multiple sclerosis and dental caries. *Journal of Epidemiology and Community Health*, **32**, 155–165

Dean, G. (1967). Annual incidence, prevalence and mortality of multiple sclerosis in White South-African-born and in White immigrants to South Africa. *British Medical Journal*, **2**, 724–730

Dean, G. and Kurtzke, J. F. (1971). On the risk of multiple sclerosis according to age at immigration to South Africa. *British Medical Journal*, **3**, 725–729

Dean, G., McLoughlin, H., Brady, R., Adelstein, A. M. and Tallett-Williams, J. (1976). Multiple sclerosis among immigrants in Greater London. *British Medical Journal*, **1**, 861–864

Frazer, K. B. (1977). Multiple sclerosis: a virus disease? *British Medical Bulletin*, **33**, (I) 34–39

Halliday, A. M. and McDonald, W. I. (1977). Pathophysiology of demyelinating disease. *British Medical Bulletin*, **33**, (I) 21–27

Hornstra, G., Lewis, B., Chait, A., Turpeinen, O., Karvonen, M. J. and Vergroesen, A. J. (1973). Influence of dietary fat on platelet function in men. *Lancet*, **i**, 1155–1157

Hutt, M. S. R. and Burkitt, D. P. (1977). Epidemiology of cancer. In: *Recent Advances in Medicine*. Editors D. N. Baron, N. Compston and A. M. Dawson. Churchill-Livingstone, Edinburgh, London and New York

Kurtzke, J. F., Beebe, G. W. and Norman, J. E. Jr. (1975). *Neurology*, **25**, 356. Cited in Acheson, E. D. (1977). Epidemiology of multiple sclerosis. *British Medical Bulletin*, **33**, (I), 9–14

Kurtzke, J. F. and Hyllested, K. (1975). Multiple sclerosis: an epidemic disease in the Faröes. *Transactions of the American Neurology Association*, **100**, 213–215. Cited in Nathanson, N. and Millar, A. (1978). Epidemiology of multiple sclerosis: critique of the evidence for a viral etiology. *American Journal of Epidemiology*, **107**, 6, 451–461

Leibowitz, U., Kahana, E. and Alter, M. (1972). Population studies of multiple sclerosis in Israel. In: *Multiple Sclerosis Progress in Research*. Editors E. J. Field, T. M. Bell and P. R. Carnegie. North-Holland Publishing Company, Amsterdam, London

Mertin, J. and Meade, C. J. (1977). Relevance of fatty acids in multiple sclerosis. *British Medical Bulletin,* **33,** (I) 67–71

Millar, J. H. D. and Allison, R. S. (1954). Familial incidence of disseminated sclerosis in Northern Ireland. *Ulster Medical Journal,* Supplement 2, **23,** 29. Cited in D. McAlpine, C. E. Lumsden and E. D. Acheson, (1972). *Multiple Sclerosis, a Reappraisal.* Churchill-Livingstone, Edinburgh

Millar, J. H. D., Zilka, K. J., Langman, M. J. S., Wright, H. P., Smith, A. D., Belin, J. and Thompson, R. H. S. (1973). Double blind trial of linoleate supplementation of the diet in multiple sclerosis. *British Medical Journal,* **1,** 765–768

Poskanzer, D. C., Schapira, K. and Millar, H. (1963). Hypothesis: multiple sclerosis and poliomyelitis. *Lancet,* **ii,** 917–921

Swank, R. L. (1961). *A Biochemical Approach to Multiple Sclerosis.* Thomas, Springfield

Swank, R. L. (1970). Multiple sclerosis: twenty years on a low fat diet. *Archives of Neurology,* **23,** 460–473

Symonds, C. P. (1975). Multiple sclerosis and the swayback story. *Lancet,* **i,** 155–156

Westlund, K. B. and Kurland, L. T. (1953). (i) Prevalence, comparison between the patient groups in Winnipeg and New Orleans. (ii) A controlled investigation of factors in the life history of the Winnipeg patients. *American Journal of Hygiene,* **57,** 380. Cited in D. McAlpine, C. E. Lumsden and E. D. Acheson, (1972). *Multiple Sclerosis, a Reappraisal.* Churchill-Livingstone, Edinburgh

Wolfgram, F. (1975). Similar geographical distribution of multiple sclerosis and cancer of the colon. *Acta Neurologica Scandanavica,* **52,** 294–302

6

Arthritides in the negroid peoples of southern Africa

Peter Beighton and Louis Solomon

Introduction

There are marked discrepancies in the geographical and ethnic distribution, prevalence and severity of many disorders of bones and joints. The arthritides, including rheumatoid arthritis, ankylosing spondylitis, osteoarthritis and gout are noteworthy in this context. The differences are not solely due to genetic factors, as variations occur in members of the same racial group who are exposed to different environments. This is clearly seen in southern Africa where the circumstances of the Negro population range from an unsophisticated tribal to a fully westernized urban lifestyle. However, the situation is far from static and there is a trend to rapid acculturalization, with a consequent change in diet and exposure to a different pattern of exogenous factors, including stress and infectious diseases. With this alteration in lifestyle, certain 'Western disorders', which are rare or absent in tribal communities, are emerging, or becoming increasingly common, in urban groups.

During the last decade a number of surveys have been carried out to determine the pattern of change in the arthritides among populations in southern Africa. Wherever relevant, these observations have been related to dietary and environmental influences. The findings are described in the present chapter.

Population surveys

The Negro population of southern Africa numbers approximately 16 million and the various subgroups such as the Tswana, Xhosa and Zulu are all closely related, sharing a common genetic heritage. Our studies were carried out in the following Negro groups in South Africa. The geographic locations of all survey areas are shown in Fig. 6.1.

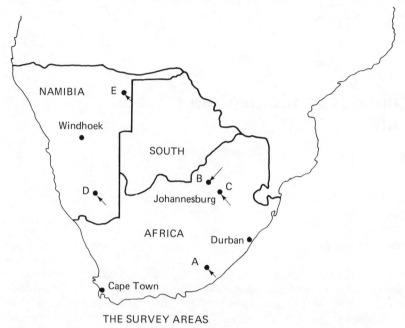

THE SURVEY AREAS

Fig. 6.1   Sketch map of South Africa and Namibia showing survey areas.
A (Negro, tribal); B (Negro, rural); C (Negro, urban); also D Nama (Hottentot)
and E San (Bushmen)

A   A Xhosa Negro community living under traditional tribal conditions
     near Tsolo in the Transkei (Beighton *et al.*, 1976).
B   A rural Negro community, intermediate in social development between
     the traditional tribal and the fully urbanized Africans. This was the
     Tswana population of Phokeng, a village in the north-western
     Transvaal (Beighton *et al.*, 1973).
C   An urban Negro community living in Soweto, Johannesburg (Solomon
     et al., 1975c).

In each of these surveys clinical, radiographic, serological and biochemical
investigations were carried out on between 700 and 1200 volunteers, who
were selected according to strict epidemiological principles. Background
data concerning diet and environmental factors were also recorded. Where
relevant, findings from these surveys will be referred to.

Similar epidemiological surveys were carried out in two non-Negro
indigenous populations in Namibia:

D   Nama (Hottentot) (Beighton *et al.*, 1974b) and
E   San (Bushman) (Beighton and Solomon, 1975) and

Finally, a comparable survey was conducted in a White suburban community
in Johannesburg.

Rheumatoid arthritis

For epidemiological purposes the diagnosis of rheumatoid arthritis (RA) was based on a modification of the Rome criteria (Kellgren, Jeffrey and Ball, 1963a, b):

1. a history of polyarthritis;
2. symmetrical deformity of peripheral joints including the hand or foot;
3. radiographic changes of RA;
4. positive serological tests for rheumatoid factor.

There was a striking difference in both the prevalence and the appearance of RA in the Negro rural and urban populations of South Africa (Solomon *et al.*, 1975b, c; Meyers *et al.*, 1977). Combined 'definite' and 'probable' RA occurred in only 0·87 per cent of the rural Tswana, and even then such changes as were present were invariably mild with none of the classical deformities of RA. By contrast, RA was diagnosed in 3·3 per cent of the urban inhabitants of Soweto—a prevalence similar to that in Johannesburg Caucasian whites. The difference between rural and urban Negroes was highly significant ($P < 0·01$).

Such marked differences in genetically closely related Negro communities must be determined by environmental factors; what these are remains unknown, but they may include differences in diet or exposure to stress and endemic infections. It is tempting to postulate that survival itself is a selective determinant of disease in later life. The mortality rate from minor infections in childhood is much higher in tribal and rural Negroes than in urban populations; possibly the survivors include those who will be more prone to autoimmune disorders like RA in adult life.

Ankylosing spondylitis

In ankylosing spondylitis the major clinical features are progressive pain and rigidity of the spine and the diagnosis is confirmed by the recognition of characteristic radiological changes. In the white population of Europe and the USA, the prevalence of the condition is about 1 in 2000, with a ten-fold preponderance of males. By contrast, out of a Negro population of 16 million in South Africa, only 6 cases have been described, in spite of a careful search for affected individuals (Solomon *et al.*, 1975b; Klemp and Meyers, 1976; Chalmers *et al.*, 1977). Similarly, there have been very few reports of the disorder from other parts of Africa south of the Sahara.

In view of the association of ankylosing spondylitis with the HLA–B27 antigen, the relative infrequency of this antigen in the South African Negro might, in fact, be responsible for the rarity of the condition in this group. However, it is likely that additional environmental factors are necessary for the development of the disease and it will be of fundamental importance to observe whether the prevalence in South Africa rises as acculturalization continues.

Other non-infective arthritides

There are no prevalence figures for systemic lupus erythematosus (SLE) in South Africa other than those derived from a hospital-based survey by Jessop and Meyers (1973). In this investigation the usual 10 to 1 female:male sex ratio was maintained, and there was no bias to any South African ethnic group and no obvious relationship with lifestyle.

Osteoarthrosis

In contrast to inflammatory polyarthritis, which shows clear-cut differences in prevalence and clinical expression in rural and urban Negroes, osteoarthrosis manifests a more complex pattern in these populations.

Generalized osteoarthrosis and Heberden's nodes

These occurred in only 3 per cent of the Negro women over 35 years, compared with an expected 40 per cent in a similar Caucasian population; moreover, there was no significant difference in prevalence between Negro men and women, whereas it is well known that Heberden's arthropathy is at least twice as common in female as in male Caucasians (Solomon et al., 1975a; 1976). However, when one compared tribal and rural Negroes with the urban community, there was no appreciable difference in the general pattern of disease. One feature, though, is worthy of particular comment: our surveys showed an extraordinarily high prevalence of metacarpophalangeal osteoarthrosis in Negro men (five times as high as the expected prevalence in Caucasian men), and comparison of the urban and rural populations showed that the latter were more severely affected. We have attributed this finding to differences in occupation of the various communities; the Negroes are essentially a labouring people and the men, in particular, continue to do rough manual work well into old age. This is a changing social pattern and a greater proportion of urban Negroes now have occupations which do not require heavy manual work. Our findings could thus be explained on the basis of differences in mechanical stress and loading of the metacarpophalangeal joints in the different groups of men.

Osteoarthrosis of the first metatarsophalangeal joints

This is generally associated with hallux valgus; both are much less common in Negroes than in Caucasians: a prevalence of 24 per cent in Tswana females over 35 years, compared with an expected 50 per cent in Caucasians. Measurement of the metatarsal and hallux angles throughout the age range in the populations studied has shown that the most significant anatomical determinant of hallux vulgus is a wide first metatarsal angle (metatarsus primus varus) in childhood; this, together with shoe-wearing, leads to hallux vulgus in later life. A highly significant finding was that not one of the 200 totally unshod San (Bushmen) whom we examined had any tendency to hallux valgus (or metatarsophalangeal osteoarthrosis); even those who had broad feet and wider-than-normal metatarsal angles did not have the expected big toe deformity.

Knee joint

In these surveys radiographs of the knees were not obtained and osteo-arthrosis was evaluated on clinical examination alone. Firm comparisons with other surveys of White populations are, therefore, not possible. However, there was no doubt that osteoarthrosis of the knee is common in all the Negro populations studied by us. Indeed, among females it appears to be more common in Negroes than in Caucasians, 40 per cent of the women over 35 years showing some clinical evidence of involvement of the knee; there was no difference between rural and urban communities. This unexpected frequency may be related to the high incidence of obesity and knock-knee deformity in older Negro women.

Osteoarthrosis of the hip

This provides one of the most striking examples of population differences in disease incidence. It is generally held that the condition is uncommon in Negroes, and this contention was borne out by the Phokeng (Tswana) and Soweto surveys; only 3 per cent of males and less than 1 per cent of females over 55 years showed any radiological evidence of osteoarthrosis of the hip (Solomon *et al.*, 1975a). Expected prevalence for White males and females of any Caucasian community would be 7 per cent and 15 per cent respectively. A similar finding in the Chinese of Hong Kong was ascribed to the 'protective' effect of squatting, which is commonly practised in that population (Hoagland *et al.*, 1973). It might be thought that the same reasoning would hold for our Negro populations. However, squatting is not particularly common in the urban Negro, and among the tribalized Xhosa who do spend considerable time squatting the prevalence of osteoarthrosis of the hip was higher than in the other groups. We are more inclined to believe that the low prevalence in South African Negroes is directly related to the rarity of predisposing disorders such as congenital subluxation, acetabular dysplasia, femoral head deformity, Perthes' disease and slipped epiphysis. There *is* a significant predisposing factor in some Negro populations—protrusio acetabuli. This condition was present in no less than 13 per cent of the Xhosa women over 55 years and in this particular population radiographic osteoarthrosis was present in 4 per cent. The cause of the protrusio acetabuli is unknown.

Gout and hyperuricaemia

It has long been recognized that both environmental and genetic factors play a part in the aetiology of gout, and a direct relationship with hyperuricaemia is well established. For instance, the Maoris of New Zealand are susceptible to gout and it has been shown that mean serum uric acid (SUA) levels tend to be high in this population (Prior *et al.*, 1964). Environmental circumstances including diet have an important influence on SUA concentrations, as shown by Ford and de Mos (1964) in their comparative study of Chinese emigrants to British Columbia and Malaya and their relatives who remained behind in Taiwan.

Gout is very uncommon in the Negro population of South Africa and the condition was not encountered in any respondent in the three Negro groups whom we studied (Beighton *et al.*, 1973; 1974a; 1976). Similarly, there was no clinical evidence of gout in the Nama (Hottentot) or San (Bushmen) populations (Beighton *et al.*, 1974b; Beighton and Solomon, 1975). By contrast, a prevalence similar to that of other Caucasian populations was established in the white population of Johannesburg (males 13/1000, females 3/1000).

SUA concentrations were measured in specimens from several hundred respondents in men and women of the three Negro populations, tribal, rural and urban (page 84) and in the urban white group (Table 6.1) (Beighton *et al.*, 1977). In each instance the mean SUA level rose with age, concentrations in males always being higher than those in females. Frequency distribution was consistently unimodal, the curves for the female being shifted to the left with respect to those for the males. The age–sex relationship is demonstrated in Fig. 6.2.

The relationship between mean population SUA levels in Negro men and women, age and lifestyle is also shown in Fig. 6.2. It is readily apparent that

Table 6.1   Mean serum uric acid (SUA) concentrations in males and females of South African populations, three Negro and one White, having different lifestyles

Population	Lifestyle	Age group (years)	Number	SUA(mmol/l) mean	range
Males					
Negro	tribal	18–75+	80	0·27	0·17–0·43
Negro	rural	14–84	128	0·29	0·17–0·63
Negro	urban	15–90	144	0·36	0·06–0·59
White	urban	16–95	213	0·37	0·18–0·64
Females					
Negro	tribal	15–75+	399	0·23	0·10–0·44
Negro	rural	14–96	242	0·27	0·07–0·67
Negro	urban	15–90	280	0·31	0·15–0·57
White	urban	16–28	298	0·30	0·12–0·50

Conversion 1 mmol/l SUA ≈ 16·8 mg/dl
Normal range 0·15–0·48 mmol/l ≈ 2·5–8·0 mg/dl

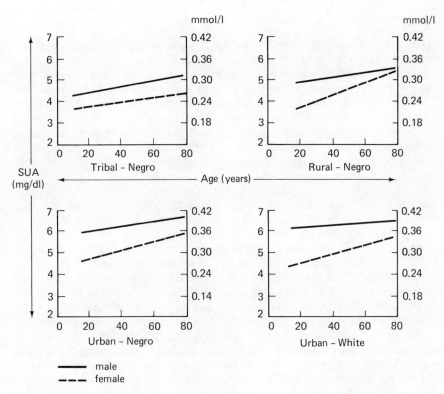

Fig. 6.2 Mean serum uric acid (SUA) concentrations in men and women of South African populations, three Negro (tribal, rural and urban), also of urban Whites, in relation to sex, age, and lifestyle

mean SUA concentrations tended to rise with acculturalization and that the sex-specific SUA concentrations of the urban dwellers were similar in both ethnic groups. The reason for this very significant trend in Negroes is unknown, but in terms of aetiological factors, it is likely that diet, and possibly stress, are involved.

In the Nama (Hottentot) population, where gout was absent, mean SUA levels were 0·34 mmol/l (5·7 mg/dl) for the males and 0·30 mmol/l (5·0 mg/dl) for the females. Analysis of data from the San (Bushmen) group is incomplete, but preliminary findings indicate that mean SUA levels are very low, in spite of their high protein diet.

Apart from gout, hyperuricaemia may be involved in the pathogenesis of potentially lethal conditions such as hypertension, myocardial infarction and diabetes mellitus. These disorders are unusual in rural Negro groups, but they are being encountered with increasing frequency in the urban population. The rise in population mean SUA concentrations which occurs with acculturalization may prove to be of importance in this situation.

Diet

Diet may well play an important role in determining the prevalence and severity of some of the arthritides, either in simple mechanical terms of body weight and its relationship to osteoarthrosis, or in more complex ways such as the effect on purine metabolism and the development of hyperuricaemia.

The transition from a Negro tribal to an urban lifestyle has important implications for nutrition. Overall nutritional status is not necessarily better in urban communities, and it is likely that more specific changes in dietary habits may explain the emergence of previously uncommon disorders in urban Negroes. The serum albumin level, which is one index of nutritional status, was compared in the populations in our surveys. The values in the rural Tswana group compare favourably with those in urban whites; values for the urban Negro community suggest a marginal situation, while those in the tribal Xhosa group indicate malnutrition (Watermeyer et al., 1977).

We have already alluded to the fact that the common occurrence of osteoarthrosis of the knee in Negro women may be related to obesity and genu valgum. As a measure of body weight we have used the Ponderal Index (Acheson and Chan, 1969). This was calculated by dividing the height in inches by the cube root of the weight in pounds; a value of 10 would be indicative of gross obesity, while that of 14 would denote a very thin individual. The Ponderal Indices of the three South African Negro populations—tribal, rural and urban—together with those of South African urban Whites, are shown in Table 6.2. In any group, females are usually fatter than males and the most weighty group of all are the urban Negro women: they had the lowest Ponderal Index. This corresponds closely to the race and sex distribution of knee arthrosis in the populations studied.

From the foregoing it seems that body weight and serum albumin con-

Table 6.2   Ponderal indices[1] of three Negro populations, tribal, rural and urban, also of urban Whites in South Africa

Population	Sex	Number	Ponderal index[1] mean ± s.d.
Negro, tribal	male	65	12·92 ± 0·93
Negro, rural	male	140	12·99 ± 0·64
Negro, urban	male	151	12·63 ± 0·63
White, urban	male	210	12·48 ± 0·69
Negro, tribal	female	400	12·44 ± 0·93
Negro, rural	female	278	12·06 ± 0·92
Negro, urban	female	292	11·56 ± 0·87
White, urban	female	288	12·13 ± 0·76

[1] The lower the ponderal index the greater the obesity—see text

centrations reflect different facets of nutritional status. However, it must be emphasized that the interpretation of dietary data, in terms of its influence on the pathogenesis of disease, must be viewed with caution.

Acknowledgements

The early population surveys were undertaken while P. B. was in receipt of a Geigy fellowship awarded by the Arthritis and Rheumatism Council of Great Britain.

Financial support for the investigations was provided by the University of the Witwatersrand Orthopaedic Chair Trust Fund, the Carl and Emily Fuchs Foundation, the South African Medical Research Council and the University of Cape Town Staff Research Fund.

References

Acheson, R. M. and Chan, Y. K. (1969). New Haven survey of joint diseases. Prediction of serum uric acid in a general population. *Journal of Chronic Diseases*, **21**, 543–553

Beighton, P., Daynes, G. and Soskolne, C. L. (1976). Serum uric acid concentrations in a Xhosa community in the Transkei of Southern Africa. *Annals of the Rheumatic Diseases*, **35**, 77–80

Beighton, P. and Solomon, L. (1975). Serum uric acid levels in the populations of Southern Africa. *Rheumatology*, **5**, 407–410

Beighton, P. H., Solomon, L., Soskolne, C. L. and Sweet, B. (1973). Serum uric acid concentrations in a rural Tswana community in Southern Africa. *Annals of the Rheumatic Diseases*, **32**, 346–350

Beighton, P., Solomon, L., Soskolne, C. L. and Sweet, M. B. E. (1977). Rheumatic disorders in the South African Negro. Part IV: Gout and hyperuricaemia. *South African Medical Journal*, **51**, 967–972

Beighton, P., Solomon, L., Soskolne, C. L., Sweet, B. and Robin, G. (1974a). Serum uric acid concentrations in an urbanized South African Negro population. *Annals of the Rheumatic Diseases*, **33**, 442–445

Beighton, P. H., Soskolne, C. L., Solomon, L. and Sweet, B. (1974b). Serum uric acid levels in a Nama (Hottentot) community in South West Africa. *South African Journal of Science*, **70**, 281–283

Chalmers, I. M., Seedat, Y. K. and Muduliar, M. Y. (1977). Ankylosing spondylitis in three Zulu men negative for the HLA–B27 antigen. *South African Medical Journal*, **52**, 567–569

Ford, D. K. and de Mos, A. M. (1964). Serum uric acid levels in healthy Caucasian, Chinese and Haida Indian males in British Columbia. *Canadian Medical Association Journal*, **90**, 1295–1297

Hoaglund, F. T., Yan, A. C. M. C. and Wong, W. L. (1973). Osteoarthritis of the hip and other joints in Southern Chinese in Hong Kong. Incidence and related factors. *Journal of Bone and Joint Surgery*, **55A**, 545–550

Jessop, S. and Meyers, O. L. (1973). Systemic lupus erythematosus in Cape Town. *South African Medical Journal,* **47,** 222–225

Kellgren, J. H., Jeffrey, M. R. and Ball, J. (1963a). Proposed diagnostic criteria for use in population studies. In: *The Epidemiology of Chronic Rheumatism,* Vol. 1, 324. Editors J. H. Kellgren, M. R. Jeffrey and J. Ball. Blackwell, Oxford

Kellgren, J. H., Jeffrey, M. R. and Ball, J. (1963b). *The Epidemiology of Chronic Rheumatism.* Editors J. H. Kellgren, M. R. Jeffrey and J. Ball. Vol. 2. Atlas of Standard Radiographs of Arthritis. Blackwell, Oxford

Klemp, P. and Meyers, O. L. (1976). Ankylosing spondylitis in a Xhosa father and daughter. *South African Medical Journal,* **50,** 1439–1441

Meyers, O. L., Daynes, G. and Beighton, P. (1977). Rheumatoid arthritis in a tribal Xhosa population in the Transkei, Southern Africa. *Annals of the Rheumatic Diseases,* **36,** 62–65

Prior, I. A. M., Rose, B. S. and Davidson, F. (1964). Metabolic maladies in New Zealand Maoris. *British Medical Journal,* **1,** 1065–1070

Solomon, L., Beighton, P. and Lawrence, J. S. (1975a). Rheumatic disorders in the South African Negro. Part II. Osteo-arthrosis. *South African Medical Journal,* **49,** 1737–1740

Solomon, L., Beighton, P. and Lawrence, J. S. (1976). Osteoarthrosis in a rural African Negro population. *Annals of the Rheumatic Diseases,* **35,** 274–278

Solomon, L., Beighton, P., Valkenburg, H. A., Robin G. and Soskolne, C. L. (1975b). Rheumatic disorders in the South African Negro. Part I. Rheumatoid arthritis and ankylosing spondylitis. *South African Medical Journal,* **49,** 1292–1296

Solomon, L., Robin, G. and Valkenburg, H. A. (1975c). Rheumatoid arthritis in an urban South African Negro population. *Annals of the Rheumatic Diseases,* **34,** 128–135

Watermeyer, G. S., Solomon, L., Daynes, G., Soskolne, C. L. and Beighton, P. (1977). The changing epidemiology of serum albumin levels in Southern Africa. *South African Medical Journal,* **51,** 614–616

7

Cancer

Sir Richard Doll and Bruce Armstrong

It is now clear, as a result of the work of cancer registries in many different countries, that cancer is not a disease of Western societies alone. When the effect of differences in age distribution is taken into account, the incidence of cancer in some economically underdeveloped countries is seen to be as high as in parts of the developed world. Economic development, however (or, more correctly, factors associated with it), has a potent influence on the types of cancer that predominate. For, whereas the total incidence of cancer varies less than four-fold from one part of the world to another, the incidence of cancer at individual body sites may vary a hundred times more. Study of this variation and its change with time has led to an understanding of the role of the environment in the aetiology of human cancer and has implications for cancer prevention in both Western and non-Western countries alike.

Geographic variations in cancer incidence

In the most recent collection of cancer incidence data from around the world, the highest incidence from all forms of cancer is recorded for black African males in Bulawayo, Rhodesia, while the next highest is recorded for blacks in the San Francisco Bay area of the USA (Waterhouse *et al.*, 1976). Both groups have a 'cumulative rate', that is a chance of developing cancer in the absence of other causes of death, of about 19 per cent by the age of 65 years. At the other end of the scale, males in Ibadan, Nigeria, have only a 6 per cent chance of developing cancer by the same age. These data are shown in Fig. 7.1 with those of other populations with high rates and the ten populations with the lowest rates. In females, the highest cumulative rate of cancer is in the white population of the USA, but women from less affluent countries, such as Colombia and Brazil, also experience high rates. Some of this variation may be due to differences in the completeness of registration; but most of it is probably real. Data have been included only for registries that are known to have a high standard of recording and the less reliable data for men and women over 65 years of age have been omitted.

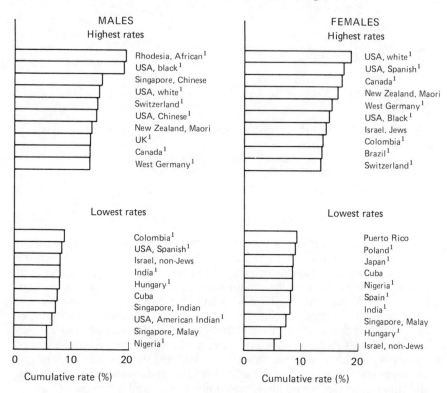

¹ Rate from a Registry covering part of the population

Fig. 7.1 Populations with the highest and lowest cumulative rates of cancer to age 65 years (as reported in Waterhouse *et al.*, 1976)

While the total rates of cancer in black males in Rhodesia and the USA and in females in North and South America are similar, the organs in which cancers occur are quite different (Table 7.1). Cancers of the liver and oesophagus rank highest among black males in Rhodesia, where they are, respectively, fifteen and three and one-half times more common than in the USA. Cancer of the cervix is five times more common in Colombian women than in women in the USA and cancer of the breast is three times more common in the USA than in Colombia. In both sexes cancers of the colon and rectum occur between four and six times more frequently in the USA than in either Rhodesia or Colombia. Contrasts of this sort are by no means extreme and similar contrasts are found whenever comparisons are made between populations at substantially different levels of economic development.

Table 7.1 Cumulative rates to age 65 years of the seven most common sites of cancer in underdeveloped populations with high overall rates of cancer

MALES				FEMALES			
Rhodesia, Africans		USA, blacks		Colombia		USA, whites	
Site	Cumulative rate (%)	Site	Cumulative rate (%)	Site	Cumulative rate (%)	Site	Cumulative rate (%)
Liver	4·3	Lung	5·3	Cervix	4·9	Breast	6·0
Oesophagus	3·5	Prostate	2·7	Breast	1·8	Corpus uteri	2·4
Lung	3·2	Colon	1·2	Stomach	1·2	Lung	1·4
Bladder	1·6	Stomach	1·1	Ovary	0·7	Colon	1·1
Prostate	1·1	Oesophagus	1·0	Corpus uteri	0·4	Ovary	1·0
Stomach	0·7	Larynx	0·8	Thyroid	0·4	Cervix uteri	0·9
Pancreas	0·7	Pancreas	0·7	Lung	0·3	Rectum	0·6

Changes in cancer incidence with time

The incidence of cancer has also changed with time in association with increasing affluence. An increase in incidence of cancer of the lung in both black and white males was the greatest change to be observed in the 32 years (1937–39 to 1969–71) spanned by three National Cancer Surveys in the USA (Devesa and Silverman, 1978). In white males, the sum of this and other increases, particularly in colorectal, prostate, and bladder cancer, was greater than the sum of all the decreases, although appreciable reductions were observed in the incidence of cancers of the mouth, pharynx, oesophagus, stomach, and liver and biliary tract. The total increase was even greater in black males because they shared only the fall in stomach cancer. During this period the women of both major ethnic groups fared rather better with net declines in total cancer incidence, mainly because there was also a sharp drop in the incidence of cancer of the cervix and the increase in cancer of the lung was less. Similar changes were observed in cancer mortality and have been reported in other countries. In Britain, notable recent changes include an increase in the mortality from myelomatosis and melanoma in both sexes (Doll, 1979).

Changes in cancer incidence in Britain and North America between 1940 and 1970 probably had their origin in changes that took place in the early part of the century and might reasonably be attributed to the rapid economic development that occurred at that time. In contrast, Japan has developed mainly since 1930 and, until recently, has had patterns of cancer incidence similar to those of underdeveloped countries. These patterns are, however, now changing towards those that prevail in the Western world.

In 1959–60, cancer of the stomach was (and probably still is) the commonest cancer in both sexes in Japan, cancer of the oesophagus was among the most common, cancer of the cervix occurred more frequently than cancer of the breast in women, and cancer of the colon was not among the seven commonest cancers in either sex. The changes that are now occurring in this pattern are precisely those expected from the experience of Britain and the United States (Table 7.2). The incidence rates of cancers of the stomach, oesophagus, and liver and biliary passages are declining while the rates of cancers of the lung, pancreas, colon and rectum are increasing. Cancer of the colon has increased at a rate of about 5 per cent per annum in the past 20 years and the incidence of cancer of the breast has begun to increase recently (Hirayama, 1978). The sum of these changes has been a net *decline* in the incidence of all cancers. Similar changes in cancer incidence have also been observed with the migration of Japanese to Hawaii and the US mainland (Haenszel and Kurihara, 1968).

These various lines of evidence are all consistent in suggesting that westernization or economic development tends to increase the incidence of some cancers and to decrease the incidence of others.

Table 7.2 Cumulative rates to age 65 years of the seven commonest cancers in each sex in Miyagi, Japan in 1959–60, with mean annual change in incidence between 1959–60 and 1968–71.

MALES

Cancer site	Cumulative rate (%)	Mean annual change (%)[1]
Stomach	5·5	−1·6
Lung	0·8	+0·5
Oesophagus	0·7	−2·8
Liver and biliary passages	0·3	−2·7
Pancreas	0·3	+1·3
Rectum	0·3	+4·0
Bladder	0·2	0·0
All sites	10·7	−1·2

FEMALES

Cancer site	Cumulative rate (%)	Mean annual change (%)[1]
Stomach	2·9	−2·2
Cervix	1·8	−3·9
Breast	1·1	0·0
Lung	0·3	+1·5
Liver and biliary passages	0·3	−2·7
Oesophagus	0·3	−4·3
Rectum	0·2	+2·4
All sites	10·0	−2·3

[1] Refers to changes in incidence rates standardized in the age range 35–64 years

Factors responsible for associations between westernization and cancer incidence

In considering the associations between economic development and cancer incidence, it is reasonable to believe that development *per se* is involved only indirectly. In parallel with economic development have come industrialization, the increasing production and use of chemicals, pollution of the environment, social change, and changes in diet and lifestyle. It is in these changes that the explanations for changes in the incidence of cancer can most probably be found.

Occupational exposure to chemicals

The change from a predominantly rural agricultural economy to an urban industrial economy is characteristic of economic development. This change has led, historically, to increasing exposure of workmen to carcinogenic chemicals and to an increased incidence of cancer among them, particularly of cancers of the skin and bladder. Occasionally, otherwise rare cancers have been rendered common, as in the case of mesothelioma of the pleura and peritoneum in asbestos workers and cancer of the nasal sinuses in nickel refiners (Doll, 1977).

The exact proportion of cancers in Western countries which could be due to industrial chemicals is the subject of some dispute. Estimates vary from 1–3 per cent of cancers due to occupational exposure to all chemicals (Higginson and Muir, 1976) to 13–18 per cent due to work exposure to asbestos alone (Bridford *et al.*, 1978). In England and Wales cancer mortality is 24 per cent higher in manual than in non-manual workers. It has been estimated, however, that nearly nine-tenths of this difference can be attributed to social factors (such as cigarette smoking) rather than to occupation (Fox and Adelstein, 1978). Adjustment for this effect leaves manual workers only 3 per cent more at risk than non-manual workers. This accords well with the lower estimates of total cancer mortality due to occupational factors and suggests that direct occupational exposure to carcinogens has contributed little to increases in total cancer incidence—at least in Britain. It is likely, however, that some occupational hazards have yet to be discovered and the exact proportion due to such factors is uncertain.

Environmental pollution

The effect of pollution of the environment by the products of industrialization is even more difficult to assess. Air pollution as a result of the burning of fossil fuels has almost certainly contributed to the incidence of lung cancer in urban areas. The effect has been small, however, accounting possibly for less than 5 deaths per 100 000 per year, and then largely dependent on an interaction with cigarette smoking (Doll, 1978). Very low levels of other carcinogens such as asbestos and vinyl chloride have also become widespread in the environment of developed countries and may cause occasional cases.

Mesothelioma has been reported in women having household contact with asbestos workers (Vianna and Polan, 1978) and angiosarcoma of the liver has occurred in individuals resident near vinyl chloride manufacturing or polymerization plants (Brady *et al.*, 1977). From the concentrations of the carcinogens involved, it is doubtful whether the incidence of any cancer other than lung cancer due to pollution from the burning of fossil fuels has been increased to any appreciable degree by such exposure.

Reproductive and sexual behaviour

Reproductive and sexual behaviour both influence the incidence of some cancers and have changed with economic development. For example, both early first childbirth and increasing total parity reduce the incidence of breast cancer (MacMahol *et al.*, 1973; Tulinius *et al.*, 1978). From the mid-nineteenth century until the mid-1930s there was, in Britain, a progressive decline in fertility with, probably, increasing postponement of first childbirth. Associated with this there was a rise in breast cancer mortality (Armstrong, 1976). Subsequently there has been an increase in fertility, followed in the early 1960s by a sharp decline in fertility in most developed countries and the effects of this on breast cancer incidence are yet to be seen.

Decreasing fertility has, in general, paralleled economic development, with some perturbations in the decline due to temporary economic depression and global war. At the present time, early childbirth and high fertility is more prevalent in underdeveloped than in developed societies (Loraine, 1976). It appears, however, that these geographic variations in fertility can explain only a small part of the geographic variation in breast cancer incidence (Hems, 1978). Moreover, in Iceland breast cancer incidence has increased more than three-fold in cohorts of women born between 1900 and 1949 when a decline might have been expected from the reduction in age at first birth and the proportion of nulliparous women (Tulinius *et al.*, 1978). It is likely, therefore, that declining fertility is not the main factor behind the recent increase in breast cancer incidence in many Western societies.

Cancer of the ovary is also associated with reduced fertility. In both England and Wales and in North America there is a close inverse correlation between the average completed family size of cohorts of women and their mortality from this disease (Beral *et al.*, 1978) and a similar association is observed in case-control studies of individual women. A decrease in fertility appeared to explain most of a three-fold increase in ovarian cancer mortality in cohorts born between 1866 and 1906. Taken with evidence of a strong inverse correlation between average completed family size and mortality from cancer of the ovary world-wide, these observations suggest that the rise of ovarian cancer with westernization has been due largely to reductions in fertility.

In contrast to cancers of the breast and ovary, cancer of the cervix increases in incidence with increasing fertility. This effect is almost certainly secondary to associations between cervical cancer and early and promiscuous sexual intercourse. The reasons for these associations are not established, although it has been variously suggested that smegma and/or spermatozoa may be carcinogenic to the cervix or that cancer is induced by a venereally trans- mitted agent, such as herpes simplex virus type 2. Genital cleanliness and the use of occlusive types of contraceptives may also reduce the likelihood that frequent or promiscuous intercourse will lead to cancer (Wright *et al.*, 1978). Early and promiscuous sexual activity is characteristic of some primitive societies and changes in both sexual behaviour and standards of personal cleanliness may have been responsible for the decline in incidence of cancer of the cervix associated with affluence. There is some evidence that the recent 'sexual revolution' in Western societies may, perhaps, be leading to a recrudescence of the disease (Beral, 1974), but if it is, the increase should be susceptible to control by cytological screening.

Hygiene

The decline in incidence of primary cancer of the liver may be a result, in part, of improved personal and community hygiene. There is increasing evidence that persistence of hepatitis-B infection is an important factor in the produc- tion of liver cancer, possibly through induction of liver cell necrosis and regeneration. Not only is the incidence of liver cancer in different countries closely associated with prevalence of hepatitis-B infection, but for each population for which adequate data are available the prevalence of hepatitis-B antigen in the serum of patients with liver cancer is substantially greater than in control patients. Both the incidence of liver cancer and the prevalence of persistent hepatitis-B infection are particularly high in underdeveloped populations such as New Guinea, Senegal, and Mozambique. Although originally thought to be transmitted only by passage of infected serum it now appears that hepatitis-B is also spread by the faecal–oral route and by close personal contact. It may also be spread by insect bites and by social customs involving ritual injury with a common instrument (Blumberg, 1977). It is likely that improvements in hygiene in developed societies have reduced or eliminated some ways in which hepatitis-B infection is spread and conse- quently have reduced the incidence of liver cancer.

Cancer of the penis is associated predominantly with the lack of circumci- sion and lack of personal hygiene, both of which would increase exposure to carcinogens formed in smegma by bacterial action. Both the widespread adoption of circumcision by Western societies (a trend which is now being reversed) and greater personal cleanliness have probably contributed to a reduction in this disease.

Tobacco and alcohol

Increasing use of tobacco has paralleled economic development in almost all countries and is the main explanation for the rise in incidence of cancers of the lung and bladder and perhaps also cancer of the pancreas. Until 1973, tobacco consumption in most underdeveloped countries was at a relatively low level (for example about 1 lb per adult per year in most African countries) and had been stable for the preceding ten years (Lee, 1975). It appears, however, that with reduction in growth of cigarette smoking in developed countries cigarette manufacturers are now looking to developing countries for new markets (Muller, 1978). Such moves must be expected to lead to increases in the incidence of respiratory cancer.

Traditional forms of smoking and tobacco chewing, with or without betel, probably resulted from a complex of factors including disappearance of the some developing countries (Jayant *et al.*, 1977). Edentia and poor oral hygiene have also been related to the development of oral cancer (Graham *et al.*, 1977). The decline in these cancers in developed countries has, therefore, probably resulted for a complex of factors including disappearance of the habit of tobacco chewing, improvements in oral hygiene and dental care, and, possibly, a reduction in consumption of alcohol.

Alcohol interacts strongly with tobacco in the production of cancers of the upper alimentary tract, oesophagus, and larynx and, independently of tobacco, increases the incidence of primary liver cancer through the induction of cirrhosis. In contrast to tobacco consumption there is no consistent relationship between economic development and alcohol consumption. In Britain alcohol consumption fell progressively from the beginning of the eighteenth century until about 1950; thereafter it has increased. The fall appeared to be due mainly to progressively increasing taxation of alcohol and the rise of the temperance movement. In the last 30 years the price of alcohol has declined relative to personal income and consumption has risen (Spring and Buss, 1977).

The falling consumption of alcohol may have contributed to reductions in incidence of cancers of the buccal cavity and oesophagus which have followed economic development. There is evidence, however, that the incidence of cancer of the oesophagus may be rising again perhaps as a result of the recent increases in alcohol consumption (McMichael, 1978). The use of traditional alcoholic beverages may contribute to the high incidence of cancer of the oesophagus in parts of the underdeveloped world such as the Transkei region of South Africa (Warwick and Harrington, 1973) but it has certainly not played any part in other areas (Joint Iran-International Agency for Research on Cancer Study Group, 1977).

Diet

The composition of the diet has been greatly affected by westernization. Correlations between several dietary variables and gross national product in 32 countries are shown in Table 7.3. Generally, a high consumption of animal protein, fat, sugar, total protein, and total food energy is characteristic of wealthy countries and a high consumption of cereals, pulses, nuts, and seeds is characteristic of poor countries. In developed countries, increases in sugar consumption, fat, and animal protein (mainly red meat, eggs, and milk) and decreases in cereal consumption have paralleled economic development (Armstrong *et al.*, 1975). Examination of cancer incidence rates in relation to these geographic variations in diet and to changes in diet with time has led

Table 7.3   Coefficients of linear correlation between food and nutrient intake in 1963–65 and gross national product in 1965 in 32 countries

Food or nutrient	Correlation coefficient
Fish	−0·01
Eggs	+0·69
Meat	+0·75
Fruits	+0·38
Vegetables	+0·03
Pulses, nuts, and seeds	−0·34
Sugar	+0·66
Potatoes	+0·09
Cereals	−0·71
Fats and oils	+0·64
Total fat	+0·82
Animal protein	+0·85
Total protein	+0·53
Total food energy	+0·57

to hypotheses that dietary energy and fat are major aetiological factors for cancers of the breast and corpus uteri, that dietary meat and fat contribute to the aetiology of cancers of the colon and rectum, and that dietary fibre may act as a protective factor (see Armstrong and Doll, 1975). Recent studies have lent support, in varying degrees, to these hypotheses.

Several studies have shown that tall obese women are the most likely to develop breast cancer (de Waard and Baanders-van Halewijn, 1974), which suggests that there may be an association between total food intake and the risk of developing the disease. Studies of Japanese women have implicated diet more directly by indicating positive associations between the consumption of meat, eggs, butter, and cheese and breast cancer incidence (Hirayama, 1978) and, in a Canadian study, women with breast cancer were shown to consume more fat than control patients (Miller *et al.*, 1978). Experimental studies have supported the idea that dietary fat may have a causal effect by showing that fat increases prolactin secretion and hence the incidence of breast cancer in rodents (Chan *et al.*, 1977). There is some evidence that dietary fat may influence prolactin levels in humans (Hill *et al.*, 1977); but there is no convincing evidence that prolactin plays any part in the induction of breast cancer in women.

Cancer of the corpus uteri is more strongly associated with obesity, and therefore with dietary excess, than is breast cancer. Corpus cancer is also associated with early menarche, late menopause, mature-onset diabetes, and hypertension which are secondary to obesity itself or to excessive consumption of energy-producing foods or fat (Armstrong, 1977). These associations are probably explained by the excessive conversion of adrenal and ovarian androgens to oestrogens in adipose tissue in obese postmenopausal women. There is evidence from case-control studies that both endogenously produced and exogenously administered oestrogens increase the risk of endometrial cancer and it seems probable that persistent stimulation of the endometrium unopposed by progestagens favours the development of the disease. Excessive production of oestrogens could also provide a means by which diet could affect the incidence of breast cancer, but the evidence for a casual role for oestrogens in this disease is much less strong.

Unlike breast and endometrial cancer, cancer of the colon is correlated geographically equally or more strongly with meat and animal protein consumption than with fat. The majority of case-control studies, however, have not shown evidence of this association. An exception is the study of Japanese migrants to Hawaii, which found that patients with cancer of the large bowel were more likely than control subjects to have adopted a Western-style diet and some two and one-half times more likely to have eaten regularly legumes and meat, particularly beef (Haenszel *et al.*, 1973). Further support for this association comes from the comparatively low mortality from colorectal cancer in Seventh Day Adventists (about 50 per cent of whom are vegetarians) and in some other vegetarian groups (L. J. Kinlen, personal communication, 1979). Mormons, however, who are among the biggest beef eaters in the United States, have colon cancer rates as low as those in Seventh Day Adventists (Lyon and Sorenson, 1978).

The world-wide incidence of cancer of the colon is also correlated strongly, but inversely, with cereal consumption. Burkitt (1975) has suggested that dietary fibre, particularly that contained in cereals, may protect against cancer of the large bowel by increasing stool volume and decreasing bowel transit time, thus reducing both the time available for bacterial production of carcinogens and their ultimate concentration. This hypothesis has gained some support from recent studies which have shown that two populations at high risk of colon cancer (Japanese in Hawaii and men in Copenhagen) have more bulky stools than corresponding populations at low risk (Japanese in Japan and men in rural Finland). There was, however, no difference in stool transit time between the high and low risk populations studied (Glober *et al.*, 1977 and MacLennan *et al.*, 1978). In addition to these indirect studies, there is also evidence that patients with colon cancer in Israel had consumed fewer foods with a high fibre content than had appropriately matched control subjects (Modan *et al.*, 1975).

Hypotheses involving meat, fat, or fibre in the aetiology of colon cancer are all consistent with the effects of westernization on the incidence of bowel cancer and are not necessarily in conflict one with the other. Dietary fat may, through an effect on the nature and concentration of biliary steroids, provide a substrate from which colonic bacteria produce carcinogens. Dietary meat is known to influence the bacterial flora of the large bowel and may produce a flora which is more active in carcinogen production. In the relative absence of dietary fibre, greater concentrations of carcinogens may result from this activity. Experimental support is available for each component of this unifying hypothesis.

Most hypotheses relating diet to cancer of the large bowel do not distinguish cancer of the rectum from cancer of the colon. Cancer of the rectum has not, however, increased as consistently or to the same degree with westernization as has colon cancer. Nor does it show the same degree of geographic variation. It is probably reasonable, however, to attribute cancer of the rectum to the same factors as cancer of the colon. These factors would be weakened in their effect by the less continuous exposure of the rectal mucosa to faecal carcinogens.

The emphasis so far has been on dietary changes occurring in parallel with economic development and increasing the incidence of cancer. Changes that decrease cancer incidence may, however, be at least as important. One of the biggest changes in cancer associated with westernization has been the fall in incidence of cancer of the stomach. The reasons for this fall are unknown. In Japan a decline in mortality from stomach cancer has occurred in parallel with increasing consumption of milk, meat, eggs, oil, and fruit. Studies of individual Japanese have shown that the risk of stomach cancer is some 40 per cent less in those who drink two glasses of milk daily than in those who do not (Hirayama, 1977). The daily eating of green or yellow vegetables also appears to confer a protective effect. Other studies have shown evidence of protection from a variety of vegetables and fruit in Japanese, American, and Norwegian populations.

While it may be reasonable to suggest that dietary change has produced the recent decline in incidence of gastric cancer in Japan, the specific dietary components that are responsible have not been identified. Possible candidates include the better preservation of food (with a reduction in carcinogenic metabolites) and increased consumption of vitamins A and C. Vitamin A and its analogues have been shown to reduce the risk of several experimentally induced cancers in laboratory animals (Sporn, 1977) and vitamin C can block the formation of carcinogenic nitrosamines in the stomach. There are now also several observations which suggest that vitamin A can reduce the incidence of cancer of the lung in man (Bjelke, 1975; Mettlin *et al.*, 1979). The protective effect of vegetables against gastric cancer could, therefore, be due either to vitamin A or to vitamin C, although there is no direct evidence of an effect of either substance at the present time. In Japan, where a protective effect of green or yellow vegetables has been observed, 40 per cent of dietary vitamin A and 23 per cent of vitamin C are supplied by these foods.

Given that vitamin A may protect against human lung cancer and, possibly, cancer of the stomach, and the generality of its effect on epithelial cancer in animals, it might be expected to protect against other cancers in man. Increasing vitamin A consumption associated with economic development and adoption of a Western-style diet may, therefore, have contributed to the falling incidence of other cancers such as cancers of the cervix uteri and the upper alimentary tract.

Dietary factors probably also contribute to the negative association between westernization and the incidence of primary cancer of the liver. Aflatoxins, produced by the mould *Aspergillus flavus*, have been found in appreciable concentrations in the diet of populations of tropical Africa and

Asia which have a high incidence of liver cancer. Studies in several countries have shown that the level of contamination of foodstuffs with aflatoxins correlates closely with the incidence of liver cancer (see for example Peers and Linsell, 1977) and human liver cells contain the enzymes that convert aflatoxin to its carcinogenic epoxy metabolite. The growth of *Aspergillus flavus* depends on warmth and moisture and can be prevented by methods of harvesting and storage which ensure that food crops remain dry. Increasing affluence permits the use of such methods and also the rejection of food that is obviously mouldy. It has yet to be shown, however, that such measures will reduce the incidence of liver cancer in areas where it is currently high.

Other factors

The increasing availability and use of medications is characteristic of economic development and several drugs have been found to cause human cancer. It is doubtful, however, whether the use of any of them, apart from oestrogens, has been sufficient to produce detectable changes in cancer rates in whole populations. In the case of oestrogens, recent increases in the incidence of cancer of the corpus uteri in the United States have been attributed to their widespread use for the relief of menopausal symptoms (Weiss *et al.*, 1976). This increase is fairly recent and has occurred against a background of comparatively high rates due, probably, to the dietary factors previously described.

There are some associations between westernization and cancer incidence for which no adequate explanation has been offered in the preceding discussion. It is doubtful, for example, whether the increases in the incidence of cancer of the pancreas can be attributed entirely to cigarette smoking, or increased consumption of fats, and better diagnosis and other factors may be involved (Wynder, 1975). Dietary influences, mediated through hormonal changes analogous to those affecting cancers of the breast and endometrium, may have contributed to the increased incidence of cancer of the prostate which is associated geographically with westernization. Available data do not, however, consistently suggest a role for hormones in the genesis of this disease (Higgins, 1975). Nor is the amount of cadmium pollution, which has produced cancer of the prostate under industrial conditions (Owen, 1976), adequate to account for the association between economic development and prostatic cancer.

Conclusion

The common cancers that tend either to increase or decrease with westernization are listed in Table 7.4 together with the factors that are thought to explain these effects. Overall, there are many different factors and, for some individual cancer sites, several independent agents are possibly involved. Although exposure to these agents usually changes with economic development this is not in all cases or, perhaps, in any case, a necessary association.

Table 7.4   Suspected causes of the changes in incidence of common cancers which occur with economic development

EXPECTED CHANGE WITH ECONOMIC DEVELOPMENT

Increase		Decrease	
Cancer	Suspected cause of change[1]	Cancer	Suspected cause of change[1]
Colon/rectum	Dietary meat or fat Decreased dietary fibre	Mouth	Improved oral hygiene Decline in some forms of tobacco use (e.g. chewing)
Pancreas	Cigarette smoking Dietary fat (?)		Decline in alcohol consumption
Lung	Cigarette smoking Some occupations Air pollution	Oropharynx/ oesophagus	Decline in some forms of tobacco use Decline in alcohol consumption Improved diet (?)
Breast	Declining fertility Dietary fat or total energy	Stomach	Vitamin A or C(?) Improved preservation of food (?)
Corpus uteri	Dietary fat or total energy Oestrogen therapy	Liver	Improved hygiene Improved food quality and storage
Ovary	Declining fertility	Penis	Circumcision Personal cleanliness
Prostate	Dietary change (?)	Cervix uteri	Delayed intercourse Reduced promiscuity Improved sexual hygiene (?)
Bladder	Cigarette smoking Some occupations		Improved diet (?)

[1] (?) Indicates speculative associations

Westernization is not, therefore, an indivisible package. There is no necessary set of cancer outcomes that must follow economic development. Depending on the presence or absence of individual components of Western lifestyle, the overall incidence of cancer may either rise (as it has in black Americans) or fall (as it is now doing in Japan). A population could retain a high incidence of a cancer rare in affluent societies (such as primary liver cancer) because the relevant aspects of the environment remain unaltered, while acquiring a high incidence of another cancer, such as lung cancer, by adoption of exposure to the responsible agent. The key to cancer prevention in non-Western societies is not, therefore, total acceptance or rejection of westernization but the selection or avoidance of components of Western technology and lifestyle as they are relevant to the elimination of existing hazards, or the avoidance of new ones.

References

Armstrong, B. K. (1976). Recent trends in breast-cancer incidence and mortality in relation to changes in possible risk factors. *International Journal of Cancer*, **17**, 204–211

Armstrong, B. K. (1977). The role of diet in human carcinogenesis with special reference to endometrial cancer. In Hiatt, H. H., Watson, J. D. and Winsten, J. A. (eds.) *Origins of Human Cancer*, 557–565. Cold Spring Harbor Laboratory, New York

Armstrong, B. and Doll, R. (1975). Environmental factors and cancer incidence and mortality in different countries with special reference to dietary practices. *International Journal of Cancer*, **15**, 617–631

Armstrong, B. K., Mann, J. I., Adelstein, A. M. and Eskin, F. (1975). Commodity consumption and ischaemic heart disease mortality with special reference to dietary practices. *Journal of Chronic Diseases*, **28**, 455–469

Beral, V. (1974). Cancer of the cervix: a sexually transmitted infection? *Lancet*, **i**, 1037–1040

Beral, V., Fraser, P. and Chilvers, C. (1978). Does pregnancy protect against ovarian cancer? *Lancet*, **i**, 1083–1087

Bjelke, E. (1975). Dietary vitamin A and human lung cancer. *International Journal of Cancer*, **15**, 561–565

Blumberg, B. S. (1977). Australia antigen and the biology of hepatitis B. *Science*, **197**, 17–25

Brady, J., Liberatore, F., Harper, P., Greenwald, P., Burnett, W., Davies, J. N. P., Bishop, M., Polan, A. and Vianna, N. (1977). Angiosarcoma of the liver: An epidemiologic survey. *Journal of the National Cancer Institute*, **59**, 1383–1385

Bridford, K., Decoufle, P., Fraumeni, J. F., Hoel, D. G., Hoover, R. N., Rall, D. P., Safiotti, U., Schneiderman, M. A. and Upton, A. C. (1978). *Estimates of the Fraction of Cancer in the United States Related to Occupational Factors*. National Cancer Institute, National Institute of Environmental Health Sciences, National Institute for Occupational Safety and Health, Washington

Burkitt, D. P. (1975). Large-bowel cancer: An epidemiologic jigsaw puzzle. *Journal of the National Cancer Institute*, **54**, 3–6

Chan, P. C., Head, J. F., Cohen, L. A. and Wynder, E. L. (1977). Influence of dietary fat on the induction of mammary tumors by N-nitrosomethylurea: Associated hormone changes and differences between Sprague–Dawley and F344 rats. *Journal of the National Cancer Institute*, **59**, 1279–1283

Devesa, S. S. and Silverman, D. T. (1978). Cancer incidence and mortality trends in the United States: 1935–74. *Journal of the National Cancer Institute*, **60**, 545–571

DeWaard, F. and Baanders-van Halewijn, E. A. (1974).A prospective study in general practice of breast-cancer risk in post-menopausal women. *International Journal of Cancer*, **14**, 153–160

Doll, R. (1977). The prevention of cancer. *Journal of the Royal College of Physicians*, **11**, 125–140

Doll, R. (1978). Atmospheric pollution and lung cancer. *Environmental Health Perspectives*, **22**, 23–31

Doll, R. (1979). The pattern of disease in the post-infection era: national trends. *Proceedings of the Royal Society of London B*, **205**, 47–61

Fox, A. J. and Adelstein, A. M. (1978). Occupational mortality: Work or way of life? *Journal of Epidemiology and Community Health*, **32**, 73–78

Glober, G. A., Nomura, A., Kamiyama, S., Shimada, A. and Abba, B. C. (1977). Bowel transit-time and stool weight in populations with different colon cancer risks. *Lancet*, **ii**, 110–111

Graham, S., Dayal, H., Rohrer, T., Swanson, M., Sultz, H., Shedd, D. and Fischman, S. (1977). Dentition, diet, tobacco and alcohol in the epidemiology of oral cancer. *Journal of the National Cancer Institute*, **59**, 1611–1618

Haenszel, W., Berg, J. W., Segi, M., Kurihara, M. and Locke, F. B. (1973). Large-bowel cancer in Haiwaiian Japanese. *Journal of the National Cancer Institute*, **51**, 1765–1779

Haenszel, W. M. and Kurihara, M. (1968). Studies of Japanese migrants. I. Mortality from cancer and other diseases among Japanese in the United States. *Journal of the National Cancer Institute*, **40**, 43–68

Hems, G. (1978). The contributions of diet and childbearing to breast-cancer rates. *British Journal of Cancer*, **37**, 974–982

Higgins, I. T. T. (1975). The epidemiology of cancer of the prostate. *Journal of Chronic Diseases*, **28**, 343–348

Higginson, J. and Muir, C. S. (1976). The role of epidemiology in elucidating the importance of environmental factors in human cancer. *Cancer Detection and Prevention*, **1**, 79–105

Hill, P., Chan, P., Cohen, L., Wynder, E. and Kuno, K. (1977). Diet and endocrine related cancer. *Cancer*, **39**, 1820–1826

Hirayama, T. (1977). Changing patterns of cancer in Japan with special reference to the decrease in stomach cancer mortality. In Hiatt, H. H., Watson, J. D. and Winsten, J. A. (eds.) *Origins of Human Cancer*, 55–75. Cold Spring Harbor Laboratory, New York

Hirayama, T. (1978). Epidemiology of breast cancer with special reference to the role of diet. *Preventive Medicine*, **7**, 173–195

Jayant, K., Balakrishnan, V., Sanghvi, L. D. and Jussawalla, D. J. (1977). Quantification of the role of smoking and chewing tobacco in oral, pharyngeal and oesophageal cancers. *British Journal of Cancer*, **35**, 232–235

Joint Iran-International Agency for Research on Cancer Study Group

(1977). Esophageal cancer studies in the Caspian Littoral in Iran: results of population studies—a prodrome. *Journal of the National Cancer Institute,* **59,** 1127–1138

Lee, P. N. (ed.) (1975). *Tobacco Consumption in Various Countries.* Research Paper 6, fourth edition. Tobacco Research Council, London

Loraine, J. (1976). The global population, 1976. *Lancet,* **ii,** 621–622

Lyon, J. L. and Sorenson, A. W. (1978). Colon cancer in a low-risk population. *American Journal of Clinical Nutrition,* **31,** S227–S230

MacLennan, R., Jensen, O. M., Mosbech, J. and Vuori, H. V. (1978). Diet, transit time, stool weight and colon cancer in two Scandinavian populations. *American Journal of Clinical Nutrition,* **31,** S239–S242

MacMahon, B., Cole, P. and Brown, J. B. (1973). Etiology of human breast cancer: a review. *Journal of the National Cancer Institute,* **50,** 21–42

McMichael, A. J. (1978). Increases in laryngeal cancer in Britain and Australia in relation to alcohol and tobacco consumption trends. *Lancet,* **i,** 1244–1247

Mettlin, C., Graham, S. and Swanson, M. (1979). Vitamin A and lung cancer. *Journal of the National Cancer Institute,* **62,** 1435–1438

Miller, A. B., Kelly, A., Choi, N. W., Matthews, V., Morgan, R. W., Munan, L. Burch, J. D., Feather, J., Howe, G. R. and Jain, M. (1978). A study of diet and breast cancer. *American Journal of Epidemiology,* **107,** 499–509

Modan, B., Barell, V., Lubin, F., Modan, M., Greenberg, R. A. and Graham, S. (1975). Low-fibre intake as an etiologic factor in cancer of the colon. *Journal of the National Cancer Institute,* **55,** 15–18

Muller, M. (1978). Cigarettes kill the poor and black. too. *New Scientist,* **78,** 679–681

Owen, W. L. (1976). Cancer of the prostate: A literature review. *Journal of Chronic Diseases,* **29,** 89–114

Peers, F. G. and Linsell, C. A. (1977). Dietary aflatoxin and human primary liver cancer. *Annales de la Nutrition et de l'Alimentation,* **31,** 1005–1017

Sporn, M. B. (1977). Prevention of epithelial cancer by vitamin A and its synthetic analogs (retinoids). In Hiatt, H. H., Watson, J. D. and Winsten, J. A. (eds.) *Origins of Human Cancer,* 801–810. Cold Spring Harbor Laboratory, New York

Spring, J. A. and Buss, D. H. (1977). Three centuries of alcohol in the British diet. *Nature,* **270,** 567–572

Tulinius, H., Day, N. E., Johanesson, G., Bjarnason, O. and Gonzales, M. (1978). Reproductive factors and risk for breast cancer in Iceland. *International Journal of Cancer,* **21,** 724–730

Vianna, N. J. and Polan, A. K. (1978). Non-occupational exposure to asbestos and malignant mesothelioma in females. *Lancet,* **i,** 1061–1063

Warwick, G. P. and Harrington, J. S. (1973). Some aspects of the epidemiology and etiology of esophageal cancer with particular emphasis on the Transkei, South Africa. *Advances in Cancer Research,* **17,** 82–232

Waterhouse, J., Muir, C., Correa, P. and Powell, J. (eds.) (1976). *Cancer Incidence in Five Continents,* Volume III. International Agency for Research on Cancer, Lyon

Weiss, N. S., Szekely, D. R., and Austin, D. F. (1976). Increasing incidence of endometrial cancer in the United States. *New England Journal of Medicine,* **294,** 1259–1262

Wright, N. H., Vessey, M. P., Kenward, B., McPherson, K. and Doll, R. (1978). Neoplasia and dysplasia of the cervix uteri and contraception: A possible protective effect of the diaphragm. *British Journal of Cancer,* **38,** 273–279

Wynder, E. L. (1975). An epidemiological evaluation of the causes of cancer of the pancreas. *Cancer Research,* **35,** 2228–2233

Part III

Hunter-gatherers

8

Eskimos (Inuit)

Otto Schaefer

Traditional diet

Epidemics of acute and chronic infections, such as measles and tuberculosis, brought by Western man to the Arctic, played an overwhelming role in the life of Eskimos during the early post-contact period, and these diseases are still important. This experience has not been peculiar to Eskimos, but has been the common lot of nearly all isolated aboriginal populations; these matters are therefore not discussed further. On the other hand Eskimos are particularly interesting because of their traditional diet, environment and relatively recent acculturation. Among the few remaining communities who were hunter-gatherers in the middle of the present century, the Eskimos relied least on food-gathering in their barren Arctic land; instead their food came almost exclusively from hunting and fishing.

This chapter outlines the unique features of their traditional diet, and the metabolic responses to this diet, also the subsequent changes consequent on acculturation, together with changes in the pattern of disease. Traditionally Eskimos, more than any other community, were carnivorous, although, contrary to popular belief, not exclusively so. They consumed, with instinctive relish, vegetable material present in the contents of the stomach and gut of slaughtered caribou, Arctic hare and ptarmigan, also plant and root stores of lemmings, called lemming-nuts, as well as berries, plants and roots collected during the short summer and autumn, likewise seaweed scraped at low tide from coastal cliffs even in midwinter (Schaefer, 1977a).

Consumption of this plant material was too small in quantity and irregular in time, especially in the far north of the Arctic Archipelago, to supply adequately certain vitamin requirements, especially those of vitamins A, C and folic acid; also perhaps it was inadequate in certain minerals. A critical situation arose concerning a possible deficiency of vitamin C. Here, once more, the traditional dietary habits of the Eskimo were beneficial. They were accustomed to eat a large proportion of fish and of meat either raw or raw-frozen. This caused their neighbours the Naskapi Indians to call them 'Askimowet', i.e. 'raw-meat-eaters'. This word became our 'Eskimo', while their own preferred, and increasingly accepted name in Canada, is Inuit, i.e. 'Men'. Eating meat raw preserved the marginal amounts of ascorbic acid present in it. Likewise their traditional preference for internal organs, such as liver, can be understood in terms of a rich source of vitamin C, 8–12 times more than that present in muscle tissue. Eskimos partook of half-digested willow buds, reindeer moss and other herbs present in the stomach of slaughtered caribou. These were important sources of vitamin C and folic acid. Spongy bones were their main source of calcium and were chewed assiduously, while cortical bones were used for weapons and tools. To use all parts of their prey, and to waste nothing, was regarded as part of the reconciliation of hunter and quarry: it ensured a healthy *modus vivendi* for both.

Eskimos appear to have been well adapted to their traditional diet, consumed by them for some thousands of years, even if it contained only small amounts of certain vitamins, and was low in plant fibre and very low in plant carbohydrate. Their traditional diet contained no added sugar or salt. Salt was not added to preserve meat or fish, which was preserved by being frozen or dried. Stefansson (1946) wrote: 'It is here (among the Eskimos) that I learned from experience . . . that (added) salt is not necessary for health and the desire for it disappears after about three months.'

Little is known concerning the pathology of the liver enlargement reported some 20–30 years ago in many healthy Eskimo hunters (Brown, 1955; Hildes, 1958; Schaefer, 1959). It was observed to disappear when more carbohydrate was eaten (Schaefer, 1971). The hepatic enlargement may have reflected increased gluconeogenesis from protein because of the relative deficiency of dietary carbohydrate in the traditional Eskimo diet. The high consumption of protein necessitated high urinary excretion of nitrogen. The increased consumption of carbohydrate and decreased intake of protein in the modern Eskimo diet lessened the metabolic load on kidneys and liver.

Transitional diet after contact

Naturally there does not exist any exact measurement of the composition of the traditional Eskimo diet in the precontact period or even in very early transitional times. The earliest estimates and detailed measurements of the Eskimo diet were made only after the introduction of Western foods, staples such as wheat, white flour and rolled oats, also sugar and lard, by whalers and fur traders.

Trends towards increasing westernization of the Eskimo diet can be seen in the dietary surveys presented in Table 8.1. These data have been collected from the literature and from my own surveys: the table compares data from Canadian Arctic Eskimos during the mid-1960s from four fairly traditionally living groups and a relatively acculturated one in a large urbanized settlement (Frobisher Bay); then contrasts data from diet surveys conducted in North Alaska and NW Greenland in the 1950s and early 1970s. The change in the dietary pattern is shown in the change in the relative consumption of the main nutrients; it has moved towards the characteristic Western pattern of diet

Table 8.1 Eskimo diets: energy, protein, fat and carbohydrate (CHO), also US diets, daily average per capita

Year	Place	Energy (megajoules)[1]	Protein	Fat	CHO	Author
			(energy percentages)			
1965	Cumberland Sound	11·5	46	17	37	Schaefer (1964–66)
1965	Holman Island	11·5	41	26	33	Schaefer (1964–66)
1965	Coppermine	10·1	43	23	34	Schaefer (1964–66)
1967	Lake Harbour	11·2	44	23	33	Kemp (1971)
1965	Frobisher Bay	8·5	25	25	50	Schaefer (1964–66)
1956–61	Alaska	8·3	28	37	35	Heller and Scott (1967)
1971–72	North Alaska	10·4	20	39	4	Draper (1977)
1955	NW Greenland	NA[3]	36	25	39	Uhl (1955)
1974	NW Greenland	11·8	26	37	37	Bang et al. (1976)
1955	United States	13·3	13	43	44	Agric[2] (1956)

[1] Conversion SI to traditional units—1 MJ ≈ 240 kcal
[2] Agricultural Marketing Service, see references
[3] Not available

exemplified at the bottom of Table 8.1 from data gathered in a United States urban household consumer survey (Agricultural Marketing Service, 1956).

Energy

Total energy intake of all Eskimo groups listed in Table 8.1 was lower than that reported by the USDA Urban Household Survey (Agricultural Marketing Service, 1956). Lower total energy intakes recorded in Alaskan natives in the late 1950s, and in urbanized Canadian Eskimos in the 1960s, may be explained as an appropriate response to decreased energy expenditures due to reduced or motorized hunting activities and living in heated houses. Increases of energy intakes in later surveys may have reflected greater affluence and the effect of further acculturation leading to excessive energy intakes most markedly shown in the USDA data.

Round mongoloid faces and bulky caribou fur clothing led to the popular but mistaken notion that a substantial subcutaneous fat layer enabled Eskimos better to withstand the cold. Estimates of prevalence of obesity based on weight/height formulae (Mann *et al.*, 1962; Nutrition Canada, 1973) contributed to this impression. They were proved false by comparing skinfold measurements and weight/height in over a thousand Canadian Eskimos (Schaefer, 1977b). Eskimos had, as Burton and Edholm (1955) postulated, and Schaefer *et al.* (1974) elaborated, created with fur clothing their own microclimate and had a greater physiological problem with heat dispersal than with heat conservation. Gross obesity was rarely seen in traditional-living Eskimo adults of either sex. It would have been a heavy liability in nomadic hunters. However, with progressive westernization of the diet and less energy expenditure in permanent settlements obesity (page 119), as reflected in skinfold measurements, has become prevalent in both sexes, and is compatible with survival.

Protein

In the hunting camps protein intakes were very high. In more acculturated Eskimo populations protein intakes fell to the third place among major nutrients, lower than either carbohydrates or fat, as evident from data recorded in recent surveys in Frobisher Bay, Alaska and Greenland (Table 8.1).

Fat

In the transitional Eskimo diet fat intakes have been moderate, even low (Table 8.1), in spite of access to large amounts of blubber from sea mammals, often available to coastal Eskimos. This is contrary to popular opinion. A moderate intake is understandable if the stimulating effect of these poly-unsaturated long chain fatty acids on gut motility is recognized. Indeed, I found that Eskimos used to regulate the frequency of their bowel movements by varying the amount of consumed blubber. It is probable that the laxative action of the blubber fat compensated for the constipating effect of a very low intake of plant fibre in the traditional diet. It is regretted that there are no data concerning stool weights of Eskimos consuming either their traditional diet or the semi-westernized transitional diet of the more modern settlements. More than half of the fat consumed by Alaskan (Heller and Scott, 1967) and Canadian Eskimos (Schaefer, 1964–66) came from imported sources. Eskimos who move to the larger settlements and eat Western shop foods often complain of constipation and take laxatives. This observation probably reflects decreased physical activity and less laxative blubber in the diet rather than a decreased intake of dietary fibre.

Complex carbohydrates

In the transitional Eskimo diet carbohydrates have moved ahead of fat as a source of energy even in the more traditional-living Eskimo groups listed in Table 8.1. Most of the carbohydrate consumed by these, and almost all of it in the larger settlements, was derived from imports such as white flour, rolled oats and sugar (page 114). Traditional taste preference secured for animal polysaccharides such as glycogen and glycoproteins a declining but still important place in the diet, especially in smaller settlements. Internal organs are rich in glycogen and skin and gut epithelium are composed largely of glycoproteins. Muktuk, the thick skin of whales, was and still is in high demand as a delicacy, perhaps explained by relative scarcity of carbohydrates in their traditional diet. Vegetable sources, such as berries, plants and roots collected in summer, or derived throughout the year from the intestines of their prey, contributed very minor amounts of carbohydrate and are very little used nowadays.

Sugar

There has been a phenomenal increased consumption of sugar in recent years. The traditional Eskimo diet contained no shop sugar. Table 8.2 reports a four-fold increase of sugar consumption in Pangnirtung–Cumberland area from 1959 to 1967. This coincided with accelerated growth and maturation, as discussed later, and has affected endocrine function in a manner for which the Eskimos, as discussed later, may have been ill-prepared.

Carbohydrate metabolism

Approximately half of randomly selected adult Eskimos, with no signs of metabolic disease, have a diabetic-type oral glucose tolerance curve, but react normally to an intravenous glucose load. The release of insulin, which follows carbohydrate ingestion and anticipates the rise in blood glucose levels in persons adapted to a high intake of carbohydrate, is lacking in a high proportion of Eskimos. If a protein meal precedes by one hour the oral glucose tolerance test, then the blood sugar and serum insulin response are normalized (Schaefer *et al.*, 1972). This alteration may be due to changes in the response of gut glucagon or other gut hormones.

Table 8.2   Sugar and cereal annual consumption in Pangnirtung, per capita, and percentage of total carbohydrate (CHO)

Year	Sugar per capita (kg)	total CHO (%)	Cereals per capita (kg)	total CHO[1] (%)
1959	11·8	18	71·0	82
1960	17·1	22	72·5	78
1964	30·0	30	92·0	70
1967	47·4	44[2]	77·3	56

[1] Total carbohydrate: CHO of cereals average 75%
[2] Comparable recent figures for Canada 47%, USA 51%

Western diseases

Diabetes mellitus

In Canadian Eskimos no case of diabetes mellitus has yet been reported in the traditional-living central and eastern Arctic regions; but an increasing number of diabetics have been reported from the Western Arctic, especially in the more acculturated Eskimos living in the Mackenzie delta. Age-adjusted prevalence rates even in this area are less than one-third of those reported in most Western nations. Comparable upward trends in prevalence have been reported in Alaska and Greenland Eskimos. The prevalence of diabetes is reported to be rising slowly in Alaska Eskimos (Mouratoff and Scott, 1973). Recently a very high prevalence rate was reported in an Eskimoid population subjected to a long period of acculturation, the Aleuts of the Pribilof Islands (Dippe *et al.*, 1976).

Recent surveys

Recent survey examinations of two Eskimo populations at different stages of acculturation provided data concerning the prevalence of certain Western diseases in very different circumstances. One group of Eskimos was examined in the large western Arctic town of Inuvik in the Mackenzie River delta. They had moved from hunting camps into permanent settlements a generation earlier and were much more acculturated than the other group of Eskimos examined in Arctic Bay in the northernmost part of the Canadian eastern Arctic on Baffin Island.

To simplify terminology these two groups will be called in this chapter the western Eskimos (Inuvik town) and the eastern Eskimos (Arctic Bay settlement). The increasing prevalence of maturity-onset diabetes mellitus in the former population has been mentioned already (page 118). Large significant differences in growth and development of children, also differences in the prevalence of certain diseases of Western civilization, were noted as acculturation influenced diet and lifestyle (Schaefer *et al.*, 1980).

Obesity and serum cholesterol

Maturity-onset diabetes, gallstones and hypertension are closely associated with obesity and also, but less closely, with high serum cholesterol levels. The skinfold thickness of the eastern Eskimo men aged 20–50 years and women aged 20–40 years was only one-third of the thickness of their more acculturated western counterparts, and serum cholesterol levels followed a similar pattern (Fig. 8.1). Differences of both parameters were largest, and most significant, in middle-aged men and women.

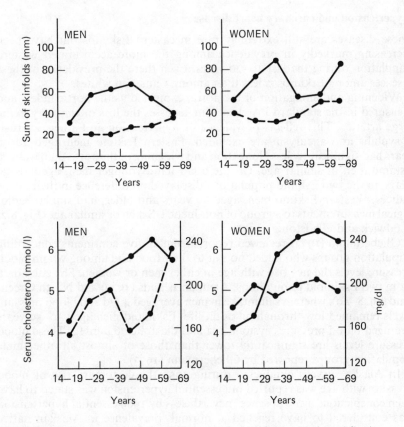

Fig. 8.1 Eskimo mean skinfold thickness (sum of arm, back and flank skinfolds), also of serum cholesterol levels, of traditional-living Eastern (–•– –•– –•–) and accultured Western (•—•—•) populations

Gallstones

These surveys of the two populations reported that western Eskimos had 10 times more persons having gallstones than members of the eastern population; 47 per cent of the western Eskimo women aged 30 years or more had proven gallstones but only 5 per cent of the eastern Eskimo women of similar age had gallstones. 10 per cent of the western Eskimo men aged 30 years or more had gallstones removed at operation, but no gallstones had been removed at operation among eastern Eskimo men of similar age.

Gallstones and maturity-onset diabetes, the emergence of the latter disease being perhaps later than the former, appear among Eskimos to follow a changing pattern similar to that reported in North American Indians, especially those of the US southwestern States, wherein these diseases have a higher prevalence than in almost any other community in the world.

Hypertension and coronary heart disease

These diseases are still extremely rare in eastern Eskimos but have been increasing markedly in prevalence among the more acculturated western population during the last 10–20 years. Even there the prevalence of these diseases among Eskimos is less than among Canadian whites.

Widening and elongation of the aorta, expressed as the aortic index, and measured in the standard PA chest film, assesses the loss of elasticity in the large arteries. This reflects prevalence of hypertension and atherosclerosis if syphilis and aneurysm are excluded. Eastern Eskimo men aged 40–70 years had significantly less elongation and widening of the aorta than western Eskimo men of similar age. On the other hand younger men, aged 18–39 years, in the two Eskimo populations displayed no difference in their aortic indices. Western Eskimo men, aged 40 years and older, had similar radiological measurements to a group of non-luetic US men of similar age (Fig. 8.2) (Lodwick and Gladstone, 1957).

Gliebermann (1973) reviewed reports from all five continents concerning population groups who added no salt to their food and among whom blood pressure levels did not rise with age in either men or women. She cited data from two Eskimoid populations, Aleutian Islands (1949) and North Greenland (1948–49), wherein salt intake in men averaged 4 g/d and blood pressure levels remained low throughout adult life. Eskimoid men aged 50–59 years averaged blood pressures systolic 102 and diastolic 76 mmHg. These blood pressure levels are significantly lower than those of almost all other male population groups reported by Gliebermann (1973).

In Alaska surveys conducted during 1958 the customary rise of blood pressure with age was reported but essential hypertension was stated to have been conspicuous by its absence; nevertheless by 1969 essential hypertension was considered to have reached a 'normal' prevalence in Alaskan native women (Mann *et al.*, 1962; Colbert *et al.*, 1978).

In Canadian Eskimos the virtual absence of essential hypertension and low salt intake have been noted (Schaefer, 1959). Low mean blood pressures and

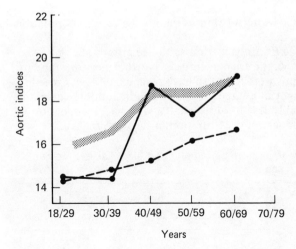

Fig. 8.2 Eskimo male mean aortic indices of traditional-living Eastern (—●— —●— —●—) and acculturated Western (●——●——●) populations compared with the 'normal' US male data of Lodwick and Gladstone (1957) (▓▓▓▓▓▓)

no increase with age in either sex were found in a little-acculturated group of eastern Arctic Eskimos (Hildes and Schaefer, 1973). This was reported to be still present in Arctic Bay men, but not women, examined in 1976; on the other hand age-related increase of blood pressure was reported in 1977 in both men and women of the more acculturated Inuvik Eskimos (Schaefer *et al.*, 1980).

Growth and sexual maturation

Secular acceleration of growth and earlier sexual maturation in both sexes during the past 100 years has been well documented in the children of Europe and North America; it has been observed during the last generation in non-European countries, which have experienced recent modernization and affluence, such as Japan. These changes are not regarded as pathological but are considered to be beneficial consequences of better nutrition. Mean age of menarche has fallen by more than two years during the past 100 years in these countries.

Table 8.3 reports the age of menarche in young and old Eskimo women in the western Arctic town (Inuvik) and in the eastern Arctic Bay settlement. Secular acceleration of growth, and an earlier age of menarche, had occurred more among the Western women, among whom acculturation had occurred earlier and more intensely, than among the Eastern women. The gradual disappearance of the traditional short Eskimo stature, namely shortness for age in comparison with North American standards, is of particular interest (Heller *et al.*, 1967; Schaefer, 1970; Sayed *et al.*, 1976). This trend was found to be more in the western Eskimos than in the eastern population (Schaefer *et al.*, 1980).

Eastern male and female Eskimos in almost all age groups above 6 years of age remained at, or below, the 5th percentile of North American standard height, but western Eskimos were found to have reached, or even exceeded, the 25th percentile of height in all age groups of children, adolescents and young adults, but noticeably less in older adults, who had their period of growth before the main impact of acculturation in the western Arctic.

Table 8.3 Age of menarche in groups of young and older Eskimo women, age of menarche in years, mean ± s.d.

Group		Young ≤ 30 years	Older > 30 years
		Age of women	
Western	No.	34	15
	Age of menarche	13·4 ± 1·1—**	14·9 ± 1·7**
	Range	11·5–155	13·5–18·0
Eastern	No.	*** 35	35 N.S.
	Age of menarche	14·4 ± 1·3— *	15·2 ± 1·3*
	Range	12·5–17·5	13·5–18·5

* $P < 0.05$
** $P < 0.01$
*** $P < 0.001$

This secular acceleration of growth of Eskimos has coincided both in time and in place with a marked increased consumption of sugar, but decreased consumption of protein; it has also been accompanied by certain signs of ill-health, such as decreased haemoglobin levels (Schaefer, 1970). These observations confirm the view of Ziegler (1967), who reviewed data from many parts of the world. One must, therefore, question the prevailing assumption that the marked secular acceleration of growth is mainly due to better nutrition, and that it is in all respects a healthy phenomenon. Indeed, the association of this phenomenon with the appearance of a number of Western diseases is too regular in time and place to be attributed to chance.

Appendicitis

Acute appendicitis was formerly a rare disease among traditional-living Eskimos. From 1928 to 1958 no case of appendicitis was reported in a mission hospital at Pangnirtung caring for 4000–5000 Canadian eastern Arctic Eskimos. However in 1964, in an eight-week journey aboard a supply ship visiting these parts, three emergency acute appendicectomies had to be performed; also in the new Frobisher Bay hospital in this area acute appendicitis has become the commonest cause of admission for acute abdominal pain. In the early 1950s I saw only three cases of acute appendicitis during two years caring for more than 3000 Eskimos and Indians in the western Arctic Region. 'Epidemics' of appendicitis began to be noted in northern Alberta Indians in the 1950s, in the western Arctic Eskimos in the 1960s, and in the eastern Arctic Eskimos in the 1970s. This corresponded in each population group with westernization of diet and lifestyle (Schaefer, 1979).

Diverticular disease

The only source of information concerning the incidence of this disease is derived from our search of patients' records, the discharge diagnosis and the reports on barium enemata, at various hospitals and clinics both in the northern and southern regions of Canada. Diverticular disease had been rarely diagnosed among traditional-living eastern Arctic Eskimos. On the other hand this disease had been diagnosed in a fair number of more acculturated western Arctic Eskimos, although probably less frequently than in the whites.

Varicose veins

Traditional-living eastern and central Arctic Eskimos are almost completely free of varicose veins; more acculturated western Arctic Eskimos may develop varicose veins, but even among them the condition remains uncommon compared to the incidence among whites of comparable age and sex.

Phleboliths

During my examination of more than a hundred abdominal radiographs for evidence of diverticular disease, only one pelvic phlebolith was seen. Phleboliths appear to be a rare condition among all Eskimos.

Colorectal cancer

Among Eskimos in Alaska colorectal cancer rates have risen and approximate nowadays to those of whites. Lanier *et al.* (1976) stated that '. . . the proportion of (Alaskan) natives with colorectal cancer has risen sharply since previous studies, due perhaps to westernization of dietary and life-style patterns. It is now the most common site of cancer, accounting for 22 per cent of the tumours in this site.'

Amongst Canadian Eskimos colorectal cancer is less common than among other North Americans. This form of cancer accounted for only 6 per cent of 180 malignant tumours during the period 1950–74; this is about half the proportion observed in most Western countries. Age-adjusted incidence of colorectal cancer more than doubled also in Canadian Eskimos in a recent (1967–74) compared with an earlier period (1950–66) even if their proportion of total malignancies observed increased only from 5 to 7 per cent during the same period of time. This was due to a markedly increased incidence of a number of other types of neoplasm, especially cancer of the lung and cervix (Fig. 8.3).

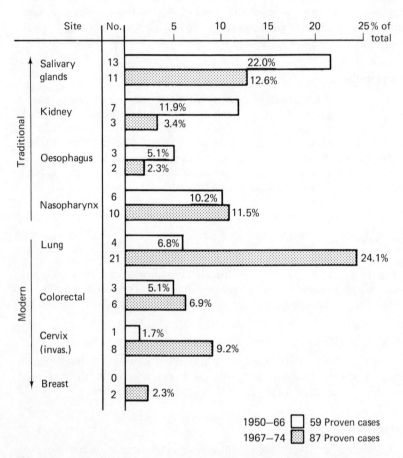

Fig. 8.3   Changing pattern of cancer in Eskimos from 1950 to 1974 in traditional-living central Arctic and modern-living western Arctic populations

Colonic disease and the Eskimo diet

Traditional-living Eskimos were less constipated and had shorter transit times than Eskimos who eat modern low fibre Western diets (Schaefer, 1979). Their soft stools and fast transit times, due to the laxative action of the polyunsaturated fatty acids in their traditional diet rather than the differences in the fibre content, probably account for their remarkably lower, but recently rising, incidence of appendicitis, diverticular disease and possibly also varicose veins, phleboliths and colorectal cancer.

Cancer of the breast and corpus uteri

The frequency of these tumours, like that of large bowel carcinoma, is closely related in many countries to economic development. In earlier periods breast cancer was extremely rare, reported almost as non-existent, among both Canadian, Alaskan and Greenland Eskimos. By 1976 it had become one of the commonest malignant tumours in Alaskan Eskimo women (Fortuine, 1969; Lanier *et al.*, 1976). While rates of breast cancer are still much lower in the more recently acculturated Canadian Eskimos, an upgoing trend can be detected when comparing an earlier and recent period (Schaefer *et al.*, 1975). The Canadian study compared Eskimo women with breast cancer and healthy cohorts in regard to factors considered likely to contribute to breast cancer epidemiology and found no difference in age at first pregnancy, or in parity, or in diet, but a difference in the history of lactation. Each of the later cancer-developing breasts had functioned either not at all or only for short periods compared to prolonged lactation—traditionally children were nursed for three years—recorded for most non-affected breasts.

Cancer of the corpus uteri is rare among Eskimos; even in 1976 the observed to expected ratio was only 0·3 in Alaskan women (Lanier *et al.*, 1976), while none had been found in Canadian Eskimos (Schaefer *et al.*, 1975).

Cancer of lung

The incidence of lung cancer has increased considerably in recent years. The accepted role of cigarette smoking may explain some, but not all, of the changes in lung cancer incidence. In earlier years half of all lung cancers in Alaskan Eskimos (Hurst, 1964) and all of those observed in Canadian Eskimos before 1967 (Schaefer *et al.*, 1976) occurred in women. Traditionally Eskimo women tended day and night lamps which emitted much heavy sooty smoke from the seal and fish oils. This practice continued in the central Arctic until the mid-1960s. Smoking, especially that of factory-made cigarettes, increased drastically in both sexes with the construction of the Distant Early Warning Line in 1955. There was, therefore, an overlapping period of heavy smoking and soot inhalation for central Arctic women and the epidemic of lung cancer recorded in this group in the late 1960s and early 1970s may relate to this historical sequence.

Cancer of cervix uteri

The even greater increase in the incidence of cervical cancer, and its appearance at an earlier age, may be indirectly related to the tremendous social problems that have attended the modern lifestyle. Since the mid-1950s specific and non-specific venereal diseases have become more common, and increased promiscuity has occurred among adolescents and young adults.

Conclusion

During the last generation Eskimos have had a drastic change of diet from a traditional diet to more westernized food; their lifestyle also has changed profoundly. Acceleration of growth and earlier sexual maturation have occurred; obesity and maturity-onset diabetes have appeared, the incidence of gallstones, hypertension and degenerative cardiovascular diseases have increased. Records from Alaskan Eskimos in particular suggest that increases in cancer of the lung, large bowel and breast have followed contact with westernization of diet and lifestyle.

Marked regional differences noted in the time of emergence and magnitude of secular growth acceleration, together with the incidence of Western diseases and certain varieties of cancer, appear to reflect closely the duration and intensity of changes in nutrition and lifestyle produced by the penetration of Western civilization.

References

Agricultural Marketing Service and Agricultural Research Service (1956). *Dietary Levels of Households in the United States.* Report No. 6, Washington, DC

Bang, H. O., Dyerberg, J. and Hjørne, N. (1976). The composition of food consumed by Greenland Eskimos. *Acta Medica Scandinavica,* **200,** 69–73

Brown, G. M. (1955). Metabolic studies of the Eskimo. In: *Cold Injury Transactions of the Third Conference,* 1954, Fort Churchill, Manitoba, 52. Editor M. I. Ferrer. Josiah Macy Jr. Foundation, New York

Burton, A. C. and Edholm, O. G. (1955). *Man in a Cold Environment.* Edward Arnold, London

Colbert, M. J., Mann, G. V. and Hursh, L. M. (1978). Nutrition studies: clinical observations on nutritional health in Eskimos of Northern Alaska. In: *A Biological Perspective.* Editors P. L. Jamison, S. L. Zegura and F. A. Milan. Dowden, Hutchinson and Ross, Strondsburg

Dippe, S. E., Bennett, P. H., Dippe, D. W., Humphrey, J., Burks, J. and Miller, M. (1976). Glucose tolerance among Aleuts on the Pribilof Islands (abstract). *Third International Symposium on Circumpolar Health.* Editors R. J. Shepherd and S. Iroh. Toronto University Press, Toronto

Draper, H. A. (1977). The Aboriginal Eskimo diet in modern perspective. *American Anthropologists,* **78,** 309–316

Fortuine, R. (1969). Characteristics of cancer in the Eskimos of Southwestern Alaska. *Cancer,* **23,** 468–474.

Gliebermann, L. (1973). Blood pressure and dietary salt in human populations. *Ecology of Food and Nutrition,* **2,** 143–156

Heller, C. A. and Scott, E. M. (1967). *The Alaska Dietary Survey, 1956–61.* Public Health Service Publication No. 999–AH–2. Anchorage, Alaska

Heller, C. A., Scott, E. M. and Hammes, L. M. (1967). Height, weight and growth of Alaskan Eskimos. *American Journal of Diseases of Children*, **113**, 338–344

Hildes, J. A. (1958). Cold war medicine. *Medical Services Journal of Canada*, **14**, 24–32

Hildes, J. A. and Schaefer, O. (1973). Health of Igloolik Eskimos and changes with urbanization. *Journal of Human Evolution*, **2**, 241–246

Hurst, E. E. Jr. (1964). Malignant tumours in Alaskan Eskimos: Unique predominance of carcinoma of the esophagus in Alaskan Eskimo women. *Cancer*, **17**, 1187–1196

Kemp, W. B. (1971). The flow of energy in a hunting society. *Scientific American*, **225**, 105–115

Lanier, A. P., Bender, T. R., Blut, W. J., Fraumeni, J. F. Jr. and Hulbert, W. B. (1976). Cancer incidence in Alaskan natives. *International Journal of Cancer*, **18**, 409–412

Lodwick, G. S. and Gladstone, W. S. (1957). Correlation of anatomic and roentological changes in arteriosclerosis and syphilis of ascending aorta. *Radiology*, **69**, 70–78

Mann, G. V., Scott, E. M., Hursh, L. M., Heller, C. A., Youmans, J. B., Consolazio, C. F., Bridgforth, E. B., Russell, A. L. and Silverman, M. (1962). The health and nutritional status of Alaskan Eskimos. *American Journal of Clinical Nutrition*, **11**, 31–76

Mouratoff, G. J. and Scott, E. M. (1973). Diabetes mellitus in Eskimos after a decade. *Journal of the American Medical Association*, **226**, 1345–1346

Nutrition Canada (1973). *National Survey*. Information Canada, Ottawa

Sayed, J. E., Hildes, J. A. and Schaefer, O. (1976). Feeding practices and growth of Igloolik infants. In: *Proceedings of the Third International Symposium on Circumpolar Health*, 254–259. Editors R. J. Shepherd and S. Iroh. Toronto University Press, Toronto

Schaefer, O. (1959). Medical observations and problems in the Canadian Arctic. Part 2. *Canadian Medical Association Journal*, **81**, 383–393.

Schaefer, O. (1964–66). Report on nutrition surveys in five Arctic trading districts (unpublished). Data published in *Canadian Medical Association Journal* (1968), **99**, 252–262; (1970), **103**, 1059–1068; (1972), **107**, 733–738

Schaefer, O. (1970). Pre- and post-natal growth acceleration and increased sugar consumption in Canadian Eskimos. *Canadian Medical Association Journal*, **103**, 1059–1068

Schaefer, O. (1971). Physiological and pathological effects of nutritional changes in the Canadian Arctic (abstract). *Second International Symposium on Circumpolar Health*, 1971. Oulu

Schaefer, O. (1977a). Changing dietary patterns in the Canadian North: health, social and economic consequences. *Journal of the Canadian Dietetic Association*, **38**, 17–25

Schaefer, O. (1977b). Are Eskimos more or less obese than other Canadians? A comparison of skinfold thickness and ponderal index in Canadian Eskimos. *The American Journal of Clinical Nutrition*, **30**, 1623–1628

Schaefer, O. (1979). Aetiology of actue appendicitis (letter). *British Medical Journal*, **1**, 1215

Schaefer, O., Crookford, P. M. and Romanowski, B. (1972). Normalization effect of preceding protein meals on 'diabetic' oral glucose tolerance in Eskimos. *Canadian Medical Association Journal*, **107**, 733–738

Schaefer, O., Hildes, J. A., Greidanus, P. and Leung, D. (1974). Regional sweating in Eskimos compared to Caucasians. *Canadian Journal of Physiology and Pharmacology*, **52**, 960–965

Schaefer, O., Hildes, J. A., Medd, L. M. and Cameron, D. G. (1975). The changing pattern of neoplastic disease in Canadian Eskimos. *Canadian Medical Association Journal*, **112**, 1399–1404

Schaefer, O., Timmerans, J. F. W., Eaton, R. D. P. and Matthews, A. R. (1980). General and nutritional health in two Eskimo populations at different stages of acculturation. *Fourth International Symposium on Circumpolar Health, Novosibirsk, 1980. Canadian Journal of Public Health* (in press)

Stefansson, V. (1946). *Not by Bread Alone*, p. 50. Macmillan, New York

Uhl, E, (1955). Cited by Bang *et al.* (1976).

Ziegler, E. (1967). Secular changes in the stature of adults and the secular trend of the modern sugar consumption. *Zeitschrift für Kinderheilkunde*, **99**, 146–166

9

North American Indians

Kelly West

Introduction

Knowledge of previous and present disease patterns in North American Indians is quite incomplete. Nevertheless, available information is sufficient to show that changes in ways of life have been attended by profound changes in disease patterns.

Most of the published data concerns Indians who reside in the United States, but this presentation will also include some discussion of Indians in other parts of the northern hemisphere. In this vast area there are many hundreds of tribes. Among these tribes there is a considerable degree of genetic heterogeneity (Neel and Salzano, 1964), but the tribes have many genetic features in common (e.g., blood group O is regularly common and group B usually quite uncommon). Physical characteristics differ somewhat among tribes. In general, however, intertribal similarities in appearance are more impressive than the differences. On the other hand, intertribal differences in environmental factors were and are great, including substantial differences of diet. There have also been profound changes in diet with time in many tribes. All degrees of acculturation may be found. In some tribes, life differs little from that which prevailed before the time of Columbus. This is particularly true in rural areas of Central America, Mexico and Alaska. One of our Oklahoma Indians has recently retired, having served as President and Chairman of the Board of one of the world's largest corporations. But even in the United States a majority of Indians still live in rural areas, leading ways of life that are still quite different from those typical of white Americans. By US standards most Indians are poor and levels of education are, in general, lower than in whites. Generalizations are subject to exceptions because of inter- and intratribal differences. Even so, it will be possible to summarize below some patterns applicable to most or many US tribes.

In the United States there are still several hundred tribes. Some consist of only a few families. In the largest tribe, the Navajo, there are more than 100 000 people. The total Indian population is now about one million. This is approximately the same number as were present in the fifteenth century. The

Indian populations of Mexico and Central America were far greater. The present population estimate for US 'Indians' of one million does not include people of Mexican descent who live in the United States. Most of these have some Spanish blood, but a substantial majority are more Indian than European.

There are still a few small Indian tribes in the eastern United States, but a substantial majority of US Indians now reside in the central and western portions of the country. These include many tribes that lived in the east before the arrival of Europeans. Some tribes live on special reservations, others do not. In Oklahoma there are no reservations but there is still a considerable amount of social segregation with tribal governments, Indian churches, tribally owned lands, Indian schools, and so forth. The Pimas live on a large reservation just south of Phoenix, Arizona.

Disease patterns before acculturation

Data are quite incomplete but there is fairly strong evidence that obesity and diabetes were rare before the twentieth century (West, 1974). In fact these conditions are still rare in a few US tribes that are extremely poor or very primitive (e.g., in Alaskan Athabascans). Diabetes and obesity are rife in all of the many tribes of modern Oklahoma. These conditions are still rare, however, in anthropologically related tribes living elsewhere in a more primitive state (West, 1974). Diabetes was rare in all Oklahoma tribes prior to 1940.

Before 1940, coronary heart disease and gallbladder disease were probably uncommon in most, if not all, American tribes. Little is known about previous cancer rates but, in general, cancer seems to have been less common than in North American whites.

In the early part of the twentieth century, malnutrition and infectious diseases were particularly common and tuberculosis a major cause of morbidity and mortality. It has long been known that congenital dislocation of the hip is especially common in American Indians. Rates of this disorder remain high in modern times.

Present disease patterns

For many reasons the toll from infectious disease has been greatly reduced in North American Indians. Tuberculosis is still more common than in whites, but this disease is no longer a leading cause of morbidity and mortality. In US Indians the spectrum of diseases is beginning to resemble that in whites. There are, however, several interesting peculiarities.

Coronary heart disease and atherosclerosis

In Indians south of the Rio Grande rates of coronary heart disease and atherosclerosis tend to be low. In our studies in rural Guatemala we found electrocardiographic abnormalities suggestive of coronary disease were much less frequent than in US whites (West and Kalbfleisch, 1970). Pathologists in Central America also have the impression that clinically significant atherosclerosis is uncommon in Indians. According to Conner *et al.* (1978) significant atherosclerosis is rare in the primitive Tarahumara Indians of Mexico in whom serum cholesterol levels average 3·2 mmol/l (125 mg/dl)! Intakes of saturated fat and cholesterol are very low in these Indians. Serum cholesterol values are not quite so low in members of this tribe who consume amounts of cholesterol that are higher than the average levels for this tribe. Exercise levels are, in general, very high in Tarahumaras.

Rates of coronary heart disease also appear to be low in most US tribes (Sievers, 1967), although these rates are increasing (West, 1978b; 1979b). Among the US tribes there appears to be considerable variation in rates of vascular disease (West, 1974). It is not yet clear to what extent these differences are the result of genetic or environmental factors. Probably Indians have lower levels of serum cholesterol even when consuming levels of saturated fat equivalent to those in whites. In several of the Oklahoma tribes we have found blood cholesterol values to be about 15 per cent lower than in local whites despite levels of dietary saturated fat that were at least as high as in the whites. In Pimas blood cholesterol values are even lower than in the Oklahoma Indians (Hamman *et al.*, 1975) even though the diets of Pimas now contain about as much fat as that of US whites (Reid *et al.*, 1971). Rates of coronary heart disease in Pima non-diabetics are lower than in US white non-diabetics (Ingelfinger *et al.*, 1976).

In diabetic Oklahoma Indians coronary heart disease has become progressively more common, but rates are still lower in Indian non-diabetics than in white non-diabetics. In Oklahoma Indian diabetics rates of coronary heart disease are now similar to those in diabetics of Europe (Keen and Jarrett, 1979, West, 1979a). These diabetic Indians are very fat; levels of serum cholesterol are modest (averaging about 5·4 mmol/l (210 mg/dl)); control of blood glucose levels tends to be mediocre, and serum triglyceride values are very high. Despite the great fatness of these diabetic Indians, blood pressure levels were about the same as in European diabetics, and stroke is not common (Keen and Jarrett, 1979). Peripheral vascular disease is common. They do not smoke as much as US whites.

Oklahoma Indians have about three times as much coronary heart disease as Pimas. Pimas now consume almost as much fat, but 20 years ago the Pima diet was very much lower in fat than that of Oklahoma Indians.

Diabetes and obesity

Prior to 1940 diabetes was probably uncommon in all American Indian tribes (West, 1974). Rates of diabetes are now markedly excessive in most US tribes. Typically, prevalence is about three times as great as in US whites. The prevalence in older Pima Indians is from 35 to 50 per cent depending on the diagnostic criteria employed. Similarly high rates prevail in each of the 20 largest Oklahoma Indian tribes. In recent years approximately half of deceased Oklahoma Indians have had clinically diagnosed diabetes.

In contrast, rates of juvenile-onset diabetes are peculiarly low in US Indians. In Oklahoma, where there are about 125 000 Indians and 50 000 Indian children, we have identified only two cases of diabetes with onset in the first decade of life, despite the huge number of diabetics. At present there are 8000 Indians in Oklahoma who are known to have diabetes. This paucity of juvenile-onset cases might be related to the differences between whites and Indians in the frequency of certain HLA histocompatibility antigens or geographically proximal genes. These Indians migrated from north-east Asia many centuries ago. Juvenile-onset diabetes is rare in some other Asian populations (e.g. in Japan), in which the frequencies of certain histocompatibility antigens differ from those in Europeans or white Americans. About 20 per cent of the diabetic Oklahoma Indians took insulin, but these insulin-takers were almost as fat at onset of diabetes as those who were not taking insulin. In Oklahoma the elderly Indians were never as fat as the present generation of middle-aged adults, and incidence rates of diabetes were considerably higher between ages 40 and 59 than in older people. This is also true in Pima Indians (Hamman *et al.*, 1978).

Bennett *et al.* (1976) published a review of the excellent studies of diabetes in the Pima. In some respects these are the best epidemiological data available on diabetes in any race or population. Other publications have provided detailed information on diabetes in more than 100 different populations of the New World and Pacific regions, including Indians, Eskimo, Micronesians and Polynesians (West, 1974; 1978a; 1978b).

In Oklahoma and in other US Indian tribes about 58 per cent of the diabetics are female. In Oklahoma this excess is apparently attributable to the greater fatness of women. Men are very fat, women are even fatter. In the Oklahoma Indian diabetics weight at onset of diabetes is typically about 165 per cent of standard. Typically, their lifetime maximum weight has been 185 per cent of standard. In a group of 557 diabetic Oklahoma Indians we found that 18 per cent were not fat (less than 115 per cent of ideal weight), but only 1 per cent had never been fat. In this population there was no relationship of level of dietary sugar intake to fatness, risk of diabetes, level of insulin secretion or plasma triglyceride (West *et al.*, 1978). The anatomical distribution of fat is peculiarly central, with relatively modest amounts of fat on the arms and legs and large amounts on the trunk.

In our experience the hyperinsulinaemia has been explained by the degree of fatness, but in other Indian tribes in other circumstances, levels of insulin secretion seem not to be entirely explained by the degree of adiposity (West, 1978a). Lean Oklahoma Indians have excellent glucose tolerance (West, 1979a).

The Indians now living in Oklahoma had very diverse geographic origins in widely separated parts of North America. Before the twentieth century their diets differed greatly. Some were nomadic hunters of the semi-arid Great Plains, some were much less primitive with highly developed agriculture, newspapers, etc. Despite these previous environmental, cultural, and genetic differences, rates of obesity and diabetes are now very similar in all these Oklahoma tribes. Their diets are now similar. These diets do not differ greatly from those of local whites but they are now somewhat higher in fat and much higher in calories than the diets of local whites. Fibre content has not been measured, but it does not appear to be much different from that of the local white population. Sugar consumption is highly variable among individual Indians of Oklahoma, but average consumption is similar to that in whites (West *et al.*, 1978).

In Pimas there is considerable family aggregation of diabetes and some of this appears to be independent of fatness. It seems likely, however, that obesity is, by far, the main cause of the epidemic of diabetes in North American Indians. Diabetes is still uncommon in tribes that are not yet fat (West, 1978a). The reasons for the extraordinary fatness are incompletely understood. It is very interesting, however, that poor black US women are almost as fat and rates of diabetes are very excessive in these black women. The incidence of diabetes is also quite high in US white women who are poor (West, 1978a). They are also much fatter than US white women who are not poor. Our preliminary studies show that Oklahoma Indians prefer to weigh considerably more than the amounts considered to be ideal by whites. Pimas are quite fat despite a consumption of generous amounts of dietary fibre. As indicated above, intestinal transit time is brief and rates of colon disease low in Pimas.

Levels of exercise are not known precisely in any tribe. In general exercise is far less than 100 years ago, but it is not known how present levels of physical activity compare with those in American whites. Obesity was rare in US Indians before the twentieth century (West, 1974). Obesity had become fairly common in some tribes in the 1920s but long-duration obesity was not common until the 1950s at the time the epidemics of diabetes began.

The epidemic of diabetes and obesity in these western hemisphere Indians includes Mexicans and Americans of Mexican descent. Rates of diabetes are highly variable by social circumstance in Mexico but age-adjusted diabetes mortality rates are higher in Mexico than in the United States (West, 1978a). In Mexican-Americans of south Texas diabetes is rife (Stern and Gaskill, 1978).

Gallbladder disease

In many US tribes rates of cholelithiasis and biliary cancer are quite excessive. These rates are, however, highly variable by tribe. Intertribal differences in rates of cholelithiasis appear to be closely related to levels of adiposity (Niswander, 1968). But in the Pimas of Arizona it was not possible to demonstrate a relationship of gallbladder disease to degree of fatness, probably because the number of lean Pimas was very small (Sampliner *et al.*, 1970). In Micmac Indians of Nova Scotia risk of gallbladder disease was related to degree of fatness (Williams *et al.*, 1977). Gallbladder disease was already common in Pimas at a time when a large portion of their calories were derived from beans containing generous amounts of fibre (Hesse, 1959). Rates of cholelithiasis in fat US tribes appear to be about five times those of the general US population.

Probably the very excessive incidence of gallstones is not entirely attributable to obesity of these Indians. Grundy *et al.* (1972) have reported peculiarities of cholesterol metabolism. Serum cholesterol levels are low, levels of biliary cholesterol high. Most US tribes now consume diets that are very high in calories, and often high in fat and saturated fat. The extent to which qualitative features of diet influence risk of gallbladder disease in the various Indian groups is not known. Gallbladder disease was quite common in Pimas 20 years ago at a time when only about one-fourth of their calories was derived from fat. Fat consumption is now considerably higher. Sugar consumption is still low by US standards (Reid *et al.*, 1971).

Cancer

Rates of biliary cancer are excessive in US Indians by a factor of about three (Creagan and Fraumeni, 1972). It is not yet clear whether this excess is entirely attributable to the high rates of cholelithiasis.

Despite the low rates of peptic ulcer, the incidence of stomach cancer does not seem to be excessive in the US Indian population (Creagan and Fraumeni, 1972). It appears, however, that there may be some intertribal differences in rates of gastric cancer (Sievers, 1972).

Cancer of the colon seems to be about half as frequent in US Indians as in US whites (Creagan and Fraumeni, 1972; Sievers, 1976). In south-western Indians Goldman *et al.* (1972) found radiographically that intestinal transit time was considerably more rapid than in whites. These latter Indians also had particularly low rates of appendicitis and diverticulosis. Probably fibre consumption is higher in these tribes than in whites. The diet of the Pimas, for example, contains a generous mount of beans, and the popular local tortillas are probably higher in fibre than the white bread typically consumed by American whites.

Rates of cancer of the prostate and breast are also much lower in US Indians than in whites (Creagan and Fraumeni, 1972). Liver cancer is particularly common in US Indians. This is probably the result of high rates of alcoholism and liver cirrhosis. The incidence of cancer of the lung is low in US Indians. In general, cigarette consumption is lower in Indians than in whites.

Other diseases

Gout

In contrast to the Polynesians in whom obesity is attended by high rates of gout, gout is not common in fat Oklahoma Indians. Clinical gout is also uncommon in the fat Pimas (O'Brien *et al.*, 1966).

Peptic ulcer

Peptic ulcer is quite rare in US Indians. Sievers (1974) has estimated that duodenal ulcer is 73 times as frequent in local whites as in Indians of the south-west United States. Gastric ulcer was about one-ninth as frequent in south-western Indians. In these same Indians some of the other 'occidental' diseases are common (e.g., gallstones, diabetes, obesity). The mechanisms for this happy immunity are not known, but Indians probably have lower levels of gastric acid secretion (Sievers, 1966).

Lactase deficiency is more common in American Indians than in whites.

Ear wax that is particularly dry is present in a very high proportion of American Indians (Petrakis, 1969). This kind of cerumen is the type that is found in a high proportion of Asians (e.g., in Japanese). *Otitis media* is particularly common in American Indians.

References

Bennett, P. H., Rushforth, N. B., Miller, M. and LeCompte, P. M. (1976). Epidemiologic studies in diabetes in the Pima Indians. *Recent Progress of Hormone Research*, **32**, 333–337

Conner, W. E., Cerqueira, M. T., Connor, R. W., Wallace, R. B., Malinow, M. R. and Casdorph, H. R. (1978). The plasma lipids, lipoproteins, and diet of the Tarahumara Indians of Mexico. *The American Journal of Clinical Nutrition*, **31**, 1131–1142

Creagan, E. T. and Fraumeni, J. F. (1972). Cancer mortality among American Indians. *Journal of National Cancer Institute*, **49**, 959–967

Goldman, S. M., Sievers, M. L., Carlile, W. K. and Cohen, S. L. (1972). Roentgen manifestations of diseases in Southwestern Indians. *Radiology*, **103**, 303–306

Grundy, S. M., Metzger, A. L. and Adler, R. D. (1972). Mechanisms of lithogenic bile formation in American Indian women with cholesterol gallstones. *Journal of Clinical Investigation*, **51**, 164–168

Hamman, R. F., Bennett, P. H. and Miller, M. (1975). The effect of menopause on serum cholesterol in American (Pima) Indian women. *American Journal of Epidemiology*, **102**, 164–169

Hamman, R. F., Bennett, P. H. and Miller, M. (1978). Incidence of diabetes among the Pima Indians. In: *Advances in Metabolic Disorders*, **9**, 49–63. Editors R. Levine and R. Luft. Academic Press, London

Hesse, R. G. (1959). Incidence of cholecystitis and other diseases among Pima Indians of Southern Arizona. *Journal of American Medical Association*, **170**, 1789–1790

Ingelfinger, J. A., Bennett, M. B., Kiebow, I. M. and Miller, M. (1976). Coronary heart disease in the Pima Indians: Electrocardiographic findings and postmortem evidence of myocardial infarctions in a population with a high prevalence of diabetes mellitus. *Diabetes*, **25**, 561–565

Keen, H. and Jarrett, R. J. (1979). *The Complications of Diabetes*, second edition. Edward Arnold, London

Neel, J. V. and Salzano, F. M. (1964). A prospectus for genetic studies of the American Indian. *Cold Spring Harbor Symposia on Quantitative Biology*, **29**, 85–98

Niswander, J. D. (1968). Discussion on Diabetes. In: *Biomedical Challenges presented by the American Indian.* WHO, Pan American Health Organization, Publ. **165,** 133–139

O'Brien, W. M., Burch, T. A. and Bunim, J. J. (1966). Genetics of hyperuricaemia in Blackfeet and Pima Indians. *Annals of the Rheumatic Diseases,* **25,** 117–119

Petrakis, N. L. (1969). Dry cerumen—a prevalent genetic trait among American Indians. *Nature,* **222,** 1080–1081

Reid, J., Fullmer, S. D., Pettigrew, K. D., Burch, T. A., Bennett, P. H., Miller, M. and Wheedon, G. D. (1971). Nutrient intake of Pima Indian women: Relationships to diabetes mellitus and gallbladder disease. *American Journal of Clinical Nutrition,* **24,** 1281–1289

Sampliner, R. E., Bennett, P. H., Commess, L. J., Rose, F. A. and Burch, T. A. (1970). Gallbladder disease in Pima Indians. Demonstration of high prevalence and early onset by cholecystography. *New England Journal of Medicine,* **283,** 1358–1364

Sievers, M. L. (1966). A study of achlorhydria among Southwestern American Indians. *American Journal of Gastroenterology,* **45,** 99–103

Sievers, M. L. (1967). Myocardial infarction among Southwestern American Indians. *Annals of Internal Medicine,* **67,** 800–807

Sievers, M. L. (1972). Cancer mortality in Indians. *Journal of the American Medical Association,* **222,** 705

Sievers, M. L. (1974). Disease patterns of Pima Indians of the Gila River Indian Reservation of Arizona in relation to the geochemical environment. In: *Trace Substances in Environmental Health—VII. A symposium,* 57. Editor D. D. Hemphill. University of Missouri, Columbia

Sievers, M. L. (1976). Cancer of the digestive system among American Indians. *Arizona Medicine,* **33,** 15–20

Stern, M. P. and Gaskill, S. P. (1978). Secular trends in ischemic heart disease and strokè mortality from 1970 to 1976 in Spanish-surnamed and other white individuals in Bexar County, Texas. *Circulation,* **58,** 537–543

West, K. M. (1974). Diabetes in American Indians and other native populations of the new world. *Diabetes,* **23,** 841–855

West, K. M. (1978a). *Epidemiology of Diabetes and its Vascular Lesions.* Elsevier, New York

West, K. M. (1978b). Diabetes in American Indians. In: *Advances in Metabolic Disorders,* **9,** 29–48. Editors M. Miller and P. H. Bennett. Academic Press, New York

West, K. M. (1979b). Introduction. Proceedings of the Kroc Foundation International Conference on Epidemiology of Diabetes and its Macrovascular Complications. *Diabetes Care,* **2,** 63–64

West, K. M. and Kalbfleisch, J. M. (1970). Diabetes in Central America. *Diabetes,* **19,** 656–663

West, K. M., Oakley, E., Sanders, M. E. and Rubenstein, A. (1978). Nutritional factors in the etiology of diabetes and its complications. In: *Epidemiology of Diabetes Mellitus and its Vascular Complications,*

27–32. Editors H. Keen, J. D. Pickup and O. V. Talwalker. World Health Organization and International Diabetes Federation, London

Williams, C. N., Johnston, J. L. and Weldon, K. L. M. (1977). Prevalence of gallstones and gallbladder disease in Canadian Micmac Indian women. *Canadian Medical Association Journal,* **117,** 758–760

10

Amerindians of Brazil

Roberto Baruzzi and Laercio Franco

Introduction

Since the beginning of the sixteenth century, following the Portuguese discovery of Brazil, it was noted that the indigenous population was composed of heterogeneous groups that have not only differences in language, customs and habits but in some physical aspects. As time went on a new element of diversity was introduced, depending on the extent of contact with the new occupants of the territory. The major concentration of Indians are in the Amazonic region, the most sparsely populated part of Brazil, covering 60 per cent of Brazilian territory and having only 9 per cent of the country's population. The Indian population is estimated to be between 70 and 100 thousand, divided into 143 tribal groups (Melatti, 1970). Depending on the degree of contact with the Brazilian society the Indians can be roughly divided into four groups.

1. Groups of Indians in a state of relative *isolation* inhabit areas as yet untouched by the process of expansion of the Brazilian society; they may have had rare contact.
2. Other tribes are in *intermittent contact* with the civilized but this is almost exclusively restricted to personnel of FUNAI (Fundação Nacional do Indio), a federal government agency, or missionaries.
3. Those in *permanent contact* are tribal groups which are in direct and constant communication with numerous and diverse civilized groups; they have thus suffered modifications in their social structure and have become dependent upon many products of civilization.
4. *Semi-integrated or integrated groups* live in almost the same manner as the back-woodsmen that surround them, but yet continue to consider themselves as Indians (Ribeiro, 1957).

The best opportunity to study the emergence of Western diseases is given by those in intermittent contact. These are estimated to represent 30–40 per cent of the indigenous population. An Indian population representative of those in intermittent contact is found in the Parque Nacional do Xingu (PNX) in Central Brazil.

138

Parque Nacional do Xingu

The Parque Nacional do Xingu (PNX) is situated in the north of the State of Mato Grosso, Central Brazil. Its area is approximately 22 000 km^2, extending along the Xingu River. To the south lie the final stretches of 'cerrado', the immense scrubland of the central plateau; the remainder is jungle of the Amazon type with its exuberance and colouring. The existence of rapids along the course of the River Xingu, the presence of hostile tribes and the great distance to be crossed to reach this region, permitted the Indian groups to remain almost isolated until the 1950s. The PNX was created by the Brazilian government in 1961, when the existence of the tribes in the region was threatened because of land speculation.

The Indian tribes inhabiting the PNX, their linguistic groups and the number of individuals in each tribe is shown in Table 10.1.

The Indians of Upper Xingu have inhabited the area of the headwaters of the Xingu River for a long time. They were first described by Steinen (1894), who crossed that region in 1884 and 1887. The tribes of the Upper Xingu

Table 10.1 Indian tribes of the Parque Nacional do Xingu, 1979

Tribe	Linguistic family	Population
Upper Xingu		
1. Aweti	Tupi	39
2. Kamayura	Tupi	168
3. Yawalapiti	Arawak	103
4. Meinaku	Arawak	77
5. Waura	Arawak	106
6. Kalapalo	Carib	166
7. Kuikuro	Carib	169
8–9. Matipu and Nafuqua	Carib	56
10. Trumai	Isolated language	24
	Subtotal	908
Jê		
11–12. Suya and Beiços de Pau	Jê	145
13. Txukahamaye	Jê	245
14. Kren-Akarore	Jê	75
	Subtotal	465
Kayabi		
15. Various groups along the Xingu River	Tupi	330
Other groups		
16. Juruna	Isolated language	75
17. Txikào	Isolated language	102
	Total	1880

have become very similar in their customs and way of life, but each tribe has preserved its own language, which is one element of differentiation. The diet of the Indians of Upper Xingu is principally based on manioc (cassava) and fish. It includes, but to a lesser extent, corn (maize), sweet potatoes, cara, peanuts, bananas, pineapples, water-melons and also piqui—a very much appreciated fruit with a fatty pulp. They do not like game animals, but occasionally eat monkeys and, among birds, mutums (curassows) and jacus.

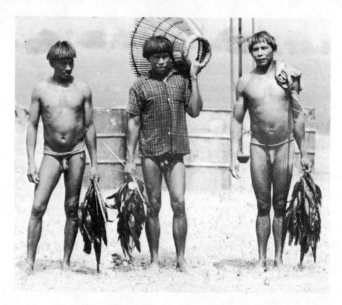

Fig. 10.1   Upper Xingu Indians, well nourished and with plenty of fish

The Indians belong to the Jê group inhabit the area north of the PNX. The presence of the Suya in this area was reported by Steinen (1894) and the Beiços de Pau (Wooden Muzzles) joined them in 1970, as they were transferred to the Park when their land was being invaded by 'civilized' groups. Both tribes have maintained some characteristics as hunter-gatherers but also cultivate some crops. The Txukahamaye, pacified in 1963, were essentially hunter-gatherers and lived in the area further north of the PNX. Now they have more fixed settlements, larger plantations of corn, manioc, sweet potatoes and bananas. The last group to enter the Park was the Kren-Akarore, in 1975, two years after first being contacted by the Villas-Boas brothers. The breaking of their state of isolation was so abrupt that it caused severe harm to them and resulted in a drastic reduction of their number. Their removal to the PNX was the alternative found to assure the survival of the tribe (Baruzzi *et al.*, 1977).

The Kayabi have entered the PNX in various groups since 1953; they originated from the region of the Rivers Teles Pires and Arinos, about

400 km to the west. They had been contacted in that region in 1926 and later were in conflict with 'civilized' groups. In the PNX they are distributed in various family groups along the course of the Middle Xingu River. Their agriculture is well developed in comparison with the other tribes in the Park and they are good hunters and fishermen.

The Juruna and Txikão are very different groups from the rest of the tribes, not only because of their separate languages but also in their physical characteristics, habits and customs. There are very frequent intratribal marriages among the Juruna, and when an Indian dies, his brother is obliged to wed the widow, even though he may already be married (Villas-Boas and Villas-Boas, 1968). They are the only Indians in the Park to make an alcoholic beverage, the caxiri, prepared through the fermentation of corn, manioc and wild fruits. The Txikão, who entered the PNX in 1967, are shorter and less robust than the rest.

Since 1965, the Escola Paulista de Medicina (one of São Paulo's medical schools) has been developing a programme of preventive medicine in the PNX which includes the determination of health conditions of the population, immunization, local medical care and removal to São Paulo of the Indians needing hospitalization. This medical programme has given us the opportunity to accumulate more experience with respect to the Indians living inside the PNX.

The Indian population of the PNX has increased in the last two decades, not only because of the entrance of new tribes, but also by the natural growth of the population. Available data regarding the Upper Xingu population growth show that in 1963 there were 623 Indians (Galvão and Simões, 1966); in 1970 the number had increased to 704 (Baruzzi and Iunes, 1970) and there were 908 Indians in 1979. These numbers show a tendency to a moderate increase in the Upper Xingu population when compared to the considerable reduction from the estimate of 3000 Indians at the end of the last century (Steinen, 1894).

A brief reference to the infectious diseases is important, since they have been until now the main causes of morbidity and mortality in the PNX.

Infectious disease

These days, among the diseases which attack the population of the PNX, malaria and respiratory infections should receive special mention. A survey made in the Upper Xingu showed the presence of *Plasmodium* in the peripheral blood in 14·3 per cent and serological antibodies against plasmodia in 98·7 per cent of the people examined. In the young children acute attacks by falciparum malaria are more severe, producing a higher mortality than in adults.

A high prevalence of gross splenomegaly was observed in 33 per cent of 730 Indians examined and diagnosed as tropical splenomegaly syndrome (TSS). During the period 1968–73, among the 22 adult deaths, 7 were due to episodes of haematemesis and melaena, probably by rupture of gastro-oesophageal varices, a complication of TSS (Baruzzi *et al.*, 1976).

Respiratory infections are quite frequent in the Indian population of PNX. These infections are sometimes considered to be influenza, but sometimes they result in more severe illness. Mortality caused by respiratory infections is relatively high in the population of the PNX.

In 1954 an epidemic of measles broke out in the Upper Xingu and affected almost the whole population of that area, estimated at 600 Indians; it caused 114 deaths among adults and children. At the beginning of 1979, there was an outbreak of measles among the Kayabi and Jê groups; 128 cases and three deaths were reported. Many of those affected had not been vaccinated, either because they were absent during the various vaccination campaigns, or because it had not been possible to reach the places where they lived. The medical assistance given to the patients during the epidemic was of major importance in reducing the measles fatality rate.

In 1968 the first cases of tuberculosis among the Indians in the Park were reported (Nutels, 1968), but its occurrence did not assume the character of an epidemic, as might have been expected. According to the same author, the cases observed in Suya and Txukahamaye Indians showed a clinical picture similar to that which occurs in civilized groups. Up to now, tuberculosis has not become a grave problem in the PNX, mainly owing to preventive measures based on BCG inoculation, and early diagnosis and treatment of cases.

Intestinal infections are not an important cause of mortality in infancy because of prolonged breast-feeding and the good nutritional state of the infant population. Intestinal parasites are common, especially in children, among whom *Ancylostoma* 67 per cent and *Ascaris* 15 per cent have been reported (Dias and Ribeiro, 1977).

Western diseases

Hypertension

For the study of blood pressure the Indians of the PNX were divided into three groups; each group includes tribes having similarity of habits, customs and dietary pattern. The first group contains the 10 tribes of the Upper Xingu, the second the Indians of the Jê group (Suya, Beiços de Pau, Txuka-hamaye and Kren-Akarore), and the third the Kayabi Indians. The Juruna and Txikão tribes were not included because of their small number and diversity in physical and cultural aspects in relation to the Indian groups mentioned above.

The blood pressure levels were determined during the general medical examination of the population made in the period 1966–71, when we tried to establish the medical priorities for the preventive programme to be followed. The Kren-Akarore were examined at the beginning of 1975 when they entered the PNX. The study of the blood pressure was made in 282 males and 245 females of 15 years of age and over.

Levels of systolic pressure $\geqslant 140$ mmHg were found in 14 males (4·9 per cent), and among them only 4 reached 150 mmHg. There were no cases of systolic pressure $\geqslant 140$ mmHg among the females. Diastolic pressure levels

Table 10.2 Blood pressure levels (mmHg) in Upper Xingu, Jê and Kayabi Indians, 1966–71

Age group[1] (years)	Males			Females		
	No.	Systolic Mean ± s.d.	Diastolic mean ± s.d.	No.	Systolic mean ± s.d.	Diastolic mean ± s.d.
Upper Xingu						
15–19	27	109·6 14·6	68·0 10·4	27	102·0 10·7	60·4 8·7
20–29	58	96·9 34·9	69·4 9·6	45	100·0 10·8	64·8 8·2
30–39	40	101·2 30·9	70·0 8·1	37	103·4 10·4	60·2 16·5
40–49	20	104·7 28·3	65·5 12·7	15	97·3 30·3	66·0 9·9
≥50	7	108·6 12·1	70·7 9·3	8	106·2 16·6	60·0 12·0
Jê						
15–19	17	117·4 14·6	69·7 9·8	12	108·7 10·5	66·2 6·4
20–29	25	117·2 11·3	73·4 10·4	32	109·4 10·1	69·4 9·0
30–39	9	111·1 8·2	69·4 7·7	14	105·0 10·7	66·4 7·7
40–49	8	108·7 14·6	65·7 7·3	8	110·0 10·7	68·7 6·4
≥50	3	120·0 10·0	76·7 5·8	2	110·0 —	70·0 —
Kayabi						
15–19	6	108·3 20·4	63·3 13·7	11	108·6 7·8	70·9 7·0
20–29	29	115·7 13·2	73·8 10·1	13	108·5 9·9	68·5 6·9
30–39	11	102·7 32·0	75·0 7·4	14	113·6 9·3	73·6 8·4
40–49	10	105·1 34·1	75·0 8·5	7	118·6 12·1	78·6 14·6
≥50	12	116·7 20·1	76·7 11·5	0	—	—

[1] Estimated age

≥90 mmHg were observed in 17 Indians, 13 males (4·6 per cent) and 4 females (1·6 per cent); in only one case the diastolic pressure reached 100 mmHg. When the systolic and diastolic blood pressure were considered together, levels ≥ 140/90 mmHg were observed only in 8 Indians, i.e. in 1·5 per cent of the total number of Indians examined, males and females (Table 10.2). In the statistical analysis of the data, the 50 years and over age group were not included, as they were few.

Age and sex
Significant differences were not observed between the mean values of the systolic and diastolic blood pressure levels of the age groups in any of the indigenous groups, either in males or females.

The mean values of the systolic and diastolic blood pressure levels were significantly higher in males than in females in the following age groups: 15–19, 20–29 and 30–39 years in each indigenous group ($P < 0·05$). In the 40–49 age group no significant differences between sexes were observed.

Various Indian groups
Comparing the Jê and Kayabi groups no significant differences were observed in the mean values of systolic and diastolic blood pressure levels within each age group in either males or females. When the Jê group was compared with the Upper Xingu, significant difference was found only in systolic blood pressure, being higher in Jê females aged 20–29 years. Between Kayabi and Upper Xingu the mean systolic blood pressure levels were significantly higher in the Kayabi group, for males in the 20–29 and for females in the 30–39 years age groups. Mean diastolic blood pressures were significantly higher in the Kayabi group only in females in the 15–19 and 30–39 age groups.

Salt intake
The PNX Indians do not use salt (sodium chloride) in their food; they do prepare a type of 'salt' obtained from plants, but use it only sporadically. This 'salt' is rich in potassium, the composition of a sample analysed was 74 g/100 g potassium chloride and 0·2 g/100 g sodium chloride. The urinary 24-hour sodium excretion was measured in 7 Indians and the levels varied from 1·8 to 16·8 mmol/l, with urinary volumes between 400 and 1800 ml. The low urinary excretion is indicative of the low intake of sodium.

Obesity

Most of the Indians included in the hypertension study had their weight and height measured at the same medical examination. There were available data for 392 Indians aged 20 years and over, 212 males and 180 females, belonging to the Upper Xingu, Jê and Kayabi groups. The means and standard deviations of the weight and height, and the percentages to 'desirable' weight standard, for the age groups 20–29, 30–39 and 40 or more years, are presented in Table 10.3 for males and Table 10.4 for females. The reference standard used was the ICNND Table (1963), which established for each height a

Table 10.3 Upper Xingu, Jê and Kayabi Indian male height, weight and percentage of 'desirable weight',[1] 1966–71

Age group (years)	No.	Height (cm) mean ± s.d.	Weight (kg) mean ± s.d.	Percentage of 'desirable weight'			
				<90	90–99	100–109	≥110
Upper Xingu							
20–29	56	161·6 6·2	62·9 5·2	1·8	30·3	51·8	16·1
30–39	44	160·8 5·3	62·6 7·9	6·8	31·8	38·6	22·7
≥40	26	160·1 5·2	63·8 7·7	15·3	15·3	38·7	30·7
Jê							
20–29	20	164·1 3·7	62·3 6·9	20·0	30·0	40·0	10·0
30–39	8	164·5 7·9	65·6 10·2	12·5	37·5	25·0	25·0
≥40	9	168·5 5·9	67·8 4·8	0·0	11·1	77·8	11·1
Kayabi							
20–29	20	155·5 4·6	55·8 5·9	20·0	45·0	30·0	5·0
30–39	10	155·3 3·3	56·3 4·5	10·0	70·0	10·0	10·0
≥40	19	158·0 4·3	54·3 5·0	52·6	21·0	26·3	0·0

[1] Jelliffe (1966)

Table 10.4   Upper Xingu, Jê and Kayabi Indian female height, weight and percentage of 'desirable weight',[1] 1966–71

Age group (years)	No.	Height (cm) mean ± s.d.		Weight (kg) mean ± s.d.		Percentage of 'desirable weight'			
		mean	± s.d.	mean	± s.d.	<90	90–99	100–109	≥110
Upper Xingu									
20–29	44	149·5	5·2	49·8	5·2	9·1	45·5	31·8	13·6
30–39	37	149·4	7·9	49·2	5·7	21·6	37·8	35·1	5·4
≥40	23	149·3	4·7	49·6	5·0	13·0	34·8	39·1	13·0
Jê									
20–29	23	152·7	8·5	55·7	7·6	0·0	26·1	47·8	26·1
30–39	14	155·1	7·2	57·5	6·3	14·3	7·1	35·7	42·9
≥40	9	152·4	5·6	53·5	4·7	0·0	44·4	44·4	11·1
Kayabi									
20–29	10	143·6	3·5	46·2	5·0	30·0	30·0	40·0	0·0
30–39	13	144·2	4·5	46·5	7·5	23·1	46·1	15·4	15·4
≥40	7	145·5	3·8	52·1	8·5	14·3	0·0	28·6	57·1

[1] Jelliffe (1966)

'desirable' weight standard considered as 100 per cent (Jelliffe, 1966). From this table individuals having percentages between 90 and 109 can be accepted as *normal*, from 110 to 119 as *overweight*, and 120 or more as *obese*.

In PNX males percentages of weight for height between 110 and 119 were found in 16·0 per cent, and equal to or above 120 on 0·9 per cent. In females the percentages were 16·7 and 5·0 respectively.

Comparing the Upper Xingu, Jê and Kayabi groups, significant differences were observed in the proportion of individuals with percentages of weight for height ⩾ 110. In the Upper Xingu and Jê groups, males had rates of percentages ⩾ 110 significantly higher than the Kayabi, while between the Upper Xingu and Jê no significant difference was found. Females of the Jê and Kayabi groups had significantly higher rates than those of the Upper Xingu, but there was no significant difference between Jê and Kayabi in this sex.

Skinfold and arm circumference measurements were made in 106 Indians from the Upper Xingu (Table 10.5).

Table 10.5 Anthropometric measurements of adult Indians of the Upper Xingu, 1979

Anthropometric data	Males (No. 59) mean ± s.d.		Females (No. 47) mean ± s.d.	
Skinfold:				
triceps (mm)	7·9	2·2	13·6	3·6
biceps (mm)	4·9	1·3	6·0	1·9
subscapular (mm)	10·4	2·5	13·0	4·7
suprailiac (mm)	7·3	3·1	11·3	3·3
Arm circumference (cm)	31·2	1·8	27·4	1·7
Arm-muscle circumference (cm)	28·8	1·6	23·1	1·4

Table 10.6 Arm-muscle circumference of adult Indians of the Upper Xingu, 1979

Sex	Percentage of normality					No.
	<90	90–99	100–109	110–119	⩾120	
Male	0	0	15	32	12	59
Female	1	24	19	2	1	47

From Jelliffe (1966)

The results of the arm-muscle circumference are presented in percentages of normality (Table 10.6), considering 25·3 cm for males and 23·2 cm for females as 100 per cent of normality (Jelliffe, 1966).

In males the skinfold thickness and the percentages of normality for the arm-muscle circumference give strong evidence that they have low subcutaneous fat and well developed musculature. Thus the values of 110 per cent or more, found in the weight for height (Table 10.3), should not be considered as representative of overweight or obesity, but as resulting from their athletic condition.

The children in the Upper Xingu are well nourished; this is being shown in a longitudinal study in progress among them. When they reach puberty, boys and girls remain in seclusion inside the hut for prolonged periods, which can amount to one or two years for males. During the periods of seclusion they are confined to a small and dimly lit place in the interior of the hut, receiving a lot of food and being introduced to the handicrafts and oral traditions of the tribe. At the end of this period, when the adolescent comes back to the community life, his physical and muscular condition are remarkably improved. He then starts to participate in corporal fights, which are very important in the Upper Xingu culture and give considerable prestige to the winners. The ritual of seclusion is a cultural characteristic trait of the Upper Xingu and it is not observed among the Jê and Kayabi groups. But all the Indians of the PNX get plenty of physical exercise in hunting, gathering, fishing, canoeing, walking long distances, and ceremonial dancing for hours.

The Indian woman does hard physical work. She prepares food, fetches water from the river and helps in the harvest. When coming back from field work, it is the woman who carries the product of the day, while the man, with his bow and arrows, must be ready to face the dangers of the forest.

Diabetes mellitus

During the 14 years of participation in medical activities in the PNX, symptoms suggestive of diabetes were not observed in the indigenous population. Among those Indians brought to São Paulo for hospitalization, the blood glucose levels were always in the range of normality.

In January 1979, a survey based on the glucose tolerance test was made on 106 Upper Xingu Indians, adults of both sexes. The Indians were submitted to a standard load of 100 g carbohydrate equivalent (Dexpak—Ames Company). Due to difficulties in assuring the fasting stage of the Indians, and for convenience in the field work, venous blood samples were taken one hour after the carbohydrate load. The plasma glucose was determined on the Auto-Analyzer using the modified Hoffman method: the results are shown in Table 10.7.

Diabetes was not shown in this investigation in the Upper Xingu, considering 10·83 mmol/l (195 mg/dl) as the critical point for normality to the plasma glucose levels one hour after 100 g of carbohydrate load, according to the United States Public Health Service (O'Sullivan and Mahan, 1968). The mean and standard deviation of the plasma glucose was 5·21 ±

1·12 mmol/l (93·7 ± 20·1 mg/dl) for males, and 5·31 ± 1·79 mmol/l (95·6 ± 32·3 mg/dl) for females.

Table 10.7 Plasma glucose levels one hour after oral carbohydrate 100 g of Indians of the Upper Xingu, 1979

Age group (years)	Plasma glucose levels (mmol/l)				
	2·22–4·43	4·44–6·66	6·67–8·88	8·89–10·56	No.
Males					
20–29	11	14	1	0	26
30–39	4	4	1	0	9
40–49	0	12	0	0	12
⩾50	2	7	3	0	12
Subtotal	17	37	5	0	59
Females					
20–29	8	10	0	0	18
30–39	5	4	1	1	11
40–49	3	2	3	1	9
⩾50	1	7	1	0	9
Subtotal	17	23	5	2	47
Total	34	60	10	2	106

Conversion: SI to traditional units—blood glucose: 1 mmol/l ≃ 18 mg/dl

Hyperlipidaemia

In the 106 Indians from the Upper Xingu, already mentioned, the serum cholesterol levels were determined by the Huang modified method, in which the normal values range from 3·88 to 6·47 mmol/l (150 to 250 mg/dl).

The mean and standard deviation of the serum cholesterol levels were 3·99 ± 0·62 mmol/l (154 ± 24 mg/dl) for males, and 4·40 ± 0·67 mmol/l (170 ± 26 mg/dl) for females.

The serum triglyceride determination was made in the 106 blood samples. The mean and standard deviation were 1·03 ± 0·41 mmol/l (91·4 ± 36·4 mg/dl) for males and 1·04 ± 0·42 mmol/l (92·1 ± 37·4 mg/dl) for females. According to the method employed, the normal values are below 1·97 mmol/l (175 mg/dl) (Bucolo and David, 1973).

Cardiovascular disease

Until now the presence of symptoms or signs suggestive of cardiomegaly, arrhythmia or congestive heart failure has not been observed at the general medical examination of the indigenous population, nor during the medical care delivered periodically since 1965 by medical teams.

Ischaemic heart disease
Complaints suggestive of angina have not been reported, nor has the occurrence of myocardial infarction been detected among the Upper Xingu, Jê and Kayabi Indians. Electrocardiographic evidence of cardiac hypertrophy, conduction disturbance and ischaemic heart disease was not found by Pazzanese *et al.* (1964).

Stroke
The occurrence of stroke was not observed and we did not find people with its sequelae, but it should be noted that there are very few Indians in the age group in which the risk of stroke is greater.

Peripheral vascular disease
Circulatory failure manifested by intermittent claudication or gangrene has not been observed in Indians from the PNX. There is a remarkable absence of varicose veins, although some tribes have the habit of tying cotton thread tightly around the upper parts of their arms and round their legs just below the knee, to show up the muscles. Varicocele, a relatively frequent finding in 'civilized' people, has not been observed among the Indians.

Gastrointestinal disorders

Complaints related to the digestive tract are uncommon among the Indians of the PNX, apart from episodes of diarrhoea which are sometimes related to the ingestion of some food such as the piqui, largely consumed from August to November. Up to date no cases of gastroduodenal ulcer, hiatus hernia, appendicitis and diverticular disease have been diagnosed. Constipation is a rare complaint, although there is a possibility that the Indians do not seek the health team for this, and use their own medicine. Haemorrhoids have not been reported or observed up to now.

Neoplastic disease

Among the Indians of the PNX, five cases of neoplasia were observed from 1965 to 1979, as follows:

1. squamous cell carcinoma of the penis of a 50-year-old patient;
2. basal cell carcinoma on the face of a 46-year-old woman;
3. carcinoma indifferentiate of the testis of a 4-year-old child;
4. gynaecological cancer with disseminated metastases in two patients, one aged 45 and the other 48 years, both of whom died.

General considerations

Tribes or tribal groups in *intermittent contact* with the Brazilian society can be found in the PNX and several other areas of Brazil. The preventive medical programme which has been carried out in the PNX from 1965 until the current year (1979) has enabled us to be in touch with all the tribes living there and to accumulate a great deal of data about the health conditions of this indigenous population. Thus it has been possible to minimize two problems involving medical research in tribal societies—the small size of the tribes and their sparse distribution in a large territory. As the age of the Indians had to be estimated because of the lack of information, there could be some margin of error, mainly for females over 30 years and for the oldest of both sexes. Three large groups can be recognized in the indigenous population of the PNX: the Upper Xingu, Jê and Kayabi groups. The pattern of Western diseases in these groups was very similar, in spite of some diversity among them.

High blood pressure was very rare among the Indians, and the blood pressure did not rise with age. The assumption that the low levels of blood pressure found in many individuals living in tribal societies in the tropics could be related to the high prevalence of malaria, or more specifically to the presence of tropical splenomegaly syndrome, has often been questioned. This association was not confirmed in the PNX when two groups of Indians, with and without gross splenomegaly, were compared (Baruzzi *et al.*, 1976). To explain the rarity of hypertension in the PNX some factors should be considered as relevant:

1. constant physical activity;
2. preservation of their traditional diet;
3. lower levels of stress.

The findings in the Upper Xingu demonstrate that the males have little subcutaneous fat but well developed musculature. Their athletic condition explains the values equal or above 110 per cent of the 'desirable' weight, found in this group, and this observation can also be extended to the Jê and Kayabi males. Among females, those from the Jê are distinguished by their athletic aspect.

Within the aetiology of hypertension it is more difficult to evaluate the importance of stress, although it has been regarded as a relevant factor to explain the increasing prevalence of high blood pressure in Western society. All the Indians participate in activities relevant to their sex. The power to make decisions is equally divided among the members of the indigenous community, without responsibility falling on a few people. Competition and strife to achieve greater socioeconomic status are not factors which influence the Indians living in the PNX.

The style of life and pattern of nutrition of these Indians also seem to protect them from the occurrence of cardiovascular disease and from some disorders of the digestive tract, which have been considered as Western diseases.

The question now is, how long can the Indians in intermittent contact preserve their present state in the face of the process of acculturation, which tends to accelerate as time goes on?

152   Chapter 10   Roberto Baruzzi and Laercio Franco

Acknowledgements

We thank Miss Yara Julian, Dr. C. Stabile Neto, Dr. L. F. Marcopito, Dr. N. Ferreira-Novo, the senior medical students B. Ciotek and F. A. Leme, and the Laboratorio Fleury for their collaboration in this work. We also acknowledge the help of Mrs. D. Hames in the English translation. The field work has been made possible with the cooperation of the Fundação Nacional do Indio (FUNAI) and the Força Aérea Brasileira (FAB).

References

Baruzzi, R. G., Franco, L. J., Jardim, J. R., Masuda, A., Naspitz, C., Paiva, E. R. and Ferreira-Novo, N. (1976). The association between splenomegaly and malaria in Indians from the Alto Xingu, Brasil Central. *Revista do Instituto de Medicina Tropical de São Paulo*, **18**, 322–348

Baruzzi, R. G. and Iunes, M. (1970). *Survey of the state of health of the native tribes of the Upper Xingu River. Application of medicoprophylactic measures for their conservation.* Parque Nacional do Xingu, Central Brazil. Escola Paulista de Medicina, São Paulo, Brasil

Baruzzi, R. G., Marcopito, L. F., Serra, M. L. C., Souza, F. A. A. and Stabile, C. (1977). The Kren-Akarore: a recently contacted indigenous tribe. In: *Health and Disease in Tribal Societies*, 179–211. Elsevier, Amsterdam, Oxford, New York. Excerpta Medica, North Holland

Bucolo, G. and David, H. (1973). Quantitative determination of serum triglycerides by the use of enzymes. *Clinical Chemistry*, **19**, 476–482

Dias, L. C. S. and Ribeiro, O. B. (1977). Prevalência de parasitas intestinais em Indios do Alto Xingu, Parque Nacional do Xingu, Brasil Central. Presented in the XIX Congresso Brasileiro de Higiene, São Paulo, Brasil

Galvão, E. and Simões, M. F. (1966). Mudança e sobrevivência no Alto Xingu, Brasil Central. *Revista de Antropologia da Universidade de São Paulo*, **14**, 37–52

Jelliffe, D. B. (1966). *The Assessment of the Nutritional Status of the Community*, 271. World Health Organization, Geneva

Melatti, J. C. (1970). *Indios do Brasil*, 208. Brasilia, Coordenadora-Editora de Brasilia, Brasil

Nutels, N. (1968). Medical problems of newly contacted Indian groups. In: *Biomedical Challenges Presented by the American Indians* (Publication No. 165), 68–76. Pan American Health Organization, Washington, DC

O'Sullivan, J. B. and Mahan, C. M. (1968). Prospective study of 352 young patients with chemical diabetes. *New England Journal of Medicine*, **278**, 1038–1041

Pazzanese, D., Ramos, O. L., Lanfranchi, W., Portugal, O. P., Finatti, A. A. C., Barreto, H. P. C. and Sustovich, D. R. (1964). Serum-lipid levels in a Brazilian Indian population. *Lancet*, **ii**, 615–617

Ribeiro, D. (1957). Culturas e linguas indigenas do Brasil. *Educação e Ciências Sociais*, **2**, 1–102. Rio de Janeiro, Brasil

Steinen, K. von den (1894). *Unter den Zentral-Brasiliens,* Berlin. Title of the Portuguese Edition: *Entre os Arborigines do Brasil Central* (1940). Departamento de Cultura, São Paulo

Villas-Boas, O. and Villas-Boas, C. (1968). Os Juruna no Alto Xingu. *Revista Reflexão de Instituto Ciencias Humanas e Letras, Universidade Federal de Goiás, Brasil,* **1,** 61–87

11

Australian Aborigines

Peter M. Moodie

Introduction

The epidemiology of Western diseases in the Australian Aboriginal population has been difficult to study in the absence of long-term and follow-up
studies in specific communities during the period after European contact,
and in the absence of reasonably accurate morbidity, mortality and population data by which secular trends can be detected.

Only the Northern Territory currently publishes comparative (but
hospital-admission-based) morbidity data, and this only since 1973. The
reasons underlying these statistical deficiencies are complex, and have been
reviewed by the writer (Moodie, 1973) to indicate that many of the problems
are virtually insoluble. It must also be pointed out that it is not now acceptable
to regard Aborigines as 'experimental subjects' for studies which do not
promise reasonably immediate benefits to the Aborigines themselves. Future
advances in this field in Australia will depend very much on the availability
of routine morbidity and mortality statistics (as available for Australia as a
whole but with Aborigines identified) supplemented by specifically oriented
surveys into contemporary lifestyle, diet and environment repeated at
appropriate intervals.

Numbers and distribution of Australian Aborigines

When Australia was first colonized from England in 1788, there were probably
about 300 000 Aborigines (Mulvaney, 1975) at an average density of one
person per 26 km². All parts of the continent were inhabited, at greater or
lesser density according to the availability of food and water. Hunting and
gathering were the universal forms of subsistence throughout, but true
nomadism was less evident with the coastal tribes. In situations where seafoods, terrestrial game, plant foods and water were plentiful throughout the
year, large groups of Aborigines might camp for weeks and possibly months
before moving to a nearby locality for another long stay, and population
densities probably reached as high as one person per km². In the central
deserts, however, irregular and unpredictable rainfall and small 'rock-hole'
stores of rainwater meant that small family groups had no option but to

cover vast areas in search of water, and to a lesser extent the rainfall-associated plant foods and animal populations. Here population densities have been estimated at around one person per 100 km^2 (Meggit, 1964; Yengoyen, 1968).

Radiometric dating indicates that the Aborigines arrived in Australia at least 30 000 years ago, and the most probable time of arrival on geological/oceanographical grounds was 50 000 years ago (White and O'Connell, 1979). With no evidence of significant contacts or admixture with other cultures, and with no plants suited to agriculture or animals suited to herding, it is a reasonable assumption that their hunting–collecting ecosystem was as highly evolved as it is possible to imagine, and exceptionally stable over millennia. The long time span also suggests strong possibilities for genetic adaptation—particularly in the harsher desert environments.

The wide variety of hunting-gathering environments implies an accompanying variety of lifestyles and physical activities within an overall hunting-gathering stereotype. These were associated with variations in foods available, in the options to follow food preferences, and in energy expenditure in the food quest. There was no single staple food, and few if any of the seasonal staples were continentally distributed. These aspects have been well researched in some areas but not in others, so that a further implication is that it would be unwise to generalize the starting points for diet or physical activity when considering the impact of westernization on Aboriginal health.

By the mid-1960s, the 'full-blood' or tribally oriented Aborigines numbered about 40 000, mainly in small communities confined within the boundaries shown in Fig. 11.1. Possibly excepting a handful of central desert nomads, none followed the traditional patterns of hunting and gathering for total subsistence, although the skills were maintained for cultural reasons and as a form of recreation.

In addition, there were about 80 000 identifiable 'part-Aborigines', mostly outside the boundary shown in Fig. 11.1, who generally followed very few hunting-gathering activities related to those of their Aboriginal forebears. Had they wished to, for subsistence, they would have had difficulties in finding suitable natural country in areas taken over for agriculture or stock raising, but in any case the majority would have lacked the skills and the inclination. It is difficult to place the larger part-Aboriginal population in a consideration of the emergence of Western diseases. In a sense, they were a new 'race' and culture dating from the early nineteenth century, but it is only very recently that any interest has been shown in their comparative health status, and part-Aborigines are not identified as such in national health and population statistics. For these reasons, the discussion that follows concentrates on the tribally oriented Aborigines of north and central Australia.

The outstation movement

A proportion of the 40 000 Aborigines have retained access to their traditional tribal lands incorporated in the few large Aboriginal reserves shown in Fig. 11.1. This has been associated with a recent movement of families and

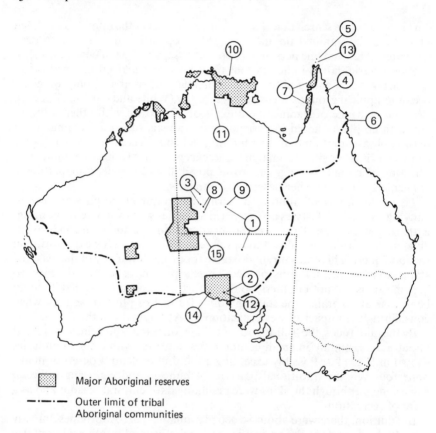

Fig. 11.1   Australia, showing major Aboriginal reserves, outer limit of tribal Aboriginal communities, and location of blood pressure surveys

larger groups away from the permanent government, mission or cattle-station settlements and a partial return to hunting and gathering for subsistence. This 'outstation movement' has gathered impetus over the past five years, precipitated by delinquent youth, alcohol-associated problems and a cultural resurgence, but is of great potential interest with respect to Western diseases and their possible regression over time—provided that an adequate epidemiological data base can be maintained.

Dietary changes since contact with Western culture

The traditional dietary patterns and practices of hunter-gatherer Aborigines have been detailed for specific groups: unfortunately these studies rarely correspond in time or locality with health studies (Moodie and Pedersen, 1971). Probably the most detailed and comprehensive study in this field was that carried out in Arnhem Land in 1948 (Macarthur, 1960); this included diet, food compositions, nutrient intakes, food-gathering practices, bio-chemical and anthropometric studies and various health parameters—mostly relating to communicable diseases.

This and other studies show the typical division of labour, with men hunt-ing the larger game (kangaroos, wallabies, emus, wombats, turtles, dugongs, crocodiles and larger fish) and women collecting all the plant foods and animal foods such as small game, lizards, insects, shellfish, crabs and small fish. The evidence throughout suggests that women provided the major part of the food and energy intake, and at the same time expended more energy in the collection and in the time-consuming labour of plant food processing and detoxification (e.g. cycad nuts). The additional energy expenditure was matched by additional food consumed during the collection—generally those foods which required little or no processing or prolonged cooking (e.g. fruits, insects, seafoods). A major consequence has been that, aside from the effects of alcohol, women have been more profoundly affected than men by the adoption of a Western diet emphasizing processed carbohydrate foods.

The change commenced with the establishment of missions and cattle stations where rations were offered in exchange for labour or provided to keep a labour pool in the area. Ration depots were also established for desert nomads and others after poor seasons or when tribal lands were being alienated. The foods provided were those which travelled well in bulk—also the staple foods of the white bushmen and stockmen—white flour, sugar and tea, plus locally killed fresh beef or mutton if available.

With the passage of time, rations provided gradually improved in variety but retained the basic pattern of highly refined carbohydrate foods. The following ration was provided on a central desert mission in the 1950s.

Weekly ration	Working men	Women/old people
White flour	4·54 kg	3·64 kg
Refined sugar	0·68 kg	0·68 kg
Golden syrup	0·45 kg	0·45 kg
Potatoes, onions or dried fruit	0·45 kg	0·45 kg
Tea	85 g	85 g
Fresh meat (issued in 3 lots)	4·08 kg	1·36 kg

Preschool children were issued 1·35 kg fresh meat per week and some fruit. School children were provided with cooked meals, as follows:

Breakfast: Porridge, bread and syrup
Lunch: Soup, meat and bread
Dinner: Liver, rice, cheese and cauliflower, stewed fruit, bread and cheese, tea (sweetened)

Experiments in the 1960s in the Northern Territory to provide balanced cafeteria-style meals failed for cultural reasons, and the next major change was to a supermarket-type store where food was bought for cash according to individual preference. A typical weekly store purchase for a family of five at a central desert mission in the 1970s (White, 1977) was as follows:

White flour	11·34 kg	Lean mutton	2·72 kg
White bread	3·63 kg	Canned meat	0·68 kg
White sugar	2·72 kg	Eggs (12)	0·66 kg
Jam	0·68 kg	Butter	0·23 kg
Canned fruit	0·85 kg	Oranges/apples	6
Semisweet biscuits	0·45 kg	Full cream dried	
Tea	230–460 g	milk	0·45 kg

In addition, families may receive around 7 kg of kangaroo meat or 4·5 kg of wombat meat or two rabbits per week; children consumed about 1 litre of canned soft drink and 3 packets of potato crisps; adults drank around 2 litres of beer and on occasions perhaps 2 litres or more of sweet 'port' in flagons.

A startling contrast in nutrient intakes is shown in Table 11.1, comparing a traditional Arnhem Land high meat diet in 1948 and a store-bought Cape York Peninsula high refined carbohydrate diet in 1972—both being coastal/ estuarine communities in similar environments. The figures indicate a pronounced reversal of carbohydrate/protein contributions and generally low vitamin and mineral intakes with the store-bought diet. It can be estimated from the Arnhem Land data that the crude fibre content of the vegetable component of the diet (itself one-third of the total by weight) averaged 1·5 per cent.

None of the ration lists or store purchases mentions salt. The fat content of the diets is difficult to estimate, but appears to be quite low.

Changes in energy expenditure following contact with Western culture

With the change to Western processed carbohydrate foods, women lost their gathering and food-processing role, and began to pass the time sitting around the camp or settlement chatting and playing cards, with less frequent recreational forays in search of favourite bush foods—if available. Men, on the other hand, were often employed in the workforce and also did not entirely lose their hunting roles. In the 1970s, however, a combination of universally available social welfare benefits (including unemployment benefits, invalid and old age pensions), a general reduction in rural employment opportunities and freely available alcohol led to a generally reduced need for physical activity by men on the Aboriginal settlements, coupled with an increased energy intake and a continued imbalance in diet, which presumably explains the increase in observable obesity among the men. Reversal of this trend would appear to be unlikely except among those involved in the 'outstation movement' or the Australian workforce. Opportunities for both these alternatives are limited.

Table 11.1 Comparison of Aborigine nutrient intakes, traditional diet in western Arnhem Land, 1948, and a store-purchased diet, Edward River, Cape York Peninsula, 1972

	Average nutrient intake as a percentage of 'average dietary requirements for Australians'	
	Traditional W. Arnhem Land, 1948[1]	Store-purchased Edward River, 1972[2]
Energy/kcal	90	117–118
Protein	338	74–92
Calcium	267	26–92
Iron	105	33
Ascorbic acid	236 ‚	28
Retinol/vitamin A	'probably adequate'	24
Thiamine	'probably adequate'	233
Riboflavin	'probably adequate'	70
Niacin	'unknown'	28

[1] Calculated from the average for four communities totalling 57 people reported by . . . . Macarthur (1960)
[2] Reported by Taylor (1977)

Western diseases in Australian Aborigines

There have been some detailed studies in respect to hypertension, diabetes and ischaemic heart disease. Information about most other Western diseases is generally anecdotal, negative (i.e. the absence of . . .) or hidden in aggregated morbidity statistics.

Hypertensive disease

The results of a number of *ad hoc* blood pressure surveys from 1926 to 1975 are depicted in Fig. 11.2, in chronological order, keyed to localities shown in Fig. 11.1, with references appended. The lowest readings were from a survey of 'primitive' central desert Aborigines surveyed in 1934 (Survey 3). The highest systolic readings were from the west coast of Cape York Peninsula in 1938—also regarded as 'primitive' (Survey 7). The highest diastolic readings were from Koonibba in the Nullarbor in 1972 (Survey 12) and although blood pressures were considerably higher than at a previous survey in 1930, a 15-years increase in average age may account for much of the difference. Another set of 'paired' results derives from the non-Australoid Torres Strait Islanders surveyed in 1938 and 1974, and showing very little change over 36 years (Surveys 5 and 13).

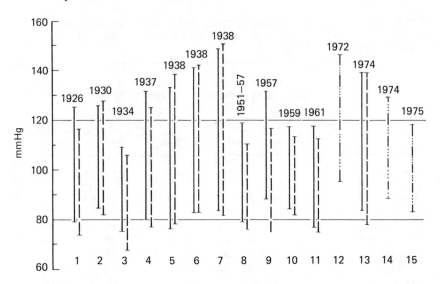

Fig. 11.2   Australian Aboriginal blood pressures, 1926–75

Locality of surveys keyed to Fig. 11.1. Males, solid line; females, broken line; males and females combined, broken/dotted line.

1   Macumba Station and Alice Springs, 1926. M × 42; F × 13. Average age 40 ± 0·5 (Ray, 1927).
2   Koonibba Station, 1930. M × 10, average age 25; F × 5, average age 21 (Pulleine and Woollard, 1930).
3   Central Australia 'primitive'—Cockatoo Creek and Mt. Liebig, 1933–34. M × 56, average age 37; F × 11, average age 31 (Casley-Smith, 1959).
4   Lockhart River 'primitive', 1937. M × 12; F × 10. Average age 45 (Nye, 1937).
5   Torres Strait Islands, 1938 (Torres Strait Islanders). M × 250, F × 328. Average age 40 (Casley-Smith, 1959).
6   East Queensland 'semi-civilized', 1938. M × 272, F × 289. Average age 40 (Casley-Smith, 1959).
7   Carpentaria 'primitive', 1938. M × 279. F × 344. Average age 40 (Casley-Smith, 1959).
8   Central Australia, 'semi-civilized', 1951–57. M × 98, F × 132. Average age 40 (Casley-Smith, 1959).
9   Central Australia, 'semi-urbanized', 1952. M × 20, F ×19. Average age 40 (Casley-Smith, 1959).
10   Maningrida 'primitive', 1959. M × 60, F × 48. Average age 40 (Abbie and Schroder, 1960).
11   Beswick Settlement, 'semi-Europeanized', 1961. M × 29, F ×32. Average age 35 (van Dongen *et al.*, 1962).
12   Koonibba, 1972. M + F × 76. Average age 39. (Edwards *et al.*, 1976).
13   Torres Strait Islands, 1974 (Torres Strait Islanders). M × 363, F × 558. Average age 40 (Nielson and Williams, 1978).
14   Yalata 'semi-civilized', 1974. M + F × 170 (Edwards *et al.*, 1976).
15   Ernabella 'semi-civilized', 1975. M + F × 56 (Edwards *et al.*, 1976).

While these results support the association between westernization and hypertension in a general way, there are several inexplicable inconsistencies. The Aborigines at Beswick (Survey 11, 1961) were described as all having lived under semi-European conditions for at least ten years, and the surveyors remarked 'an indication of the extent to which (they) had been converted to European foods was the prevalence of dental caries'. Yet their mean blood pressures were amongst the lowest in all surveys. The nearest correlation between 'civilization' and blood pressure derives from Surveys 3, 8 and 9, all in central Australia, and covering a progression from 'primitive' in 1934 through 'semi-civilized' in 1951–57 to 'semi-urbanized' in 1957.

Access to salt might explain why nearly all the surveys with elevated pressures were coastal (except Koonibba in 1972) but a further anomaly occurs in that Maningrida (Survey 10 in 1959) is coastal and also showed low mean blood pressures.

The question of salt intake is difficult to unravel. Salt does not appear to have featured in traditional diets anywhere in Australia, although it could be obtained all round the coastline and also from the numerous salt lakes throughout the interior. None of the writer's informants can recall salt being a part of the traditional diet, the 'hand-out' ration, or the supermarket store purchases, and only one can remember bulk salt being available for cooking and bread-making—at Lockhart River after World War Two. Janice Reid, who spent periods in eastern Arnhem Land collecting with the women, recalls that she felt a need to dip her cooked crab-meat in the sea to salt it, whereas her Aboriginal companions felt no such need. The traditional cooking method—all food cooked on open fires or in the embers—is still generally followed today by tribal Aborigines, and may explain why salt is not added even if available. Seafoods in themselves contain no more sodium than terrestrial flesh foods. Although Aboriginal women in central Australia preserved plant foods by drying, or making them into pastes (Meggitt, 1964), there is no evidence anywhere that foods were salted for this purpose.

The most likely sources of salt in present-day Aboriginal diets are bread, canned foods—particularly canned meat—and salted butter. The saltier foods, with one exception, do not seem to be popular dietary items. The exception is the packet of potato crisps, and its popularity with the rising generation may herald a change in tastes for the future. Each packet contains around 280 mg (4 mmolNa) of added salt.

Macfarlane (1971) has reported a study of water and salt balance in central desert Aborigines and European controls walking in summer temperatures of 38 °C. Compared with the Europeans under the same stresses, the Aborigines had 15 per cent more extracellular water; up to twice the loss of water by sweating (but with much lower sodium losses in sweat); up to five times the urine flow rate, and from five to eight times the urinary sodium excretion rate during prolonged exertion. The latter rose from initial levels about three times that of the controls, but the levels fell in the controls during prolonged exertion.

It is uncertain whether these differences in water and salt turnover were inherited or due to conditioning, but in either case they suggest that active

Aboriginal hunter-gatherers, at least in the desert, may be better able to cope with a salt loading.

There is increasing evidence of hypertensive disease among settled Aborigines today. Among 685 Bathurst and Melville Islands Aborigines (north of Darwin), 9·9 per cent had both systolic and diastolic pressures above limits of 150/90 mmHg. A further 16·6 and 2·5 per cent had raised systolic and diastolic pressures respectively (Dr. J. C. Hargrave, personal communication). Dr. D. Devenesan (personal communication) reports that in 100 central desert (Yuendumu) Aboriginal adults in 1979, 17 per cent had diastolic pressures above 94 mmHg. Wise *et al.* (1976) have reported 52 per cent of adults averaging 52 years at the Davenport Reserve near Port Augusta, South Australia, as having pressures above limits of 160/100 mmHg. The latter community is largely part-Aboriginal and has not been included in Fig. 11.2.

Northern Territory hospital diagnoses relevant to Western diseases are shown in Table 11.2. The apparently higher prevalence of essential hyper-

Table 11.2 Relative hospitalization rates, Northern Terriroty Aborigines and Whites, Jan. 1975 through June 1977 (not age-adjusted)

	Rate per 100 000 per annum			
	Males		Females	
Disease	Abor.	Whites	Abor.	Whites
Essential benign hypertension	131	124	101	93
Hypertensive heart disease	25	14	6	1
Other hypertensive disease	3	5	—	8
Acute myocardial infarction	19	111	3	38
Other ischaemic heart disease	9	95	6	33
Cerebral haemorrhage	9	9	6	1
Cerebral infarction	16	12	9	4
Acute ill-defined cerebrovascular disease	63	35	22	21
Other cerebrovascular disease	19	13	—	8
Arteriosclerosis	3	3	—	1
Other peripheral vascular disease	3	13	—	8
Pulmonary embolism and infarction	—	10	6	14
Phlebitis, thrombophlebitis, thrombosis	13	50	3	58
Varicose veins of lower extremity	3	59	9	124
Haemorrhoids	9	107	3	46
Malignant neoplasm (excluding skin)	106	92	121	117
Diabetes mellitus	63	79	127	62

Source: Commonwealth Department of Health (1977) *Northern Territory Medical Service Bulletin*, Issue No. 18, December 1977

tension and of hypertensive heart disease in Aborigines may be misleading because many non-Aborigines are diagnosed and treated by private practitioners.

Other cardiovascular diseases

Reports suggest that there was a minimal occurrence of arteriosclerotic, ischaemic heart disease and venous disease in nomadic and semi-civilized Aborigines until the 1960s. In a series of papers on biochemical risk factors, Schwartz and Casley-Smith (1958a, b) refer to a series of 44 autopsies which showed 'little or no incidence of atheroma or arteriosclerotic heart disease'. A cardiological survey of western Australian desert Aborigines by Woods (1966) reports few ECG abnormalities and no cardiovascular disease other than mild hypertension (in 9·5 per cent) and possible viral myocarditis.

Table 11.2 shows that the 'hospital' incidence in the Northern Territory in the mid-1970s for cardiovascular diseases other than hypertension was lower for Aborigines except for the categories 'cerebral infarction' and 'ill-defined cerebrovascular disease' where the Aboriginal figures were a little higher. Again this may be hospital selection bias.

At Haast's Bluff in central Australia, in the area of Survey 8 in Fig. 11.1, Schwartz and Casley-Smith (1958a, b) surveyed diets and serum cholesterol and mucoprotein levels in 'semi-civilized' Aborigines. Dietary fat was described as low and contributing less than 10 per cent of energy intake. The main fat sources were fresh meat after a large part had been used for other (non-dietary) purposes; and witchetty (moth) grubs consumed by women and children. Their comparison of serum factors, from nomadic and urban Aborigines and white controls, is in Table 11.3.

Table 11.3 Serum cholesterol and mucoprotein levels in nomadic and urban Aborigines and White controls

	Nomadic Aborigines	Urban Aborigines	White controls
Mean age (years)	32	37	35
Serum cholesterol (mmol/l)	5·47	6·27	7·54
Serum mucoprotein (mmol/l)	743	936	901

The authors attributed the lower cholesterol levels to a higher dietary ratio of vegetable to animal fat, but were uncertain of the significance of the mucoprotein levels, which they thought reflected the rate of depolymerization of intercellular ground substance. It was evidently not an inherited feature protecting Aborigines from disease because of the high levels found in urbanized Aborigines.

Edwards *et al.* (1976) have reported coronary heart disease risk factor studies on two 'near-nomadic' groups in the south Australian desert (also included in the blood pressure surveys) (Table 11.4) as well as in several partly part-Aboriginal groups not included here because of a general similarity to Western communities, and for lack of space.

Table 11.4   Coronary heart disease risk factors in two near nomadic Aboriginal groups

	Ernabella	Yalata
Number of subjects	56	170
Mean ages (years)	39	41
Serum cholesterol (mmol/l)	4·42	4·96
Serum triglyceride (mmol/l)	1·88	2·31
Hypertriglyceridaemia (%)	40	36
Activity index (0−3 scale)	1·9	1·7
Obesity (ideal weight + 20%)	16%	8%
'Probable' ischaemic heart disease	4·5%(M)	5·4%(M)
	0·0%(F)	6·5%(F)

Compared with the above, the other part-Aboriginal communities studied showed more frequent CHD (9·0–15·8 per cent); more frequent obesity (21–33 per cent); higher cholesterol levels (5·27–5·76 mmol/l; higher blood pressures (up to 146/95 mean mmHg); some higher activity levels (1·4–2·1) and similar triglyceride levels (1·84–2·23 mmol/l). The pattern is indeed confusing!

Diabetes mellitus

The first Aboriginal diabetic was diagnosed in 1923 (Cleland, 1928). He was an elderly station hand, and responded well to dietary measures and small doses of insulin. Thereafter there has been little or no mention of diabetes until the 1970s. Today, the prevalence exceeds 10 per cent in many Aboriginal communities, and Wise *et al.* (1976) have reported a prevalence of 19 per cent among part-Aborigines in the Port Augusta area of South Australia. Dr. D. Devenesan (personal communication) reports 11 per cent of Yuendumu (central Australian) Aboriginal adults with diabetic glycosuria, and similar figures have been reported from Bathurst Island. The only comprehensive report is that by Wise *et al.* (1976), to which the interested reader is referred. The 'new' diabetics were associated with a period of civilization, obesity (females predominate), frank myocardial ischaemia, higher serum cholesterol and triglyceride levels, and lower activity levels when compared with non-diabetics, but not associated with hypertension, or high intakes of energy, carbohydrate or protein. The overall prevalence of myocardial ischaemia (Minnesota coding) was about *five times* that for an Australian white community aged 21–59 using the same criteria.

Other Western diseases

Appendicitis now occurs among Northern Territory Aborigines, at an un-known but evidently low incidence. Bateson (1976, 1977 and personal communication, 1979) reports a radiographically nil occurrence of duodenal ulcer, hiatus hernia, diverticular disease and ulcerative colitis; and no renal tract calculi in the north although cases have been seen around Alice Springs in central Australia.

Although serum uric acid levels are often relatively high, there have been no reports of gout. Gallstones, of unknown chemical composition, are being detected in Northern Territory Aboriginal women.

With regard to malignant disease, the figures given in Table 11.2 suggest that overall incidence in Northern Territory Aborigines and non-Aborigines is comparable, provided that malignant skin diseases are not included (they are very common in whites but very rare in Aborigines, for obvious reasons). It will be some years before there are sufficient numbers for any differences to become statistically certain, but in any case there still remains the need for evaluating morbidity and mortality in the population as a whole, rather than through the hospitals.

Acknowledgements

The writer is indebted to Drs. E. M. Bateson, J. C. Hargrave and D. Jacobs (Darwin), Dr. D. Devenesan (Alice Springs), Mrs. H. Conn (Lake Cargelico), Mrs. F. M. Edwards (Adelaide) and Dr. J. Reid (Sydney) for information personally supplied while writing this chapter.

References

Abbie, A. A. and Schroder, J. (1960). Blood pressure in Arnhem Land Aborigines. *Medical Journal of Australia,* **2,** 493–496

Bateson, E. M. (1976). Duodenal ulcer—does it exist in Australian Abori-gines? *Australian and New Zealand Journal of Medicine,* **6,** 545–547

Bateson, E. M. (1977). Do Australian Aborigines suffer from renal tract calculi? *Australian and New Zealand Journal of Medicine,* **7,** 380–381

Casley-Smith, J. R. (1959). Blood pressures in Australian Aborigines. *Medical Journal of Australia,* **1,** 627–633

Cleland, J. B. (1928). Diseases among the Australian Aborigines: Part IV (continued). *Journal of Tropical Medicine and Hygiene,* **31,** 438–446

Edwards, F. M., Wise, P. H., Thomas, D. W., Murchland, J. B. and Craig, R. J. (1976). Blood pressure and electrocardiographic findings in the South Australian Aborigines. *Australian and New Zealand Journal of Medicine,* **6,** 197–205

Macarthur, M. (1960). Report of the nutrition unit. In: *Records of the American-Australian Scientific Expedition to Arnhem Land: 2: Anthro-pology and Nutrition,* 1–194. Editor C. P. Mountford. Melbourne University Press, Melbourne

Macfarlane, W. V. (1971). Ecophysiology of water: mammalian functions in arid areas. In: *Research in Physiology*. Editors F. F. Kao, K. Koizumi and M. Vassalle. Aulo Caggi, Bologna

Meggitt, M. J. (1964). Aboriginal food-gatherers of Tropical Australia. *Proc. Pap. I.U.C.N. 9th Technical Meeting*, Nairobi, 30–37

Moodie, P. M. (1973). *Aboriginal Health*. Australian National University Press, Canberra

Moodie, P. M. and Pedersen, E. B. (1971). *The Health of Australian Aborigines: an Annotated Bibliography*, 219–220. Australian Government Publishing Service, Canberra

Mulvaney, D. J. (1975). *The Prehistory of Australia*. Penguin Books, Melbourne

Neilson, G. and Williams, G. (1978). Blood pressure and valvular and congenital heart disease in Torres Strait Islanders. *Medical Journal of Australia*, 1 (Special Supplement on Aboriginal Health: 10), 12–16

Nye, L. J. J. (1937). Blood pressure in the Australian Aboriginal, with a consideration of possible aetiological factors in hyperpiesia and its relation to civilization. *Medical Journal of Australia* 2, 1000–1001

Pulleine, R. and Woollard, H. (1930). Physiology and mental observations on the Australian Aborigines. *Transactions of the Royal Society of South Australia*, 54, 62–75

Ray, W. (1927). Adelaide University Field Anthropology, No. 2: Physiological observations. *Transactions of the Royal Society of South Australia*, 51, 76–77

Schwartz, C. J. and Casley-Smith, J. R. (1958a). Atherosclerosis and the serum mucoprotein levels of the Australian Aborigines. *Australian Journal of Experimental Biology and Medical Science*, 36, 117–120

Schwartz, C. J. and Casley-Smith, J. R. (1958b). Serum cholesterol levels in atherosclerotic subjects and in the Australian Aborigines. *Medical Journal of Australia*, 2, 84–86

Taylor, J. C. (1977). Diet, health and economy: some consequences of planned social change in an Aboriginal community. In: *Aborigines and Change*. Editor R. M. Berndt. Humanities Press, New Jersey

van Dongen, R., Davivongs, V. and Abbie, A. A. (1962). Aboriginal blood pressures at Beswick, South-Western Arnhem Land, and correlation with physical dimensions. *Medical Journal of Australia*, 2, 286

White, I. M. (1977). Pitfalls to avoid: the Australian experience. In: *Health and Disease in Tribal Societies*, 269–292. Ciba Foundation Symposium 49 (new series). Elsevier, Amsterdam

White, J. P. and O'Connell, J. F. (1979). Australian prehistory: new aspects of antiquity. *Science*, 203, 21–28

Wise, P. H., Edwards, F. M., Craig, R. J., Evans, B., Murchland, J. B., Sutherland, B. and Thomas, D. W. (1976). Diabetes and associated variables in the South Australian Aboriginal. *Australian and New Zealand Journal of Medicine*, 6, 191–196

Woods, J. O. (1966). The electrocardiogram of the Australian Aboriginal. *Medical Journal of Australia*, 1, 438–441

Yengoyan, A. A. (1968). Demographic and ecological influences on Aboriginal Australian marriage sections. In: *Man the Hunter*, 185–199. Editors R. B. Lee and I. DeVore. Aldine, Chicago

Part IV

Peasant agriculturalists

12

Papua New Guinea

Peter Sinnett and Malcolm Whyte

Environmental and cultural background

Situated in the south-west Pacific and separated from Cape York of Australia
by the Torres Strait, Papua New Guinea claims sovereignty over 462 000
square kilometres of island territory which extends from the equator to
12 degrees south. This territory includes the eastern half of the island of New
Guinea, the Bismark Archipelago, the islands of the Trobriand, Woodlark,
Louisiade and D'Entrecasteaux group, as well as Buka and Bougainville,
the northernmost islands of the Solomons (Fig. 12.1).

Papua New Guinea provides a uniquely wide range of physical environments: snow-covered peaks of Mount Wilhelm; mountain forests and
rugged, almost inaccessible highland valleys where human habitation extends
up to 2600 m and where human survival is threatened by frosts; tropical
rain forests; broad fertile valleys in the mountain folds where high population
densities can render food availability marginal; rugged foothill country
where soil and high rainfall combine to render the population susceptible to
endemic goitre and cretinism; hot, humid coastal deltas, where malaria is
endemic and where the gene for thalassaemia confers a survival advantage;
coastal plains with coconut stands, sandy beaches and rolling surf; volcanic
islands and coral atolls. All form part of the Papua New Guinea environment.
The diversity in the physical environment is matched by the ethnic and genetic
diversity that exists among the people who inhabit these islands, consisting
as they do of peoples of Melanesian, Micronesian, Polynesian and Papuan
descent.

Papua New Guinea is not only a land of environmental, genetic and
cultural diversity, it is also a land of rapid social and economic change. At
the time of independence (in 1975) no population in Papua New Guinea had
experienced sustained European contact for much longer than 100 years.
In 1874 Dr. and Mrs. Lawes of the London Missionary Society, took up
residence at Port Moresby. Ten years later in 1884 Britain annexed all the
territories subsequently known as Papua while the north-eastern section of
New Guinea and the related islands were claimed by the German Empire.

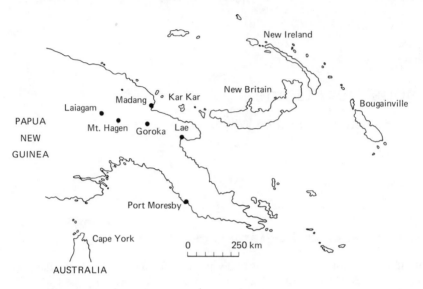

Fig. 12.1　Papua New Guinea

The First World War had little impact on Papua New Guinea apart from leading to the transfer of administrative responsibility for German territories to Australia. The Japanese invasion of New Guinea in early 1942, however, had profound social and economic consequences for the local communities involved. Although hostilities ceased on the 13th September 1945, it was not until the 1950s that effective, progressive, civil administration was re-established (Essai, 1961).

For the majority of the people living in the remote interior of the island of New Guinea, these events were of little significance. For these people sustained European contact commenced in the 1950s and they were expected to make the transition from a subsistence economy based on a stone-age technology and regulated by tribal law, to a Western, cash-based economy regulated by a Westminster parliamentary system, in less than 25 years.

The variable influence of European contact accentuated the traditional differences in environmental, genetic and cultural characteristics and in disease patterns that already existed between Papua New Guinea communities. In spite of this Papua New Guinea rural communities, especially those of the remote Western Highlands, exhibit a sufficient degree of social and economic homogeneity to serve as a model in evaluating the development of disease patterns in Western societies.

The origin of these New Guinea highlanders is obscure. It is claimed that the first human migration to Papua New Guinea occurred from South East Asia between 20 000 and 50 000 years ago (Golson, 1970). Gradually the initial hunting and gathering economy was replaced by a seminomadic agriculture based on a stone-age technology, and associated with the cultivation of taro, bananas, yams and sugar cane which, according to Brookfield (1964) restricted the population to altitudes below 2135 m.

The final stage in the agricultural development of the highlands was associated with the introduction of the sweet potato 350 years ago. This crop made possible the development of relatively large settled communities, and the colonization of altitudes up to 2700 m. The occupation of altitudes above 2000 m, presumably the result of population pressure, led to heavy dependence on the sweet potato and to a restricted range of food intake, an important factor in view of the low protein content of the sweet potato and its susceptibility to frosts.

In 1966 an epidemiological survey was commenced among a traditional Papua New Guinea highland community. The objective of this study was to investigate the influence of social, nutritional and other environmental factors on the anthropometric, biochemical and physiological characteristics, as well as on the disease pattern of a traditional Papua New Guinea population. The people selected for study form the entire membership of 'Murapin', a complete Yandapu-Enga[1] phratry, or tribal community of 1500 individuals. Their clan territory is centred on the hamlet of Tukisenta, 160 km north-west of Mount Hagen and 25 km from Laiagam (Fig. 12.1).

The people of Murapin are hamlet dwellers; their homesteads of timber and grass extend along the river valleys at an altitude of 1800–2600 m and are scattered among sweet potato gardens and beech trees which grow in the narrow river valleys and on the foothills of the mountain forests. They are preliterate farmers and pig-herders whose subsistence economy depends almost entirely on the cultivation of a single, staple food, the sweet potato. These people are polygamous and their social organization, which is based on the extended family, is overtly patrilineal in structure. The results of the study of these people which have been published as a monograph (Sinnett, 1977b) form the basis for the present discussion of the disease patterns in a traditional Papua New Guinea community.

Agriculture

Traditional agriculture is based on the intensive cultivation of a single staple food, the sweet potato (*Ipomoea batatas*). Some 24 varieties of this plant are grown within the clan's territory. Once planted, the sweet potato takes about ten months to mature. The gardens are planted in rotation to ensure a continuous supply of sweet potato. After harvesting, a garden plot is left fallow while another plot, usually adjacent to the first and within the same garden site, is cleared and planted. The period of fallow is highly variable but at Tukisenta the pattern appears to be one of continuous cultivation.

Other crops cultivated include taro (*Colocasia esculenta*), which is now grown to only a limited extent although it is claimed that one to two generations ago this crop was extensively cultivated throughout the area; pit-pit

[1] Yandapu-Enga is one of the 13 dialects of the Enga language and is spoken by 14 000 people living mainly in the area around Laiagam.

(*Saccharum spontaneum*); sugar cane (*Saccharum officinarum*) and pandanus palms (*Pandanus* sp.). Extensive herds of pigs are maintained and, during exchange ceremonies, large amounts of pork are consumed. However, in terms of overall dietary intake, meat is only a minor food source.

Dietary intake

A diet survey was undertaken involving 90 subjects, in which all food consumed by each individual was weighed over a period of seven consecutive days. Sweet potato supplied over 90 per cent of their total food intake, while non-tuberous vegetables accounted for less than 5 per cent of the food consumed and the intake of meat was negligible. A similar heavy dependence on a single vegetable staple has been reported for other Papua New Guinea Highland communities (Hipsley and Clements, 1947; Norgan *et al.*, 1974).

Chemical composition of the sweet potato varied widely. Protein content ranged from 1·01 to 1·9 per cent of wet weight, fibre content from 1·25 to 3·03 per cent wet weight and energy values varied from 470 kJ (112 kcal) to 650 kJ (155 kcal) per 100 g edible portion.

The daily energy intake was 9·6 MJ (2300 kcal) in the case of males and 7·4 MJ (1770 kcal) for females. Of these, 94·6 per cent were derived from carbohydrates, 3 per cent from protein and only 2·4 per cent from fat. Male subjects consumed 25 g and female subjects 20 g of protein per day. By contrast Australians derive 40 per cent of their energy from fat and consume approximately 100 g of protein per day (Woodhill *et al.*, 1969).

The intake of dietary fibre was high among this population. Young men in their twenties consumed 34 g of fibre per day derived from sweet potato alone while women in the same age group consumed 27 g of fibre per day. The high fibre intake of this group is in marked contrast to the situation in most Western urbanized communities in which the intake of dietary fibre is between 15 and 20 g per day. The result of the increased consumption of refined foods has led to a 37 per cent reduction in fibre intake over the past century (Burkitt *et al.*, 1972).

The dietary pattern of this New Guinea Highland population was thus characterized by a low intake of total calories, protein, fat and refined carbohydrate and a high intake of complex carbohydrate and fibre.

Demographic characteristics and health status

The population of Murapin was a young one: 43·6 per cent of subjects in this community were less than 15 years of age. By contrast 29·4 per cent of Australians were under the age of 15 years (Commonwealth Bureau of Census and Statistics, 1968). The population of Murapin was found to have a crude birth rate of 42 per 1000, a death rate of 15 per 1000 and thus a rate of annual increase of approximately 2·7 per cent per annum. In contrast the Australian population had a birth rate of 19·3 per 1000, a death rate of 9·0 per 1000 and a crude rate of annual increase of 1·03 per cent per annum (Commonwealth Bureau of Census and Statistics, 1969). The infant mortality rate for Murapin was 85 per 1000 live births. The infant mortality rate for this highland population is considerably lower than the rate of 124·7 deaths per 1000 live births reported for the highland area by Vines (1970).

The high rate of annual increase for the population of Murapin testifies to its successful biological adaptation. Further, this rate of annual increase is achieved by a high birth rate operating in spite of a high death rate and, more specifically, a high infant mortality rate. Indeed, 42·8 per cent of children in the present study died before they reached an age at which they were eligible for marriage (Sinnett and Whyte, 1973a; Sinnett, 1977b).

Delayed growth rates in both height and weight were a further characteristic of this community. The values for heights and weights of Murapin children were lower at all ages than those of Australians. Growth in height was not completed until the age of 18 years in the case of females and 24 years in the case of males. By contrast British schoolchildren reached adult stature by the age of 15 years in females and 17 years in male subjects (Tanner *et al.*, 1966). The delayed growth of the Papua New Guinea child is associated with a delayed onset of sexual maturity. A detailed study of growth and development of children in a Papua New Guinea community has been published in respect to the Bundi people of the Madang District (Malcolm, 1970).

In spite of the high infant and childhood mortality rates and the delayed growth of children, only one case of protein–calorie malnutrition was detected. Young adults were well built and physically fit and had normal levels of haemoglobin and serum albumin. Further, adult females showed no clinical evidence of malnutrition in spite of the demands by repeated cycles of pregnancy and lactation. On the basis of American standards (Society of Actuaries, 1959) both sexes were close to 100 per cent standard weight in their twenties. The Harvard Pack Test carried out on 152 consecutive subjects demonstrated a high level of physical fitness which was maintained well into middle-age. Use of a bicycle ergometer gave an estimated maximum oxygen uptake of 45·2 ml per kilogram per minute and thus confirmed the high level of cardiopulmonary fitness of this group (Sinnett and Solomon, 1968).

Age-related changes in body build

Many European populations show a progressive increase in body weight from maturity through middle-age and even into the seventh and eighth decades (Society of Actuaries, 1959). Subjects of the present study are typical of other Papua New Guinea populations in that their body weight reaches a maximum between the ages of 20 and 29 years. In this group the mean body weight is 59·8 kg in male subjects and 50·9 kg for females. Thereafter both sexes show a progressive decrease in body weight as age advances. By the seventh decade the average body weight has decreased by 13·3 kg or 23·3 per cent in the case of men and 13·5 kg or 25 per cent in the case of women.

Even in Western populations, the lean body mass in adults falls progressively with advancing age. Forbes and Reina (1970) argued that after maturity is reached anabolic processes are 'superseded by catabolic events which slowly erode the lean body mass. The adult should be looked upon as being in a continuous state of negative potassium and hence nitrogen balance.' Their figures indicate that between the third and seventh decades there should be a reduction of 16·4 per cent in the body weight of male subjects and 8·5 per cent in the body weight of females. Application of these estimations to the present New Guinea population provides insight into their nutritional status. New Guinea males lose 23·3 per cent of their body weight between the third and seventh decades in contrast to the 16·4 per cent suggested by Forbes and Reina. The contrast is more marked in the case of women, females in the present study experienced a weight reduction of 25 per cent compared with a loss of 8·5 per cent predicted on the basis of Forbes and Reina's data (Sinnett *et al.*, 1973; Sinnett, 1977a).

Disease prevalence

In view of the differences that exist between communities in Papua New Guinea in terms of climate, altitude, population density, nutritional intake, duration of Western contact and levels of urbanization, it is not surprising that regional differences exist in disease prevalence. In the highlands pneumonia, influenza and gastroenteritis are more common while malaria and tuberculosis have a lower prevalence than in other areas of Papua New Guinea. In spite of these regional differences it is, however, true that infectious diseases are a major cause of both morbidity and mortality in this country. Respiratory and intestinal infections, malaria, tuberculosis, leprosy, parasitic infestations, together with trauma, constitute the major public health problems. By contrast chronic degenerative diseases, especially those involving the cardiovascular system, are rarely encountered.

Malaria

In the present population malaria was uncommon. Examination of thick blood films yielded a parasite rate of lower than 0·4 per cent and none of these subjects had splenic enlargement or anaemia. Enlargement of the spleen occurred in only 0·9 per cent of adults. The low prevalence rate of malaria is not surprising in view of the high altitude (2600 m) at which these people live.

Leprosy and tuberculosis

Leprosy was relatively common with a prevalence rate of 2·7 per cent. In contrast to the high prevalence rate of leprosy, tuberculosis was an uncommon disease among this group. No evidence of pulmonary tuberculosis was detected among nearly 300 subjects on whom chest radiographs were taken.

Previous tuberculosis surveys through the area confirmed the rarity of this disease. Wigley (1967) makes the interesting point that tuberculosis is 'by and large' predominantly a coastal disease. He claims that the prevalence rate of the condition is proportional to the degree of urbanization.

Respiratory disease

In contrast to tuberculosis, which is claimed to be more common in coastal than in urban communities, other forms of respiratory diseases have a higher prevalence in the highlands. Between the years 1963 and 1966 pneumonia accounted for 15·7 per cent of hospital admissions in the highlands, 9·5 per cent in the mainland region and 6·1 per cent in the island region. Bronchitis showed a similar distribution accounting for respectively 5·8 per cent, 4·1 per cent and 3·7 per cent of admissions in the regions considered. Pneumonia was responsible for 45·4 per cent of all hospital deaths in the highlands, 15·8 per cent in the mainland and 12·3 per cent in the island region (Vines, 1970).

Respiratory disease was certainly the most common cause of people seeking medical treatment during the present survey; the majority of these people were suffering from acute bronchitis, pneumonia and pleurisy. Only one patient was diagnosed as having bronchial asthma. On the basis of physical examination 14 per cent of adults in the present study were diagnosed as having respiratory diseases. The prevalence increased steadily with advancing age from 4 per cent in the 15–19 years age group to 56 per cent in subjects over the age of 60.

Wright peak flow measurements were carried out on all adult subjects. Both males and females showed a significant decrease in maximum expiratory flow rate with advancing age amounting to 3·4 litres per minute per year. In association with the age-related decrease in respiratory function and increasing prevalence of respiratory diseases, electrocardiographic results indicated a higher prevalence of right axis deviation among the older group.

Environmental factors undoubtedly contributed to the respiratory problems of these people. Seventy-three per cent of adult males and 20 per cent of adult females smoked home-grown tobacco and although the method of smoking more closely resembled pipe than cigarette smoking, the proportion of male and female smokers were similar to those reported in an American community (Epstein *et al.*, 1965). Further, the people of Murapin habitually spent up to twelve hours a day inside smoke-filled houses. Cleary and Blackburn (1968) have shown that the smoke from their wood fires contain aldehydes which are extremely irritating.

Cardiovascular disease

Hospital-based studies indicate that pulmonary, rheumatic and congenital heart diseases are the most frequent cardiovascular problems encountered in Papua New Guinea, while cases of cardiomyopathy, hypertension and coronary heart disease are rarely seen among indigenous populations. Mathews (1974) in his review of patients admitted to the Lae Angau Memorial Hospital for the years 1969–73 claimed that congenital heart disease and chronic rheumatic heart disease were probably as common in Papua New Guinea as they were in Western countries. However, diseases of the myocardium, pericarditis, endocarditis and disorders of the arteries and veins were found in only a small number of Papua New Guineans.

The limited pathological studies that have been undertaken support the conclusions that atherosclerosis is uncommon among Papua New Guineans (Kariks and McGovern, 1967; Magarey *et al.*, 1969; Cooke and Kariks, 1970). Aiken *et al.* (1974) reported the result of the 146 autopsies carried out on Papua New Guineans in Port Moresby Hospital from January 1973 to April 1974. Of these, seven deaths were due to atherosclerotic heart disease. Of the atherosclerotic heart disease cases all were males, ranging in age from 28 to 45 years. The average period of urban contact was sixteen years for these subjects. These authors believe that the prevalence of atherosclerotic heart disease is increasing among urbanized Papua New Guineans.

The population-based studies on cardiovascular disease which have been undertaken in Papua New Guinea have largely concentrated on blood pressure patterns and the prevalence of hypertension. The study carried out on people of Murapin was the first comprehensive survey of cardiovascular disease to be undertaken among a defined Papua New Guinea population which included electrocardiography and in which procedures were standardized in accordance with recognized international criteria (Rose and Blackburn, 1968).

Cardiac decompensation

Only 5 cases of heart failure were detected in over 780 adults examined. One of these patients had right-sided heart-failure associated with mitral stenosis and the other 4 cases had evidence of cor pulmonale. X-ray evidence of cardiomegaly was detected in 9·1 per cent of adult males and 13·3 per cent of adult females. As none of these subjects had evidence of overt heart disease it is believed that the cardiac enlargement represented an adaptation to high altitude.

Valvular heart disease

Of the 780 adults, 16 were found to have cardiac murmurs, 3 were diastolic and 13 systolic in timing. Diastolic murmurs were attributed to mitral stanosis in 2 cases and to aortic enlargement in one subject. The 13 systolic murmurs presented a greater problem in interpretation. One 36-year-old male had a classic atrial septal defect. All the other subjects were asymptomatic and had no thrills or other abnormality of heart sounds. It was impossible to exclude a functional or haemic basis in most cases and no attempt was made to record a firm diagnosis. It was, however, felt that mitral incompetence was the most probable diagnosis in 5 of the subjects.

Blood pressure and hypertensive cardiovascular disease

Males in their twenties had a mean systolic blood pressure of 130 mmHg, mean diastolic pressure of 84 mmHg and a mean pulse pressure of 46 mmHg, while females in the same age group had a mean systolic pressure of 121 mmHg, a mean diastolic pressure of 78 mmHg and a mean pulse pressure of 43 mmHg. The blood pressure levels reached their maximum in males in the third decade, after which there was a progressive decrease in systolic and diastolic pressures, while the pulse pressure remained virtually unchanged. In females the systolic pressure increased with age, exceeding male values by the age of 35 years, while diastolic pressure remained unchanged. Thus the pulse pressure increased with advancing age in female subjects.

Similar blood pressure relationships with age have been found in other surveys in Papua New Guinea (Whyte, 1958; Vines, 1970; Hornabrook *et al.*, 1974). Indeed highly urbanized Papuans living in Hanuabada village in Port Moresby are the only group in Papua New Guinea in which a significant rise in blood pressure has been reported with advancing age (Maddocks, 1967). It is interesting that it was among this same group that Price and Tulloch (1966) reported the highest prevalence of diabetes mellitus.

These findings in Papua New Guinea are in contrast to the marked increase in blood pressure with advancing age in Western communities and emphasize the fact that a rise in blood pressure is not an inevitable accompaniment of the ageing process. Whyte (1958) found that pulse pressure increased with age in both sexes in his study and the difference in mean blood pressure between the two sexes was of the same order as found in Western populations. He suggested that 'the influence of sex on ageing of elastic arteries affected both races alike but that New Guineans lack, while Europeans acquire, the complaint of muscular arteries, which is sometimes called essential hypertension'.

Dahl (1963) suggested that differences in the consumption of salt might contribute to population differences in blood pressure. Certainly the salt intake is low among this particular New Guinea population who probably consume less than 1 g per day. The 24-hourly urinary sodium excretion for young adult subjects was 8·9 mmol (sodium chloride 0·5 g) per day for males and 18·5 mmol (sodium chloride 1·1 g) per day for females. By contrast the average daily sodium chloride intake is 10 g per day for Americans and 27 g per day for inhabitants of certain areas of Japan (Frank and Mickelsen, 1969).

While sodium excretion was low in the present population the urinary potassium output was high. The 24-hour urinary potassium values for young adults were 159 mmol per day for males and 171 mmol per day for females. These figures suggest a higher level of potassium intake than common amongst urban American subjects. Michelson *et al.* (1962) calculated that young American adults consumed 118 mmol of potassium per day. It is noted that sweet potato has a very low content of sodium and that 'native salt' is prepared from wood ash and is a potassium salt (Wills, 1958). However, as in European studies (Dawber *et al.*, 1967) no relationship was demonstrated between blood pressure and sodium output for individual subjects in this study.

Attention has been drawn to the possibility that high levels of potassium intake protects against hypertension in human beings (Trowell, 1978). In the present study a correlation between blood pressure and urinary potassium output was not demonstrated.

Accepting Rose and Blackburn's (1968) definition of hypertension as being a systolic blood pressure of 160 mmHg or more, and/or a diastolic blood pressure equal to, or greater than, 95 mmHg, then only 3 per cent of males over 40 years were hypertensive in the present population, in contrast to 20 per cent in the case of middle-aged American men (Epstein and Eckoff, 1967). Similarly there was little evidence of hypertensive cardiovascular disease.

Funduscopic examination was normal in all but 6 per cent of the population over the age of 40 years and these subjects showed no change greater than a grade 2 retinopathy. This is in contrast with a rate of 40 per cent in an American group reported by McDonough *et al.* (1965). In addition, left axis deviation was an uncommon electrocardiograph finding and no subject showed evidence of left-sided heart failure or previous cerebrovascular accident. Thus not only did blood pressure fail to rise with age but there was little evidence of either hypertension or its complications in this population.

Clinical evidence of arteriosclerosis including ischaemic heart disease

There was little evidence of the three major clinical complications of arteriosclerosis, namely ischaemic heart disease, peripheral vascular disease and cerebrovascular accident. Using the criteria of Rose and Blackburn (1968) a diagnosis of angina pectoris was made in only 2 subjects. Neither case showed any electrocardiographic abnormality. The dorsalis pedis and posterior tibial pulses were readily palpable in all subjects irrespective of age. It was possible to palpate the wall of the radial artery in only 12 subjects. Only 2 subjects gave a history suggestive of intermittent claudication but in neither was there any detectable diminution of the peripheral pulses. No subject showed evidence of Parkinson's disease or of previous cerebrovascular accident.

Despite the rarity of these complications of arteriosclerosis other degenerative changes were common, arcus senilis was present in 43 per cent of the population over the age of 40 years, cataract in 32 per cent, arthralgia in 15 per cent and greying and loss of hair were also common.

Standard resting 12 lead electrocardiographs carried out on 780 subjects over the age of 15 years, and supported by the post-exercise tracings, confirmed the rarity of ischaemic heart disease. The Q wave rate interpreted according to the Minnesota Code (Rose and Blackburn, 1968) was among the lowest so far reported for any population. In fact no large Q waves were detected among the people of Murapin. Further, unlike Western communities, ageing in this New Guinea community was associated with progressive right axis deviation and with an increasing prevalence in low voltage tracings (Sinnett and Whyte, 1973b; Sinnett, 1977b).

Population-based studies undertaken on Kar Kar Island off the coast of Madang and in Lufa in the Eastern Highlands of Papua New Guinea support the conclusions that arteriosclerosis and its complications are rare in traditional Papua New Guinea communities (Hornabrook *et al.*, 1974).

Venous varicosities

Vines (1970) in his epidemiological sample survey of Papua New Guinea claimed that varicosities of the venous system were rare in all areas, indeed, only 14 cases of lower leg variscosities were identified in 1805 subjects examined, a prevalence rate of 1·3 per cent. By contrast, Burkitt (1975a) claimed that varicose veins and haemorrhoids are among the commonest ailments in Western societies, and quotes figures showing that varicose veins affected between 10 and 17 per cent of adults in England and in North America. While the prevalence of varicose veins in Papua New Guinea is considerably lower than that in Western communities it is nevertheless above the prevalence rate of 0·12 per cent reported by Burkitt (1975a) for Ugandans as a result of a survey carried out in 1958.

Blood sugar levels and diabetes mellitus

The mean fasting blood glucose levels were 4·5 mmol per litre (80 mg/dl) for young men and 4·3 mmol per litre (77 mg/dl) for young women. Fasting blood glucose levels showed a modest rise with age in the case of male subjects but no increase was detected in the case of females. Post-prandial blood glucose estimations were carried out after an overnight fast and following the oral administration of 100 g of glucose. Only 3·8 per cent of the present population had a post-prandial blood glucose level in excess of 9 mmol per litre (160 mg/dl) in contrast to 20·9 per cent of people studied in the American National Health Survey (US Department of Health, Education and Welfare, 1964).

The clinical complications of diabetes were not detected in this population. No case of diabetic retinopathy was found and the population was free from any manifestation of peripheral vascular disease. These findings are in keeping with other population and hospital studies carried out in Papua New Guinea which indicate that diabetes mellitus is rare among rural populations and among groups which have had a relatively brief period of European contact (Hingston and Price, 1964). The low prevalence of diabetes mellitus is generally attributed to the low energy intake and to the absence of obesity in this group. However, a high intake of dietary fibre may be a significant contributing factor (Trowell, 1975).

Price and Tulloch (1966) in a study of 7512 subjects with varying lengths of residence in Port Moresby demonstrated that the prevalence of diabetes among groups with a brief period of European contact was 0·1 per cent of adult subjects. By contrast subjects living in the village of Hanuabada which has had close Western contact since 1874 and whose population has largely adopted European dietary patterns, had a 1·4 per cent prevalence of diabetes.

Serum cholesterol

Serum cholesterol levels are high in affluent communities such as the United States of America. In such populations a dietary pattern characterized by high intake of total energy, saturated fat, cholesterol, refined carbohydrate and a low intake of fibre is associated with a low level of habitual physical activity and obesity. By contrast people from Africa and the South Pacific generally have low serum cholesterol levels. These populations subsist largely on vegetable staples and have a low consumption of total energy, saturated fat, cholesterol and sugar but a high intake of complex carbohydrates and fibre (Burkitt, 1973). The people of Murapin have a low level of serum cholesterol which does not increase with age. The serum cholesterol value for young men was 4·7 mmol per litre (180 mg/dl) and for young women 5·0 mmol per litre (192 mg/dl).

There are at least four dietary factors which contribute to the low cholesterol values in this study—low energy intake, the quantity and quality of dietary fat, the low level of protein intake and the high fibre content of the diet.

Keys et al. (1950) have shown that low energy diets are associated with a reduction in serum cholesterol levels even when the intake of dietary lipids is constant. Further, Mann et al. (1955) demonstrated that an energy-induced increase in serum cholesterol could be prevented by a programme of exercise sufficient to dissipate the excess energy. Thus the high level of physical activity of these people is a significant factor contributing to their low serum cholesterol levels.

The low level of dietary fat intake is a second factor determining low serum cholesterol levels. The mean daily consumption of fat was 6·4 g for males and 9·8 g for females. The fact that this fat was derived from vegetable sources is also significant. Dietary cholesterol and saturated fats increase serum cholesterol levels while polyunsaturated fats have the reverse effect. Notable among population studies in which low levels of serum cholesterol have been reported in spite of high diet intakes of animal fat, are those of the Masai and Samburu tribesmen of Kenya. In depth metabolic studies of the Masai tribesmen reported by Taylor and Ho (1971) confirmed previous observations that the Masai were in fact consuming 12·5 MJ (3000 kcal) per day, 66 per cent of which was derived from animal fat. In spite of this the serum cholesterol levels were a modest 4 mmol per litre (150 mg/dl). These studies demonstrated that the Masai had a much greater capacity to suppress endogenous cholesterol synthesis than did North Americans.

The low protein content of the diet of the people of Murapin is another factor affecting serum lipid levels. Olson et al. (1958) demonstrated that the reduction in protein intake to 25 g a day resulted in a decrease in serum cholesterol and lipoproteins, even when the total energy and the fat intake remained constant. Thus below a critical level in protein intake there is a reduction in cholesterol levels which can be wholly corrected by protein replacement. It is interesting to note that this critical level (25 g per day) corresponds to the observed level of protein intake in the present study. Replacement of animal protein by protein derived from vegetable sources results in a decrease in serum cholesterol. Methionine is considered to be the limiting amino acid in vegetable protein and it has been postulated that low levels of this amino acid result in a decrease in available methyl groups and a subsequent reduction in choline synthesis. A further factor which has a potential influence on the serum cholesterol levels in this study is the high fibre content of the sweet potato.

Cancer

In 1958 a Cancer Register was established for Papua New Guinea. The average annual incidence rate for cancer per 100 000 subjects was 15·9 for males and 11·7 for females. Under-reporting undoubtedly contributed to these low incidence rates. In spite of this, certain trends emerge from the analysis of the data in the registry. For instance, the reported incidence rates for cancer of the lip and mouth in the highlands were low compared with other geographical areas of Papua New Guinea. Burkitt's lymphoma was present throughout Papua New Guinea in proportions as high as in West Africa and presenting with the same clinical features. Liver cancer rates were high, likewise malignant tropical ulcers and basal cell carcinoma were of frequent occurrence (Scott, 1974).

Clezy (1974) drew attention to the fact that the rate of colon and rectal cancer was low in Papua New Guinea, average annual reporting rates per 100 000 being 0·6 for males and 0·2 for females for cancers of the large bowel. By contrast Burkitt (1975b) quotes an incidence rate for cancer of the colon and rectum per 100 000 population as 41·6 in the United States of America, 51·5 for Scotland, 38·1 for England, 14 for South India and 3·5 for Uganda. Clezy believed that under-reporting alone was insufficient to account for the extremely low incidence rates for cancer of the colon and rectum in Papua New Guinea.

Conclusion

Infectious diseases presented the major health problem for the people of Murapin, a traditional Papua New Guinea community. By contrast arterio-sclerosis and its various manifestations, including coronary heart disease, cerebrovascular disease and peripheral vascular disease were rarely encountered. In keeping with the virtual absence of these conditions there was little evidence of those characteristics considered to be 'coronary risk factors' in Western societies. The diet was low in total energy, saturated fats, refined carbohydrates and salt, while the intake of complex carbohydrates, fibre and potassium was high. A high level of habitual physical activity assured that cardiopulmonary fitness was maintained well into middle-age. Obesity, diabetes and hypertension were uncommon. Although smoking was a common pastime among these people the practice resembled pipe rather than cigarette smoking. In the wider context of Western disease as defined by Burkitt (1973) carcinoma of the large bowel and varicose veins were also uncommon in Papua New Guinea.

Continued economic expansion associated with developments in education, nutrition and technology, as well as improvement in the health services, can be predicted to decrease infant mortality and to increase life expectancy. The resulting changes in the age structure of the population, together with alterations in lifestyle, including changes in physical activity, dietary patterns and psychological stress, seem likely to increase the incidence of those diseases considered characteristic of Western society. Already there is evidence that diabetes is increasing in urban areas (Price and Tulloch, 1966). Likewise there is an indication that coronary artery disease is also becoming more common (Aiken *et al.*, 1974).

References

Aiken, G. H., Lytton, D. G. and Everingham, S. (1974). Atherosclerotic heart disease in urbanised Papua New Guineans. *Papua New Guinea Medical Journal,* **17,** 248–250

Brookfield, H. C. (1964). The ecology of highland settlement: some suggestions. *American Anthropologist,* **66,** 20–38

Burkitt, D. P. (1973). Some diseases characteristic of modern western civilization. *British Medical Journal,* **1,** 274–278

Burkitt, D. P. (1975a). Varicose veins, deep vein thrombosis and haemorrhoids. In: *Refined Carbohydrate Foods and Disease: Some Implications of Dietary Fibre,* 143–160. Editors D. P. Burkitt and H. C. Trowell. Academic Press, London

Burkitt, D. P. (1975b). Benign and malignant tumours of large bowel. In: *Refined Carbohydrate Foods and Disease: Some Implications of Dietary Fibre,* 117–133. Editors D. P. Burkitt and H. C. Trowell. Academic Press, London

Burkitt, D. P., Walker, A. R. P. and Painter, N. S. (1972). Effect of dietary fibre on stools and transit-times, and its role in the causation of disease. *Lancet* **ii,** 1408–1412

Cleary, G. J. and Blackburn, R. B. (1968). Air pollution in native huts in the Highlands of New Guinea. *Archives of Environmental Health (Chicago)* **17,** 785–794

Clezy, J. K. A. (1974). Cancers of the gastro-intestinal tract. In: *The Epidemiology of Cancer in Papua New Guinea,* 76–83. Editors L. Atkinson, J. K. Clezy, P. S. Reay-Young, G. C. Scott and S. C. Wigley. Department of Public Health, Konedobu, Papua New Guinea

Commonwealth Bureau of Census and Statistics (1968). *Age Structure of the Population Excluding Aborigines at the Census of 30th June, 1966, Adjusted for Misstatement of age*. Canberra

Commonwealth Bureau of Census and Statistics (1969). *Summary of Vital and Population Statistics: June Quarter, 1969*. Canberra

Cooke, R. A. and Kariks, J. (1970). Myocardial infarction in Papua New Guinea. *Medical Journal of Australia*, **2**, 1242–1244

Dahl, L. K. (1963). Metabolic aspects of hypertension. *Annual Reviews of Medicine*, **14**, 69–98

Dawber, T. R., Kannel, W. B., Kagan, A., Donabedian, R. K., McNamara, P. M. and Pearson, G. (1967). Environmental factors in hypertension. In: *The Epidemiology of Hypertension*, 255–257. Editors J. Stamler, R. Stamler and T. H. Pullman. Grune and Stratton, New York

Epstein, F. H. and Eckoff, R. D. (1967). The epidemiology of high blood pressure—geographic distributions and etiological factors. In: *The Epidemiology of Hypertension*, 155–166. Editors J. Stamler, R. Stamler and T. H. Pullman. Grune and Stratton, New York

Epstein, F. H., Ostrander, L. D., Johnson, B. C., Payne, M. W., Hayner, N. S., Keller, J. B. and Francis, T. (1965). Epidemiological studies of cardiovascular disease in a total community—Tecumseh, Michigan. *Annals of Internal Medicine*, **62**, 1170–1187

Essai, B. (1961). *Papua and New Guinea: a Contemporary Survey*, 1–12. Oxford University Press, Melbourne

Forbes, G. B. and Reina, J. C. (1970). Adult lean body mass declines with age: some longitudinal observations. *Metabolism*, **19**, 653–663

Frank, R. L. and Mickelsen, O. (1969). Sodium–potassium chloride mixtures as table salt. *American Journal of Clinical Nutrition*, **22**, 464–470

Golson, J. (1970). *Foundations for New Guinea Nationhood*. Presidential Address, ANZAAS, August, 1970, Port Moresby, Papua

Hingston, R. G. and Price, A. V. G. (1964). Diabetic surveys in Papua. *Papua New Guinea Medical Journal*, **7**, 33–35

Hipsley, E. H. and Clements, F. W. (1947). *Report of the New Guinea Nutrition Survey Expedition, 1947*. Department of External Territories, Canberra

Hornabrook, R. W., Crane, G. G. and Stanhope, J. M. (1974). Karkar and Lufa: an epidemiological and health background to the human adaptability studies of the International Biological Programme. *Philosophical Transactions of the Royal Society of London, B*, **268**, 293–308

Kariks, J. and McGovern, V. J. (1967). Heart disease in the Territory of Papua-New Guinea: a preliminary report based on a necropsy study. *Medical Journal of Australia*, **1**, 176–177

Keys, A., Brozek, J., Henschel, A., Michelsen, O. and Taylor, H. L. (1950). *The Biology of Human Starvation*, Vol. 1. University of Minnesota Press, Minneapolis

Maddocks, I. (1967). Blood pressures in Melanesians. *Medical Journal of Australia*, **1**, 1123–1126

Magarey, F. R., Kariks, J. and Arnold, L. (1969). Aortic atherosclerosis in Papua and New Guinea compared with Sydney. *Pathology*, **1**, 185–191

Malcolm, L. A. (1970). *Growth and Development in New Guinea—a Study of the Bundi people of the Madang Subdistrict*. Institute of Human Biology Monograph Series No. 1, Madang, New Guinea

Mann, G. V., Teel, K., Hayes, O., McNally, A. and Bruno, D. (1955). Exercise in the disposition of dietary calories. Regulation of serum lipoprotein and cholesterol levels in human subjects. *New England Journal of Medicine*, **253**, 349–355

Mathews, C. L. (1974). Cardiovascular disease in Lae—a five year review. *Papua New Guinea Medical Journal*, **17**, 251–262

McDonough, J. R., Hames, C. G., Stulb, S. C. and Garrison, G. E. (1965). Coronary heart disease among negroes and whites in Evans County, Georgia. *Journal of Chronic Diseases*, **18**, 443–468

Michelson, I., Thompson, J. C., Hess, B. W. and Comar, C. L. (1962). Radioactivity in total diet. *Journal of Nutrition*, **78**, 371–383

Norgan, N. G., Ferro-Luzzi, A. and Durnin, J. V. G. A. (1974). The energy and nutrient intake and the energy expenditure of 204 New Guinean adults. *Philosophical Transactions of the Royal Society of London, B*, **268**, 309–348

Olson, R. E., Vester, J. W., Gursey, D., Davis, N. and Longman, D. (1958). The effect of low protein diets on the serum cholesterol of man. *American Journal of Clinical Nutrition*, **6**, 310

Price, A. V. G. and Tulloch, J. A. (1966). Diabetes mellitus in Papua and New Guinea. *Medical Journal of Australia*, **2**, 645–648

Rose, G. A. and Blackburn, H. (1968). *Cardiovascular Survey Methods*. World Health Organization Monograph Series No. 56, Geneva

Scott, G. C. (1974). Some epidemiological features of the Papua New Guinea cancer survey. In: *The Epidemiology of Cancer in Papua New Guinea*, 16–23. Editors L. Atkinson, J. K. Clezy, P. S. Reay-Young, G. C. Scott and S. C. Wigley. Department of Public Health, Konedobu, Papua New Guinea

Sinnett, P. F. (1977a). Nutritional adaptation among the Enga. In: *Subsistence and Survival: Rural Ecology in the Pacific*, 63–90. Editors T. Bayliss-Smith and R. Feachem. Academic Press, London

Sinnett, P. F. (1977b). *The People of Murapin*. Institute of Medical Research, Monograph Series No. 4, Papua New Guinea. E. W. Classey Ltd., Oxford

Sinnett, P., Keig, G. and Craig, W. (1973). Nutrition and age-related changes in the body build of adults: studies in a New Guinea Highland community. *Human Biology in Oceania*, **II**, 50–62

Sinnett, P. F. and Solomon, A. (1968). Physical fitness in a New Guinea population. *Papua New Guinea Medical Journal*, **11**, 56–59

Sinnett, P. F. and Whyte, H. M. (1973a). Epidemiological studies in a Highland population of New Guinea: environment, culture, and health status. *Human Ecology*, **1**, 245–277

Sinnett, P. F. and Whyte, H. M. (1973b). Epidemiological studies in a total

Highland population, Tukisenta, New Guinea. Cardiovascular disease and relevant clinical, electrocardiographic, radiological and biochemical findings. *Journal of Chronic Diseases,* **26,** 265–290

Society of Actuaries. (1959). *Build and Blood Pressure Study. Chicago,* **1,** 16

Tanner, J. M., Whitehouse, R. H. and Takaishi, M. (1966). Standards from birth to maturity for height, weight, height velocity and weight velocity for British children, 1965. *Archives of Disease in Childhood,* **41,** 454–613

Taylor, C. B. and Ho, K. J. (1971). Studies on the Masai. *American Journal of Clinical Nutrition,* **24,** 1291–1293

Trowell, H. (1975). Diabetes mellitus and obesity. In: *Refined Carbohydrate Foods and Disease: Some Implications of Dietary Fibre,* 227–249. Editors D. P. Burkitt and H. C. Trowell. Academic Press, London

Trowell, H. C. (1978). Hypertension and salt. *Lancet,* **ii,** 204

US Department of Health, Education and Welfare. (1964). *Glucose Tolerance of Adults.* United States, 1960–1962. National Center for Health Statistics, Series 11, No. 2, Washington

Vines, A. P. (1970). *An Epidemiological Sample Survey of the Highlands, Mainland and Island Regions of the Territory of Papua and New Guinea.* Department of Public Health, Territory of Papua and New Guinea, Port Moresby.

Whyte, H. M. (1958). Body fat and blood pressure of natives of New Guinea: reflections on essential hypertension. *Australasian Annals of Medicine,* **7,** 36–46

Wigley, S. (1967). Personal communication

Wills, P. A. (1958). Salt consumption by natives of the Territory of Papua and New Guinea. *Philippine Journal of Science,* **87,** 168–188

Woodhill, J., Palmer, J. and Blackett, R. (1969). Dietary habits and their modification in a coronary prevention programme for Australians. *Food Technology in Australia,* **21,** 264–271

13

Uganda West Nile district

Edward Williams and Peter Williams

West Nile district and Kuluva Hospital

From 1941 one doctor (E. H. W.), and from 1948 the second doctor (P. H. W.), have treated Ugandans at Kuluva Hospital, Arua, the administrative head-quarters of the West Nile district of Uganda. This district lies on the border of Uganda with the Sudan to the north and Zaire to the west. Communications with the central more populated districts of Uganda have always been difficult and lengthy: the river Nile separates the two regions. Economic development started only in the 1930s, later than in other areas of Uganda. Cash income per head is lower in this district than in other parts of Uganda. A mixture of Nilotic tribes, principally Alur, Madi, Lugbara and Kakwa, live as peasant agriculturalists; they came as a part of the Nilotic invasion of Uganda and Kenya several hundred years ago.

Kuluva Hospital has 108 beds for Ugandans. During the past 38 years over 150000 Ugandan patients have been treated as inpatients or out-patients. An inpatient's record is filed with the outpatient's notes, thus providing a single continuous account of the various illnesses of each person. Both of us speak fluently one or more of the local languages: this has obviated the limitations imposed by interpreters; it has also gained the confidence of patients. All outpatients and inpatients are seen by a doctor; none is left to be treated exclusively by a nurse or medical assistant.

About 50 Europeans and 150 Asians, and in recent years a few Arabs, have been treated each year at the hospital. They suffer from infections, often tropical in character. Europeans and Asians also suffer from the usual pattern of diseases encountered in all Western countries; Arabs occupy an intermediate position.

Diagnostic facilities have included the normal instruments used by a clinician, also specialized ophthalmological instruments, portable x-rays, electrocardiograph and laboratory equipment for the examination of blood and excreta, also a rocking microtome. An operating theatre has permitted the treatment of the common surgical diseases. Autopsies have not been performed because of considerable public feeling.

Life and diet of West Nile Ugandans

Formerly all West Nile Ugandans were peasant agriculturalists. Latterly a small but increasing proportion have regular employment locally as artisans, clerks and other occupations. Even nowadays almost all Ugandan men and women have much physical activity every day; they dig by hand their food-producing land, all work demands much muscular exertion, and they walk or cycle long distances. Many of the young men travel to the more developed and richer districts of Uganda and obtain work as labourers or in more skilled occupations; then they return home years later.

The diet of these peasants reflects their background and the small amount of cash that they can spend in purchasing food. Home-grown grain, usually some of the millets, provide the staple crop and food; they are processed at the homestead and provide fibre-rich starchy food, also vegetable protein and vitamins. Cassava flour may be mixed with the ground cereal meal; a little cassava was added in the 1940s, this increased in the 1950s, but was found to be of low nutritional value and has decreased in recent years. Maize meal has become increasingly popular. Lentils, groundnuts and green vegetables of the spinach variety, also cabbage recently, all provide relish to the basic starchy foods. Green vegetables are boiled thoroughly and their water is not consumed. Sweet bananas are plentiful and many of them are eaten raw.

Owing to the low cash income bought foods constitute only a small portion of the total diet, but nowadays even the poorest purchase all necessary salt and at least some sugar. The traditional 'salt' in the West Nile was similar to that described by the first governor of Uganda, Johnston (1902), who wrote: 'Salt is made by burning reeds and water-plants.' This salt substitute is rich in potassium but contains very little sodium. In 1941, when one of us (E. H. W.) arrived, shop salt had already come into fairly general use for some time. During the past four years of increasing economic difficulty in Uganda shop salt has been in short supply and there has been some attempt to revive the traditional method of preparing the plant salt substitute.

Sugar has become very popular; increasing amounts were being purchased until the price became prohibitive during the past four difficult years. It was being purchased in large amounts to make very sweet milky tea, drunk early in the day and at evening festive occasions. Those able to afford it, traders, artisans, government officials and church workers, purchased large amounts, such as those revealed by a dietary survey in Kampala, capital of Uganda, in the early 1960s. There the average daily intake of a Ugandan adult was reported to be 100 g and the level of consumption has probably risen to approximate that of the West. Tea is purchased and is the favourite drink. Nile fish is purchased; much of this has been salted to aid preservation. Fresh meat is only an occasional luxury. Simsim oil and cotton seed oil, both usually of local East African manufacture, are purchased by those able to afford them, to aid cooking and palatability. In the diet of the upper socioeconomic groups sugar, cooking oils, milk, fish and meat all increase, with a decrease in the proportion of the home-grown starchy staple foods. This reduces the intake of minerals, vitamins and fibre. During the recent economic difficulties there has been a change back towards the local produced home-grown foods and a decrease of all purchased foods. Cigarette smoking has increased during recent decades but remains low in comparison with Western levels. Western-type beer and spirits show increased consumption in the wealthier classes.

Unusual pattern of disease

Obesity

Unless the rains fail, West Nile peasants have always grown more than enough of their staple foods, but storage can mean that a variable amount is lost. In the 1940s it was quite unusual to see a stout man or woman. In recent years, however, a fair number of upper-class middle-aged West Nile women have begun to look rather stout, and some men have become very obese, especially those who hold lucrative posts and can purchase whatever food they like.

Hypertension

Essential hypertension, displaying itself in one of its accompanying complications, was not diagnosed among hospital patients for the first 19 years; it began to be diagnosed in the 1960s. One of us (P. H. W.), with special interests in ophthalmology, worked at Kuluva Hospital for ten years before the typical fundal changes of hypertension began to make their appearance in the 1960s, together with very high systolic and diastolic blood pressures. Stroke and resultant hemiplegia are encountered, but it is not possible to compare the incidence of these diseases with that prevailing in Western nations, as a smaller proportion of West Nile Ugandans are elderly, even if the proportion, to judge from our clinical impression, is increasing. The clinical manifestations of essential hypertensive disease appeared to be restricted almost exclusively to upper socioeconomic groups. An increased consumption of sugar was a recent feature of their diets, so that patients were advised to reduce severely its consumption. Patients appeared to benefit from this reduced intake of sugar and it proved possible to decrease the dosage of hypotensive drugs.

Diabetes

The emergence of the mature type of diabetes mellitus has been followed with considerable interest by one of us (E. H. W.), who, although he had previous experience of this disease in Britain, failed to diagnose a single case in his first nine years' residence at Kuluva Hospital in the 1940s. Meanwhile several cases of diabetes were diagnosed and treated in the small Asian communities resident in the West Nile district. In the 1950s typical cases of the mature type of diabetes mellitus began to be diagnosed in West Nile Ugandans. They complained of polyuria, thirst and lassitude; many were thin, and only a minority were overweight. In the early 1950s only half a dozen Ugandan diabetic patients were diagnosed each year; then the number increased until 50–70 new patients a year were diagnosed in the 1960s, but during the recent years of economic difficulties, there has been a substantial reduction in this number. Sugar consumption increased much in the 1950s, so that it was considered that this might be a causative factor. Campbell (1960) had reported a comparable association of increased consumption of sugar and a rising prevalence of diabetes in South African Bantu. The decreased consumption of sugar in recent years has coincided with a decreased number of new diabetic patients reporting for treatment. Most patients responded well to hypoglycaemic drugs, only a minority required insulin.

Ischaemic heart disease

Ischaemic heart disease, myocardial infarction, and angina remain still very rare conditions in West Nile Ugandans, as in all other East Africans (Vaughan, 1978a). These diseases, although emerging, are still uncommon in South African Bantu (Seftel, 1978).

Stool characteristics

The characteristic stool of the West Nile Ugandans is large and soft, it is passed easily, usually twice daily. If a faecal specimen is required for microscopy it can be produced immediately. If a day passes without a stool action, a West Nile Ugandan regards this as truly alarming.

Haemorrhoids

Haemorrhoids were seen only once or twice a year in the 1940s and early 1950s, have increased steadily since then so that about three or four patients each month have asked for treatment of their haemorrhoids during the past four years.

Varicose veins

The incidence of varicose veins has not been specially studied by us; they were seldom noticed during the 1960s, but are seen fairly often nowadays, although patients seldom complain about them or ask for treatment.

Appendicitis

This is certainly a very rare disease in West Nile Ugandans, even nowadays. Only three appendicectomies have been performed by us among them during the 37 years of our residence; not one of these three appendices showed evidence of acute appendicitis. Typical cases, proved at operation, have occurred in the few Europeans, Asians and Arabs resident in this district. Failure to detect this disease in our Ugandans cannot be explained by lack of transport; many cases of strangulated hernia are admitted. The hospital is situated near the district headquarters township of Arua; several thousand young Ugandans live in the vicinity; many are at school, other institutions, or in regular employment and must report sickness.

Dental caries

During the 1940s and 1950s dental caries was seen occasionally, but extractions for pain were seldom requested. At that time extractions were performed for root infections and abscess formation. At the present time caries is commonly seen in Ugandan adolescents and young adults; this occurs most frequently in the first, second and third molar teeth.

Thyrotoxicosis

Although thyrotoxicosis can often be recognized by the typical exophthalmos, we have diagnosed the disease only twice in West Nile Ugandans.

Cholesterol gallstones

Cholesterol gallstones have never been diagnosed, but the population contains fewer elderly Africans, and specialized methods of x-ray examination are seldom undertaken.

Peptic ulcer

We do not consider we are in a position to comment on the incidence of this disease, but the complications of perforation, haemorrhage or stenosis have never been diagnosed.

Other diseases

Rheumatoid arthritis has been diagnosed on only two occasions, one man and one woman.

Pernicious anaemia has never been diagnosed.

Renal calculus and ureteric colic have been diagnosed only once in a Ugandan adult male who had a large staghorn calculus.

Discussion

This seemingly peculiar pattern of non-infective disease in West Nile Ugandans is similar to that seen formerly in many rural hospitals in the less developed areas of Africa (Trowell, 1960; Gelfand, 1976). Slowly the pattern changes as development occurs: this change is not restricted to the emergence of ischaemic heart disease; it is only that this disease has been studied more than other disorders. Lifelong low blood pressure levels and the virtual absence of essential hypertension and stroke have been described in many developing communities, but always at the earliest stage of development. It is still being detected in a few undeveloped communities such as the Mzigua tribe of Tanzania (Vaughan, 1978b). The rarity of diabetes mellitus in the Bantu rural areas of South Africa has been demonstrated in careful surveys (Politzer, 1960), also in Malawi (Davidson, 1963). The virtual absence of acute appendicitis in West Nile Ugandans is paralleled by its complete absence in the first thousand Kenyan autopsies (Vint, 1936–37), although it occurs nowadays commonly in Nairobi Kenyans. In other diseases many may consider that our West Nile data are not weighty, for instance they have not been related to age and sex, and have not been verified by autopsies. This is freely acknowledged; possibly it will lead to better surveys of the prevalence and incidence of Western diseases in the future, and eventually, let it be hoped, the identification of environmental factors.

References

Campbell, G. D. (1960). The incidence of diabetes mellitus in one district of Basutoland. *South African Medical Journal*, **34**, 332

Davidson, J. C. (1963). The incidence of diabetes in Nyasaland. *Central African Journal of Medicine*, **9**, 92–94

Gelfand, M. (1976). The pattern of disease in Africa and the Western way of life. *Central African Journal of Medicine*, **21**, 145–152

Johnston, H. (1902). *The Uganda Protectorate*. Hutchinson, London

Politzer, W. M. (1960). Indicence of diabetes mellitus in Basutoland: possible nutritional factors. *South African Medical Journal*, **34**, 1037–1039

Seftel, H. C. (1978). The rarity of coronary heart disease in South African Blacks. *South African Medical Journal*, **52**, 99–105

Trowell, H. C. (1960). *Non-Infective Disease in Africa*. Edward Arnold, London

Vaughan, J. P. (1978a). A review of cardiovascular diseases in developing countries. *Annals of Tropical Medicine and Parasitology*, **72**, 101–109

Vaughan, J. P. (1978b). A cardiovascular survey in rural Tanzania. *East African Medical Journal*, **55**, 380–388

Vint, F. W. (1936–37). Postmortem findings in the natives of Kenya. *East African Medical Journal*, **13**, 332–340

14

Zimbabwe

Michael Gelfand

Zimbabwe Africans' diet and lifestyle

The country of Rhodesia became Zimbabwe in 1980, but in this chapter the shorter terms Zimbabwe Africans (or just Africans) and Rhodesian Europeans (or just Europeans) will be used to distinguish the two main ethnic groups before independence came to Zimbabwe.

Zimbabwe Africans total at present six and a half million; two million live in the townships, four and a half million in rural areas, and one and a half million live on European farms. Comparatively few of those living in the townships are true urban dwellers, for most of them retire to their rural homes after middle-age; also during their sojourn in the urban areas there is continual movement from town to country and back again. Rhodesian Europeans number at present about half a million.

Zimbabwe Africans have accepted many of the material features of Western culture, such as its dress and economic system. Western foods have come into vogue, although in both rural and urban areas traditional foods still predominate: white bread, refined sugar, jam and tea are all popular nowadays and are taken between the two main meals of lunch and dinner. These main meals consist of large portions of stiff porridge, usually made from maize meal, and eaten with a vegetable relish and some meat or fowl occasionally. Breakfast, a modern innovation, eaten even by rural inhabitants, consists largely of tea with milk and sugar and one or two slices of white bread and jam. Salt has been in common use by Africans for a long period of time.

It was commonly said that African men and women employed by Europeans, usually as cooks, were liable to indulge in rich dishes, thereby predisposing themselves to certain diseases, such as appendicitis and peptic ulcer. However, after investigating this matter closely, I am unable to prove this association, although the figures definitely showed that urban Africans were more prone to develop both these diseases than rural Africans (Gelfand, 1971).

Psychological aspects

It is often considered that a westernized way of life, with its increased tensions

194

(a rather vague term), is a factor in the increased incidence of the so-called stress diseases, seen commonly in Western Europe. The African too has his tensions and stresses: who is to judge whether his cares are greater or fewer than those experienced by the Westerner? The difference may lie in the different ways of reacting to these stresses. It is difficult to find an accurate means of measuring the state of tension in a black or a white man.

Perhaps an indication may be found in the suicide rates in the two races. Like other workers, I was able to show that suicides among Rhodesian Europeans were, relative to population numbers, about ten times more frequent than among Zimbabwe Africans, despite the many acute problems faced by the latter. We delved further into the matter in order to determine whether Africans, living in a more traditional environment in a rural tribal area, committed suicide less frequently than Africans living in urban areas under more Western conditions. To our surprise there was no difference between the two groups. Actually there were slightly more suicides in the rural than in urban areas. On the other hand, it was interesting that there were a far greater number of attempted suicides (parasuicides) amongst young Africans, especially girls, than in any other section of the African population. None the less, the frequency of parasuicides in Rhodesian Europeans is still ten times higher than in Zimbabwe Africans (Gelfand, 1976).

Cardiovascular diseases

General considerations

Autopsy evidence from South Africa has indicated that atheroma is less severe in Bantu than in whites, especially in aorta, coronary and iliac arteries. Thus Reef and Isaacson (1962) and Meyer *et al.* (1964) reported less atheroma in the aorta and coronary vessels of Bantu; but the cerebral vessels were almost equally affected in both racial groups.

In South Africa and Zimbabwe some workers consider that Africans are beginning to show more manifestations of atherosclerosis than formerly. As African ways change to a Western pattern, the diet becoming rich in refined sugar and animal fats, it has been considered that more cardiovascular degenerative disease would become manifest. This is not easy to demonstrate in Zimbabwe Africans. It would be difficult to provide proof that any cardiovascular degenerative diseases are increasing in Zimbabwe Africans, except, perhaps, myocardial infarction and angina.

Coronary heart disease and angina

Twenty-five or thirty years ago, we were aware that we were not noticing cases of myocardial infarction, or angina pectoris, conditions that are associated with atherosclerosis. When a patient was encountered with an anginal type of pain another cause was usually found, such as aortic incompetence, due to syphilis, or pericardial disease, commonly due to tuberculosis. For the first time in 1958 I met a Zimbabwe woman, employed as a nanny in a European household in Salisbury, with a typical history of anginal pain, and her ECG revealed an inversion of T waves in leads I and II (Gelfand and Kaplan, 1958).

In Salisbury during the next few years few patients, if any, were seen with this condition. At Mpilo Hospital, Bulawayo, no example of coronary heart disease (CHD) was reported in a review of 564 cases of heart disease among Africans (Baldachin, 1963). In Salisbury during the following year the second case of CHD in an African was reported (Forbes and Newey, 1964). Four years later another example of CHD in an African male, aged only 21 years, was confirmed at autopsy (Buchanan, 1968).

However, it is only within the last decade, 1968–78, that CHD has been encountered with any degree of regularity in Zimbabwe Africans in Salisbury. Thus during the three years 1975–77 (inclusive) some 44 African patients at Harare Hospital, Salisbury, were diagnosed as cases of myocardial infarction. The increased number of cases diagnosed each year may be partly explained by the great increase of the Zimbabwe population of Salisbury. In spite of this it is probable that CHD is increasing in Africans, but is still uncommon.

The Salisbury pathologists also recorded the slow emergence of CHD in Zimbabwe Africans in the 1960s. Ross (1969) reported no less than ten CHD autopsies among Africans. Over the period January 1968 to August 1969 a total of 1604 autopsies had been performed on African cases of sudden or unnatural death: among these, the CHD rate was only about 1 per cent During the same period 236 autopsies had been performed on Rhodesian Europeans and CHD had been reported in 46, a rate of nearly 20 per cent. The Africans with CHD had been mainly elderly persons; only two of them appeared to have been influenced much by westernization of diet and lifestyle, so that Ross (1969) could not decide whether westernization of the diet or the Western way of life had been responsible for the emergence of CHD.

Rhodesian Europeans suffer from the usual high incidence of CHD encountered in Western communities and among them diabetes and hypertension are strong risk factors in the production of myocardial infarction. Nearly half a million Europeans have settled for many years in Zimbabwe. A larger proportion of them, compared to the Africans, are in the older age groups; among the latter many, however, are over 55 years of age. In Salisbury during the three years 1975–77 (inclusive) there were 1103 European CHD patients in the Andrew Fleming Hospital, but only 44 African CHD patients in Harare Hospital. Among the 1103 European CHD patients 353 also had hypertension; among the 44 African CHD patients only 9 also had hypertension. During these three years at these hospitals 1227 Europeans and 1058 Africans had been treated for hypertension. It would appear therefore that essential hypertension is in Africans a much less severe CHD risk factor than in Europeans. Diabetes mellitus also does not appear to be a CHD risk factor in Africans; none of the 703 African diabetic patients treated at Harare Hospital during these three years developed myocardial infarction.

The rarity of angina pectoris in Zimbabwe Africans even at the present time is a puzzle, particularly since myocardial infarction is beginning to rise in incidence. I would have expected more cases.

Arteriosclerotic gangrene

Arteriosclerotic gangrene in the lower extremities is a well recognized disorder in Western communities. During the three years under review, 1975–77 (inclusive), only 5 cases were diagnosed in Harare Hospital (African) in contrast to 12 cases in Andrew Fleming Hospital (European), although the latter patients were derived from a much smaller population.

Essential hypertension and strokes

Essential hypertension is commonly seen in Zimbabwe in both races. During the three years under review, 1975–77 (inclusive), 1058 cases were admitted into Harare Hospital (African) compared to 1227 cases into Andrew Fleming Hospital (European). It might appear that hypertension is less common in Africans, but as this is a silent disease, until complications occur, judgement should be reserved until blood pressure surveys in the two racial groups, in terms of age, sex and body build, offer a true basis for comparison.

During the same three years under review 286 cases of stroke were diagnosed in Harare Hospital (African) compared to 308 in Alexander Fleming Hospital (European).

Diabetes mellitus

I have seen diabetes mellitus in Zimbabwe Africans ever since I started medical practice in a large urban African hospital nearly 38 years ago. It had been predicted that the Western way of life, especially dietary changes such as increased consumption of sugar, even possibly that of fats, would result in much increased prevalence of diabetes. In rural areas there have been no reports of any increased prevalence in spite of greater consumption of sugar and perhaps fats. In urban areas there may have been a slight, but insignificant, increase; certainly no striking change, especially when the enormous increase of the African urban population, and their increased life-span, is remembered.

Rural areas

In rural areas diabetes is still a rare disease among Zimbabwe Africans. For instance, during the three years 1975–77 (inclusive), the urines of all in-patients and out-patients were tested at a hospital in the former tribal trust land of Mtoko, which served a population of 40 000 Africans. Only one case of glycosuria was detected; this was a member of the nursing staff, who had arrived only recently in the district (Guidotti and Gelfand, 1976). During 1971 a similar survey had been carried out in the African hospital of the Mount Darwin district, and not a single case of glycosuria had been discovered (Wicks *et al.*, 1973).

Urban areas

In urban areas there may have been a slight, but insignificant, increased incidence of diabetes among Zimbabwe Africans. Carr and Gelfand (1961) conducted a diabetes survey in the Highfield African Township of Salisbury; they found very few cases in the general population. Ten years later a similar survey was conducted in the African population of the same township; I found more cases but the rise in the prevalence was only slight and of doubtful significance. During the three years 1975–77 (inclusive) 703 African diabetics were treated at Harare Hospital, and 529 European diabetics at Andrew Fleming Hospital, Salisbury. In attempting to compare these figures, it must be remembered that the African population of Salisbury is four to five times that of the European, but there are fewer Africans in older age groups. In spite of these uncertainties I consider that maturity-onset diabetes is still less prevalent among urban Africans than among Europeans.

During 1967, when the African population in the Salisbury district was 280 000, the Harare Hospital (African) had 137 diabetic patients. During 1977, when the Salisbury African population had increased to 480 000, the same hospital had 234 diabetic patients. One might argue that there had been no increase of diabetes during this decade, in spite of the greater consumption of sugar and perhaps fat in the urban population.

In my experience diabetes mellitus of juvenile onset is still a very rare disease in Zimbabwe African children (Gelfand, 1975).

Complications

All cardiovascular complications of diabetes are rare in Zimbabwe African patients. During the three years 1975–77 (inclusive) no case of coronary heart disease was detected among 703 African diabetics in Harare Hospital, Salisbury, compared with 42 cases of coronary heart disease among 629 European diabetics at Andrew Fleming Hospital, Salisbury. Diabetic gangrene does, however, occur in Zimbabwe Africans: during the three years of review there were 12 cases in the African diabetics and 12 cases in the European diabetics.

Gout

Although the cause of gout is not known, this metabolic disorder is associated with affluence and good living. In the three years 1975–77 (inclusive) 14 African patients suffering from gout were in Harare Hospital, compared with 67 European patients in Andrew Fleming Hospital, Salisbury. Gout is much commoner in Europeans than in Africans in Zimbabwe.

Non-infective gastrointestinal disease

Peptic ulcer

It had been feared that increasing westernization of the African diet and lifestyle, especially in urban areas, would be accompanied by an increase in these disorders. Certainly duodenal ulcer and gastric ulcer are far more commonly diagnosed in urban Africans than in rural Africans (Gelfand, 1971; Friedlander and Gelfand, 1978). However, if the total number of peptic ulcer cases at Harare Hospital, Salisbury, in 1967, drawn from an African population of about 280 000, is compared with the figures of 1977 from a population of about 480 000, there has been no significant increase. On the other hand Wapnick and Gelfand (1973) considered that peptic ulcer had been increasing in both urban and rural areas in a slow and steady manner over a long period of time.

Gastroenterologists in Britain consider that gastric ulcer and duodenal ulcer have different aetiological factors and a different epidemiology, so that they should be considered separately. In Zimbabwe there is some evidence that the incidence of duodenal ulcer has increased over the last two decades. When I carried out a prospective study of the causes of haematemesis and acute intestinal haemorrhage in 1957, and again in 1971, there appeared to have been an undue rise in the number of cases ascribed to duodenal ulcer compared with cirrhosis (Gelfand, 1965; 1974).

Acute appendicitis

Acute appendicitis certainly occurs much less often in Africans than in Europeans: there is also a lower incidence of this disease in the rural African populations compared with urban populations. In 1949 I had been able to show that the incidence of acute appendicitis was ten times less in Africans than in Europeans (Gelfand, 1950). This large difference has not decreased. For instance, during the three years 1975–77 (inclusive) there were only 277 African cases of appendicitis in Harare Hospital, compared with 1079 European cases in Andrew Fleming Hospital, Salisbury, and the latter were drawn from a population about one-quarter of the size of the former. Acute appendicitis is therefore about 17 times less common in Africans than in Europeans. I specially investigated the place of origin of these African patients and found that almost all had been working in the Salisbury urban area; very few had lived in, or been referred from, the adjoining countryside. Most had eaten the usual diet of urban Africans; only a few had been cooking for Europeans and might have eaten much European food.

In 1967 in Salisbury 51 African patients, drawn from a population of 280 000, were treated for acute appendicitis. In 1977 there were 118 African appendicitis patients from a population of 480 000. The low incidence rate of acute appendicitis in Africans therefore appears to have been stationary in the urban areas of Salisbury. Among Africans acute appendicitis is predominantly a disease of the adult, mostly between the ages of 20 and 45 years, but in Europeans it is largely a disease of children and adolescents.

The very low incidence of acute appendicitis in rural Africans is illustrated by two enquiries. I studied the incidence of acute appendicitis in a mission hospital in the tribal trust lands of Katarere, a medical centre for 30 000 Africans: one case of appendicitis had been diagnosed in the four years 1969–72 (inclusive). At all Souls Mission in Mtoko area, a medical centre for a similar number of Africans, no case of acute appendicitis had been diagnosed during the whole of 1971. By way of contrast cases of acute appendicitis were comparatively frequently diagnosed in Salisbury urban Africans during all these years.

Diverticular disease

Diverticular disease is a Western disease rarely encountered in Zimbabwe Africans, although many reach 60 or 70 years of age (Levin and Wapnick, 1972; Moffat and Gelfand, 1974). In the two years 1967 and 1968 no case was reported at Harare Hospital in Salisbury. During the three years 1975-77 (inclusive) only four African cases were admitted to Harare Hospital in contrast to 128 cases seen in the smaller European population at the Andrew Fleming Hospital, Salisbury. This may be due to the higher cereal fibre content of the African diet, derived from the maize meal, adding bulk to the stool and rendering constipation much less likely.

Carcinoma of the colon and rectum

Colorectal cancer, like diverticular disease, shows striking differences in incidence in Europeans and Africans living in Zimbabwe. During the three years 1975-77 (inclusive) Harare Hospital (African) admitted 19 patients with cancer of the colon and 36 with cancer of the rectum in contrast to Andrew Fleming Hospital (European), which admitted 110 patients with cancer of the colon and 62 with cancer of the rectum. The African diet, high in cereal fibre and low in fat, may account for this difference.

In the two-year period 1967-68 (inclusive) 14 cases of colon cancer and 14 of rectal cancer were observed in Salisbury Africans (Ross, 1967). In the two years 1976 and 1977 14 colon cancers and 27 rectal cancers were seen in Salisbury Africans. As the African population had nearly doubled between these periods there appears to have been no rise in incidence of large bowel cancer.

Ulcerative colitis

No case of ulcerative colitis was diagnosed at Harare Hospital (African), Salisbury during the two years 1967 and 1968 (Sealey and Gelfand, 1968). Again no case of ulcerative colitis was encountered at the same hospital during the three years 1975-77 (inclusive). This disease is not uncommon among Europeans; 27 patients were treated at the Andrew Fleming Hospital during the same three years, derived from a much smaller population. Our experience of the rarity of ulcerative colitis in Africans is similar to that of other parts of Africa.

Other diseases

Gallstones

Cholesterol gallstones are much less common in Africans than in Europeans in Zimbabwe. During the three-year period 1975–77 (inclusive) in Harare Hospital, Salisbury, 13 African patients, derived from a population of 480 000, were diagnosed to have gallstones. On the other hand in Andrew Fleming Hospital, Salisbury, 203 European patients, derived from the much smaller population of 105 000, were diagnosed to have gallstones.

Stones in kidney, ureter and bladder

Kidney and ureteric stones are much less common in Africans than in Europeans. During the three years 1975–77 (inclusive) in Harare Hospital, Salisbury, 54 African patients were diagnosed to have kidney and ureteric stones, but in Andrew Fleming Hospital 588 European patients were diagnosed to have these calculi. These stones are particularly common amongst Westerners living in Zimbabwe.

Bladder stone prevalence is different. During the same three years 91 patients having bladder stone were seen in the Harare Hospital (African); 20 patients having bladder stone were seen in the European hospital. As the African population of the Salisbury district is about four times that of the European, bladder stone appears to have a comparable prevalence in both communities.

Anorexia nervosa

For a long time I have been interested in this disease, which reflects the psychological strain imposed on Western adolescents, especially girls. This disorder has been encountered regularly, even if not frequently, in European girls, but I have not yet met the disorder in an African. During the three years 1975–77 (inclusive) no case of anorexia nervosa was diagnosed in Harare Hospital (African), but seven cases were treated in Andrew Fleming Hospital (European).

Autoimmune and endocrine disorders

It would prolong the scope of this chapter to produce evidence concerning the rarity of many autoimmune diseases in Zimbabwe Africans (Gelfand, 1975). Pernicious anaemia is very rare and I have never seen subacute combined degeneration, nor multiple sclerosis, in an African. The rarity of ulcerative colitis has already been discussed. Rheumatoid arthritis too is much rarer in Africans. Thyrotoxicosis was previously very rare in Zimbabwe Africans (Gelfand, 1962), but I am beginning to see a few cases of true Graves' disease nowadays. Hashimoto's thyroiditis is rare. Sjogren's disease is also seldom seen.

In fact all endocrine disorders are rarely diagnosed in Africans. Addison's disease has been encountered in Salisbury Africans, but other endocrine disorders, such as Cushing's disease, acromegaly and hyperparathyroidism, are uncommon. Endocrine diseases may be under-reported in Zimbabwe, but the apparent rarity of many endocrine disorders has made me consider that Africans have a stable endocrine system (Gelfand, 1975). Cancer of the female breast is certainly less common in Zimbabwean than in European women.

Summary

I have witnessed changes in the pattern of many non-infective diseases in Zimbabwe Africans. The prevalences of certain diseases have increased but those of others have not changed. Essential hypertension has for long been common in Zimbabwe Africans: I found the disease already present when I started medical practice in a large African hospital nearly 40 years ago. There is no evidence that the prevalence of essential hypertension has increased in Zimbabwe Africans since that time. Hypertension predisposes to cardiac failure and cerebrovascular attacks; these occur in Africans as frequently as in Western communities, but hypertension does not, at present, predispose to myocardial infarction. Coronary thrombosis has begun, only recently, to emerge in Zimbabwe Africans and angina remains a rare disease. Most coronary thrombosis patients have lived in urban areas; a minority, however, have lived in rural areas and followed a traditional manner of life.

Diabetes mellitus is still a rare disease in Africans living in certain rural areas. It is commoner in urban areas. The incidence of diabetes may be rising in urban areas, but this is doubtful.

Acute appendicitis occurs far less frequently among Africans than Europeans; among the former the incidence is much lower in rural than in urban communities. Diverticular disease is very uncommon in Africans compared with Europeans; ulcerative colitis is a very rare disease in Africans and cancer of the colon is less common. Cholesterol gallstones occur far less frequently in Africans; this is also true of kidney and ureteric stones, but not of bladder stones. Autoimmune disorders and endocrine diseases are far less commonly diagnosed in Africans than in Europeans. Thyrotoxicosis was certainly very rare in Africans but has been increasing.

Whilst there have been changes in the African diet, such as an increased consumption of white bread, sugar and animal fat, with a decreased proportion of maize meal in the diet, I find it impossible to pinpoint specific features causing the appearance of the so-called Western diseases. I consider that these changes in disease incidence reflect the reaction to the Western way of life. Both Africans and Europeans are affected by pressures resulting from working to the clock. Perhaps thyrotoxicosis and even duodenal ulcer reflect psychological pressures. There is some evidence that duodenal ulcer has been increasing in recent years, probably more in urban than in rural areas.

References

Baldachin, B. J. (1963). Cardiovascular disease in the African in Matabeleland. *Central African Journal of Medicine,* **9,** 463–469
Buchanan, W. (1968). Coronary artery occlusion in an African male of 21 years. *Central African Journal of Medicine,* **14,** 80

Carr, W. R. and Gelfand, M. (1961). The incidence of diabetes mellitus in the African. A survey carried out in Highfield, Salisbury, Southern Rhodesia. *Central African Journal of Medicine*, **7**, 332–335

Forbes, J. I. and Newey, W. (1964). Myocardial infarction in the African. *South African Medical Journal*, **38**, 786–788

Friedlander, M. and Gelfand, M. (1978). Duodenal ulcer, largely an urban disease in Africans in sub-tropical Africa. *Tropical Doctor*, **8**, 205–206

Gelfand, M. (1950). *Schistosomiasis in South Central Africa. A clinico-pathological study*, 19, 190. Juta, Cape Town

Gelfand, M. (1962). Thyrotoxicosis in the African. Report of a case. *Central African Journal of Medicine*, **8**, 123–124

Gelfand, M. (1965). Haematemesis in an African male ward. *Central African Journal of Medicine*, **11**, 366–368

Gelfand, M. (1971). The pattern of disease in Africa. *Central African Journal of Medicine*, **17**, 69–78

Gelfand, M. (1974). Haematemesis in the African. A comparison of the two main causes after a ten year interval. *Central African Journal of Medicine*, **20**, 100–101

Gelfand, M. (1975). The pattern of disease and the Western way of life. *Central African Journal of Medicine*, **21**, 145–152

Geland, M. (1976). Suicide and attempted suicide in the urban and rural African in Rhodesia. *Central African Journal of Medicine*, **22**, 203–205

Gelfand, M. and Kaplan, M. (1958). Bantu coronary insufficiency. Report of a possible case. *Central African Journal of Medicine*, **4**, 157–159

Guidotti, L. and Gelfand, M. (1976). Frequency of diabetes in Mtoko. *Central African Journal of Medicine*, **22**, 28–29

Levin, L. and Wapnick, S. (1972). Cholelithiasis, diverticular disease and hiatus hernia in the Rhodesian African. *Central African Journal of Medicine*, **18**, 25–27

Meyer, B. J., Pepler, W. J., Meyer, A. C. and Theron, J. J. (1964). Athero-sclerosis in Europeans and Bantu. *Circulation*, **29**, 415–421

Moffat, H. J. and Gelfand, M. (1974). Diverticulosis in a Rhodesian African male. *Central African Journal of Medicine*, **20**, 188–190

Reef, H. and Isaacson, C. (1962). Atherosclerosis in the Bantu. The distribution of atheromatous lesions in Africans over 50 years of age. *Circulation*, **28**, 66–72

Ross, M. D. (1967). Tumours in Mashonaland Africans (Part 1). *Central African Journal of Medicine*, **13**, 107–116

Ross, M. D. (1969). Death due to coronary atheroma in Rhodesian Africans. *Central African Journal of Medicine*, **15**, 247–249

Sealey, B. J. and Gelfand, M. (1968). Ulcerative colitis in the Mashonaland African. *Central African Journal of Medicine*, **14**, 173–175

Wapnick, S. and Gelfand, M. (1973). Peptic ulcer in the Rhodesian African. *South African Medical Journal*, **47**, 625–628

Wicks, A. C. B., Castle, W. M. and Gelfand, M. (1973). The effect of time on the prevalence of diabetes in urban Africans in Rhodesia. *Diabetes*, **22**, 733–737

15

Pacific islands of Nauru, Tuvalu and Western Samoa

Paul Zimmet and Sunny Whitehouse

'Sometimes I've thought of an island
   lost in a boundless sea,
Where I could live in some hidden valley,
   among strange trees in silence.
There I think I could find what I want.'

The Moon and Sixpence by W. Somerset Maugham (1919)

Introduction

Increasing numbers of people in developed and Western societies dream, as did Somerset Maugham, of a carefree and idyllic life on some remote South Pacific island paradise. It must come as a great surprise to these people to discover that the inhabitants of the Polynesian paradise they dream of do not necessarily share this Utopian dream. Most of the Pacific island nations are engaged in the race to get into the twentieth century—a race towards the competitiveness and technological progress that initially bypassed them. Today, the modern lifestyle has permeated into the very core of even the most isolated Pacific populations.

As many populations in the Pacific changed from subsistence to cash economies, a drastic change in lifestyle occurred. Modernization has had dramatic effects on many aspects of these societies and, in many instances, there have been major changes in the cultural, social, moral, health and economic components of their society. Arthur Koestler has labelled this process 'Coca-colonization' (Koestler, 1976).

The price paid for civilization has been high for the people who have enthusiastically embraced our Western lifestyle. Coincident with this, there has been a pronounced increase in chronic degenerative diseases such as diabetes, hypertension, gout, obesity and vascular disease—conditions previously rare in these societies but major causes of morbidity and mortality in Western populations (Prior, 1974).

Since white man first arrived in the Pacific region with his two inevitable companions—alcohol and new diseases—there have been two disastrous waves of diseases previously unknown in the Pacific islands. The first wave was that of certain infectious diseases; chronic degenerative diseases, in relation to westernization, constitute the second wave (Zimmet, 1979).

A Pacific viewpoint of epidemiological transition

The change in patterns of diseases in developing countries may best be understood by considering the concept of epidemiological transition (Leading article, *Lancet*, 1977). There are three recognizable stages in the epidemiological transition. These can be examined using the Pacific region as the model, but are equally applicable to many developing countries (Zimmet, 1979).

1. *Stage 1—era of pestilence and famine*
2. *Stage 2—receding pandemics*
3. *Stage 3—era of degenerative and man-made diseases*

It is the third stage of the epidemiological transition and its effect on Pacific populations, particularly relating to diabetes, hypertension, gout and vascular disease that will be covered in this chapter.

The problems caused by the third stage, 'era of degenerative and man-made disease', are not just Pacific ones. A global pattern of the emergence of these diseases can be clearly seen affecting many populations; for example, Yemenite Jews (Cohen *et al.*, 1961), the Indian population of South Africa (Marine *et al.*, 1969), and the American Indians (West, 1974), to mention but a few. Yet this pattern is not necessarily an inevitable consequence of modernization, and certain ethnic groups appear to have a relative protection against these diseases, e.g. Melanesians and Eskimos (Zimmet, 1979; Mouratoff *et al.*, 1967).

The concept of epidemiological transition should prove useful in our historical appraisal of population dynamics in developed and developing countries. More important, it should enable us to identify emerging patterns of disease, understand their causes and, having done so, to deal with them in their appropriate demographic, social and economic contexts.

Background information on populations studied

Over the last four years, we have had the opportunity to study several populations in the Pacific region. These include the Tuvaluans and Western Samoans (both Polynesian) and Nauruans (Micronesian). The degree of modernization varies considerably among these groups. Background information and results of these studies are reported in greater detail elsewhere (Zimmet *et al.*, 1977a, b; 1978a; Zimmet, 1978).

Tuvalu

The country of Tuvalu (formerly the Ellice Islands) is composed of a group of eight islands in the 'Polynesian Triangle' in the Central Pacific (Fig. 15.1).

The inhabitants are Polynesians, and the islands are believed to have been originally settled from Samoa. Their culture has many similarities to those of the people of Samoa, Tonga, and the Tokelau Islands. Funafuti is the main island and is famous as the atoll studied by scientists from the Royal Society of London in 1896 to determine the nature of atoll structure and the study proved Charles Darwin's theory on their origins. Fuller background and demographic information can be found elsewhere (Zimmet *et al.*, 1977a).

The atoll soil is poor and supports a limited number of crops—only coconut and pandanus grow naturally. The only economic crop is copra, but considerable foreign exchange is generated by the periodic release of attractive stamps. Of Funafuti's present population of 2000, only half are indigenous, i.e. have traditional family connections in Funafuti.

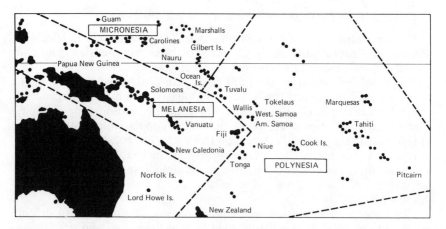

Fig. 15.1   Map of the Pacific region showing the three geoethnic areas of Melanesia, Micronesia and Polynesia

Until World War II, there was little development or European influence in Funafuti. While Western foods such as rice, flour, sugar, and canned meats were sometimes available as the result of occasional visits by trading ships, the islanders maintained a subsistence economy and a traditional diet and lifestyle. The main items of the diet were fish, coconut, breadfruit, and pulaka (*Cyrtosperma chamissonis*).

With Allied occupation and the establishment of an important naval and air base in 1943, many of the islanders entered a cash economy for the first time. The modernization of lifestyle commenced then and a growing dependence on imported goods resulted. At the present time, 85 per cent of the islanders' food requirements are imported. The lifestyle has changed as outboard motor boats replace the canoes for fishing, and motorcycles and motor cars become the main forms of land transport.

Western Samoa

Almost half way between Hawaii and Australia lies a group of islands known as the Samoas (Fig. 15.1). The islands are situated 2600 miles south-west of Hawaii and 2700 miles east of Sydney. Western Samoa consists of two large islands, Upolu and Savai'i, with several other smaller islands.

The total area of the islands is 700 000 acres and they are mountainous in character. For the most part, a dense blanket of forest covers the land, completely overshadowing the narrow coastal fringe which supports the bulk of the population and their plantations. Western Samoa possesses the world's largest Polynesian population; 90 per cent of the 150 000 inhabitants are full-blooded Polynesians.

The climate of Western Samoa favours primary production and copra and cocoa processing, fruit and fish canning and tourism are the main sources of income. As in many Pacific islands the stimulus of increasing westernization is changing the lifestyle of the Western Samoans. Apia is quite cosmopolitan, being the site of the main government offices, several luxury hotels, restaurants and nightclubs.

Many paradoxes exist as a result of conflicts between traditional Samoan cultural values and the steadily increasing modern influences. Many families still grow their own staple foods—breadfruit, bananas and taro, or these are available and inexpensive at the local market. Yet the diet is liberally supplemented with canned goods, flour, sugar, beer, and other manufactured foods from the supermarkets or village stores. In Apia, many of the people work in sedentary positions, such as clerical jobs or in the stores.

In the rural areas, the effects of westernization are now being seen in dietary changes, but not to the same extent as in Apia. While the men in Apia are predominantly sedentary workers, the rural males work in the plantations. This involves heavy labour and also gives them and their families direct access to the basic staple foods which they themselves grow.

Nauru

Nauru is situated in the Central Pacific near the intersection of the three geoethnic areas—Melanesia, Polynesia, and Micronesia (Fig. 15.1). Its area is about 6263 acres, the island being 12 miles in circumference. It is one of the most isolated islands in the Pacific, being 2500 miles from Sydney, 1600 miles from Honolulu and 3000 miles from Tokyo. Fuller background and demographic information can be found elsewhere (Zimmet *et al.*, 1977b; Zimmet and Taft, 1978).

Phosphate deposits have made Nauru the world's richest nation based on per capita income. The 4000 Micronesian inhabitants of Nauru have an annual average per capita income of US$34 000. After independence in 1968, all of the proceeds from the phosphate bonanza finally came directly to the Nauruans. Until that time, the industry was controlled by the British Phosphate Commission.

In the ensuing decade, there has been unleashed an unbelievable burst of consumerism and modernization to the point that now the Nauruans are almost totally westernized. All food requirements are imported and luxury goods are snapped up as quickly as they appear on the shelves of the local stores. There are about 2000 motor vehicles and motor cycles for the 4000 inhabitants. Most of the heavy manual labour in the phosphate mine is performed by indentured Chinese labourers from Taiwan, and by other Pacific islanders (mainly from the Gilberts and Tuvalu).

Until now, we have not had the opportunity to study a completely traditional-living Pacific population. However, several other workers have reported diabetes prevalence rates in traditional populations in Micronesia and Polynesia. However, the groups we have surveyed provide marked contrasts in the degree of modernization. There is a progressive gradient from the less affected Funafutians and rural Western Samoans to the more urbanized town-living Western Samoans and fully urbanized Nauruans.

Diabetes in Pacific populations

There are three major ethnic groups in the Pacific region—Melanesians, Polynesians, Micronesians, and the geographic locations of their populations are shown in Fig. 15.1. This accident of nature presents the epidemiologist with exciting opportunities to study genetic and environmental susceptibility to disease in these different ethnic groups. On some islands, two of these differing ethnic groups live side by side under identical environmental conditions, allowing controlled studies of the role of genetic factors and diseases such as diabetes.

Owing to lack of standardization of survey methodologies and varying diagnostic criteria for diabetes, it is difficult to compare directly the various diabetes epidemiological studies that have been carried out in the Pacific region (Zimmet, 1979). However, broad patterns have emerged and it is quite clear that the diabetes prevalence is low in Melanesians (Cassidy, 1967; Zimmet, 1979), and certainly less than the 2 per cent prevalence rates reported for New Zealand and Australian Caucasians (Prior and Davidson, 1966; Welborn *et al.*, 1968). Similarly, diabetes is almost unknown in Polynesian or Micronesian populations where traditional lifestyle has been maintained (Zimmet, 1979). On the other hand a high diabetes prevalence ranging from 8·1 to 39·8 per cent has been reported in urbanized Australian Aboriginals, Micronesians, and Polynesians. In almost all instances, the diabetes is insulin-independent in nature (i.e. maturity-onset) (Zimmet, 1979).

We have conducted epidemiological studies in a number of Pacific countries including Nauru, Tuvalu, and Western Samoa. As the methodologies and diagnostic criteria have been standardized, the opportunity exists to compare disease patterns between the populations of these countries. These three countries are all undergoing the modernization process to varying degrees and for varying reasons, as discussed earlier.

Our prevalence studies were the first performed in each country and hospital records indicated that diabetes was virtually unknown prior to 1960. Yet, in each of these countries there has been an increase in the number of cases since then. We were unable to obtain evidence of any cases of diabetes in Funafuti, Western Samoa, or Nauru before 1945.

Diabetes prevalence in Funafuti, Western Samoa, and Nauru

As the methodology and diagnostic criteria for these studies were identical, direct comparison of prevalence rates is possible. Table 15.1 shows the age-adjusted diabetes prevalence rates in these studies both for the combined sexes and for males and females separately.

Table 15.1 Age-standardized prevalence of diabetes mellitus in Funafuti, Western Samoa and Nauru islanders, aged 20 years and over

Population	Diabetes prevalence[1]		
	Male (%)	Female (%)	Combined sexes
Funafuti	5·3	15·4	10·6
Western Samoa (rural)	2·8	6·2	4·6
Western Samoa (urban)	12·6	12·2	12·4
Nauru	41·9	42·3	42·1

[1] Diagnostic criteria for diabetes: patients with documented evidence of diabetes or a 2-hour post-loading plasma glucose of 8·9 mmol/l (160 mg/dl) or more after 75 g oral carbohydrate

As the degree of modernization progressed through rural Samoans and Funafutians to the highly modernized Nauruans, so did the overall diabetes prevalence show an increase with the lowest levels in rural Samoans (4·6 per cent) and highest in the Nauruans (42·1 per cent).

Similar trends were noted in both sexes. However, while the male : female rates were similar in urban Western Samoa and Nauru, diabetes was two to three times more common in the females in rural Western Samoa and Funafuti. Possible reasons for this difference are discussed later.

Possible aetiological factors for diabetes in these populations

Possible causative factors for the high diabetes prevalence rates in these populations have been discussed in greater detail elsewhere (West, 1974; Zimmet, 1979), but they are summarized below.

A diabetic genotype
The evidence available suggests that the Polynesians and Micronesians, like certain American Indian groups, have a diabetic genotype, and that clinical diabetes is unmasked by factors related to the change in lifestyle (Prior *et al.*,

1966; Zimmet, 1979). The familial associations for diabetes are quite striking in these populations (Prior and Davidson, 1966; Zimmet *et al.*, 1977b). In the smaller island populations considerable intermarriage has occurred so that the prevalence of any hereditary disease such as diabetes would be further amplified. Prevalence rates in Nauru are nearly four times those of other Pacific islanders and this may be the reason.

The diabetes in these populations is predominantly of the non-insulin dependent (maturity-onset) form (NIDDM). While strong associations have now been noted between certain HLA antigens (B8, BW15, DW3, and DW4) and the insulin dependent form of diabetes (IDDM), no such associations are documented for NIDDM (Nerup, 1978).

We have recently reported that there is an increase in frequency of the glyoxylase-2 (GLO2) allele, and a significant disturbance in the distribution of glyoxylase (GLO) phenotypes in Caucasian NIDDM patients (Kirk *et al.*, 1979). The GLO locus is on the short-arm of chromosome 6 close to the HLA locus. These new findings raise the possibility that there is a recessive susceptibility allele for NIDDM in association with the GLO2 allele. The demonstration of a genetic marker association other than HLA in diabetics allows new approaches to test genetic hypotheses for diabetes in these high prevalence populations. We are studying both the Nauruans and Western Samoans for similar associations to define the diabetic genotype. If a genetic marker can be demonstrated, then the earlier reported bimodality in frequency distributions of glucose levels in the Nauruans and urban Western Samoans may be of more than passing interest (Zimmet and Whitehouse, 1978; Zimmet, 1979).

The phenomenon of bimodality suggests that the Nauruans and Western Samoans can be divided into two subgroups—the first component representing normal subjects and the second component constituting diabetics (Fig. 15.2). Whereas unimodality implies a multiple gene causation of a disease such as diabetes, the presence of bimodality might suggest a single gene hypothesis for the inheritance of diabetes. Thus, we are at present studying the frequencies of certain genetic markers in the normal and diabetic components of the populations of Nauru and Western Samoa.

Definition of the genotype might allow identification of the people 'at risk' of developing diabetes with respect to the environmental factors involved, e.g. the genotype for NIDDM may render an individual susceptible to such factors as obesity, dietary excess, stress, certain viruses, or other as yet undefined environmental factors. An obvious analogy is that of IDDM where it appears that in the presence of certain HLA antigens mentioned earlier, there is a much higher chance of developing IDDM in Caucasian individuals carrying these particular antigens. These antigens may render an individual susceptible to the effect of an infective pancreotrophic virus (Nerup, 1978).

Obesity
For many centuries, obesity has been regarded as a sign of high social status and prosperity in Micronesian and Polynesian societies. Data are not

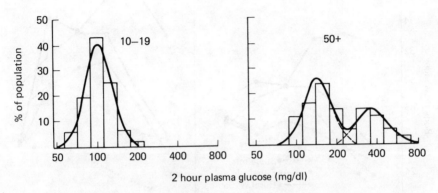

Naruan males

Fig. 15.2 Frequency distributions of the logarithms of 2-hour plasma glucose in male Nauruans 10–19 years and 50 years and over. Bimodality of glucose levels is clearly shown in the older group

available on the precise degree of obesity that existed in these societies, but pictorial records from Nauru (1925), as shown in Fig. 15.3, indicate that formerly the women were not particularly obese when compared with present-day standards. The present-day degree of obesity in Nauruans and Samoans is also very striking in comparison to Caucasian populations.

Fig. 15.4 shows the mean body mass index (weight/height^2) values by decades for males and females in the three Pacific populations compared to

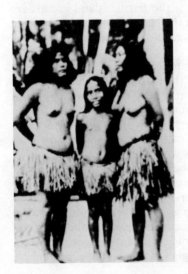 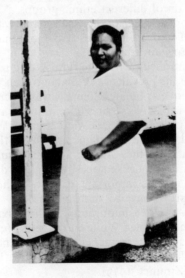

Fig. 15.3 A comparison of typical Nauruan women—1925 (left) and 1979 (right)

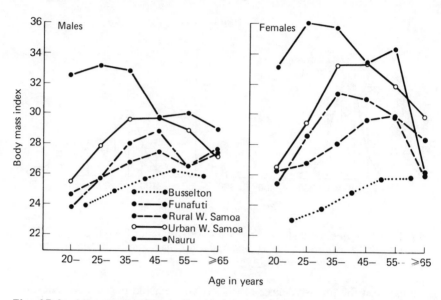

Fig. 15.4   Mean body mass index (weight/height²) by age group for males and females in Funafuti, Western Samoa and Nauru compared with the Australian Busselton (Caucasian) sample

an Australian Caucasian population (Busselton). The use of the body mass index, which takes into account weight and height, allows standardized comparison of different ethnic groups. All of the Pacific island groups are much more obese than the Caucasians, with the Nauruans showing extreme obesity. The degree of obesity is more marked in the females in all but the Australian Caucasians.

As mentioned earlier, the rural Western Samoans and Funafutian females had twice the prevalence of diabetes seen in the males. The difference in the degree of obesity, male to female, was much more marked in these two groups than the urban Western Samoan and Nauruans where the male to female diabetes prevalence rates were similar. West and Kalbfleisch (1970) have suggested that obesity in females explains the increased prevalence of diabetes in the countries they studied and our results would tend to confirm this.

In view of the marked obesity and high diabetes prevalence in the Nauruan population, it is important to assess what effect obesity has on the age-specific prevalence of diabetes in lean versus obese Nauruans. This is obviously of great importance in the debate as to the relationship between obesity and diabetes. While the diabetes prevalence for lean and obese subjects was similar in the younger (10–19 years) and older (40 years and over) groups, the prevalence rate was at least three times higher in the 20–39-year-old obese subjects (Zimmet, 1979).

This differing pattern of prevalence in relation to age suggests that the degree of obesity may influence the time at which diabetes appears rather than whether or not diabetes develops. These findings are in agreement with those of the Pima Indians (Bennett *et al.*, 1976). In both Nauruans and Pima Indians, high diabetes prevalence rates cannot be attributed solely to the marked obesity. However, the data cited here suggest that obesity may be a permissive or precipitating factor.

Dietary patterns
In each of the populations we have been studying, there has been a dramatic change in dietary patterns. Better transport facilities (both air and sea) and increasing affluence have resulted in major shifts to the consumption of foods more characteristic of the Western diet. The traditional diet (such as fish, coconuts, taro, breadfruit) has been discarded for a Western-style diet of imported goods (such as rice, sugar, flour, canned meats and vegetables, soft drinks, beer) low in dietary fibre and of dubious nutritional value.

Table 15.2 Mean nutrient intakes in Funafuti and Nauru islanders in comparison to American Caucasians

Nutrient	Funafuti		Nauru		Caucasian[1]
	Male	Female	Male	Female	General population
Energy (MJ)	13·1	11·0	30·0	22·0	13·2
(kcal)	3130	2620	7190	5220	3160
% carbohydrate	49	49	46	51	47
% fat	34	36	32	34	41
% protein	15	14	14	15	12

[1] Obtained from Reid *et al.* (1971)

As part of our studies of the health effects of modernization in Funafuti and Nauru we have carried out nutritional studies in the adult populations (Ringrose and Zimmet, 1979; Wicking *et al.*, 1980). Table 15.2 shows nutrient intakes of Funafutians and Nauruans compared to Caucasians (Reid *et al.*, 1971).

The distribution of nutrients (carbohydrate, fat and protein) of the two Pacific populations is very similar to that of Caucasians. This is in contrast to other Pacific populations where there is a higher contribution from carbohydrates (traditional foods) and lower contribution from protein (Hankin *et al.*, 1970). The energy intakes of the Nauruans are at least twice those of the Funafutians and Caucasians. However, as the Funafutians have a subsistence economy, the nutrient intakes are comparable with those of developed countries such as Australia and the United States of America. Seen in this context, they are high intakes for a developing Pacific country or, indeed, any developing country.

Reduced physical activity
In each of the countries studied, there have also been major changes in physical activity patterns with a definite tendency towards the sedentary Western style. Certainly, the high energy diet and reduced physical activity are likely culprits in relation to the marked obesity now seen in these populations. It seems more than likely that they also play major permissive roles in the high diabetes prevalence rates now being reported.

Stress—a diabetogenic factor?
Apart from changes in customs, diets and exercise patterns, the change to cash economy brings many psychosocial stresses. For many years, epidemiologists have been frustrated by the lack of an effective measure of stress to assess the psychosocial component. As a consequence, our assessment of the contributions of stress has been relatively superficial. An easy-going Pacific islander may find the change to a desk job and the responsibilities of a senior civil service post very stressful in contrast with his previous traditional lifestyle. It is almost impossible to assess what contribution stress may have in precipitating diabetes in people with a genetic susceptibility to the disease. Nevertheless, the possibility that stress may be a diabetogenic factor in this situation cannot be ignored. Proof of this hypothesis is difficult to obtain and will require the careful control of numerous other environmental determinants so that stress can be studied as a lone factor. Perhaps it is one of a number of factors which, in varying degrees of magnitude, have a role in the high diabetes prevalence.

Blood pressure studies in Funafuti, Western Samoa, and Nauru

Blood pressure studies in traditional-living populations have demonstrated that there is usually no change in systolic (SBP) or diastolic (DBP) pressure with increasing age (Lowenstein, 1961; Maddocks and Rovin, 1965; Prior, 1974; Sinnet and Whyte, 1978). However, both SBP and DBP rise with age in Caucasian populations, as well as in once traditional-living groups who have experienced the modernization process (Prior, 1974; Johnson *et al.*, 1965).

Fig. 15.5 shows mean SBP and DBP in Funafuti, rural and urban Western Samoan and Nauruan males and females. Both SBP and DBP rise with age in males and females of each population studied. The highest mean levels were seen consistently in the Nauruans and urban Western Samoans and lowest in the Funafutians and rural Western Samoans. Thus, as with the diabetes prevalence, the mean blood pressure rose in relation to the degree of modernization—lowest levels being in the less modernized groups and highest levels in the most modernized.

Table 15.3 shows the age-standardized sex specific prevalence rates for hypertension in the population studied. The lowest rates were seen in Funafuti males and rural Western Samoan females and the highest in Nauru males and urban Western Samoan females. Again, the trend in prevalence rates bears some relationship to the degree of modernization.

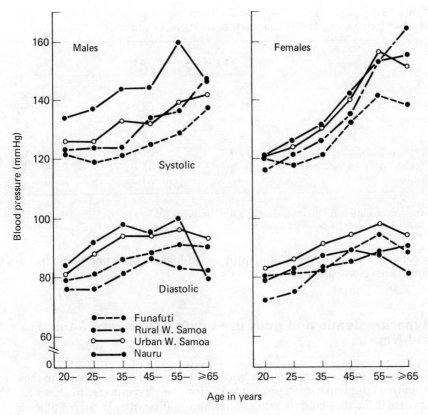

Fig. 15.5 Mean systolic and diastolic blood pressure by age group for males and females in Funafuti, Western Samoa and Nauru

Possible aetiological factors for hypertension

Our blood pressure findings are substantially in agreement with those of Prior and Tasman-Jones (see Chapter 16). They showed a progressive rise in mean blood pressure levels in Cook islanders and New Zealand Maoris with lowest levels in traditional-living islanders and highest levels in town-living subjects (Prior, 1974).

Perhaps the aetiological factors for hypertension are substantially the same as those we have already discussed for diabetes, i.e. heredity, obesity, diet, reduced physical activity, and stress.

These differing and paradoxical findings highlight the need for continued medical and anthropological research into the role of psychosocial and other factors in hypertension. Longitudinal studies such as the Tokelau Migrant Project (Beaglehole *et al.*, 1975; Stanhope and Prior, 1975) provide unique opportunities to produce such answers. They may demonstrate to what extent heredity, stress, diet, physical activity, etc., contribute, both individually and

Table 15.3 Age-standardized prevalence of hypertension in Funafuti, Western Samoa, and Nauru islanders, aged 20 years and over

Population	Hypertension prevalence[1]		
	Male (%)	Female (%)	Combined sexes (%)
Funafuti	11·6	20·2	16·1
Western Samoa (rural)	20·1	18·1	19·1
Western Samoa (urban)	35·7	37·0	36·4
Nauru	47·5	27·3	36·9

[1] Diagnostic criteria for hypertension: hypertension was defined by the World Health Organization criteria of blood pressure $\geqslant 160$ mmHg systolic and/or $\geqslant 95$ mmHg diastolic

in combination, to the escalating problem of hypertension and its complications in developing countries.

Hyperuricaemia and gout in Funafuti, Western Samoa, and Nauru

Diabetes, ischaemic heart disease, hypertension, and gout are rare in populations maintaining their traditional lifestyle and mainly appear in their urbanized counterparts (Zimmet, 1979). However, hyperuricaemia has been reported in Pacific islanders both affected and unaffected by Western influence (Prior *et al.*, 1966; Zimmer *et al.*, 1978b). Thus, the metabolic abnormality of hyperuricaemia is present in both environments.

Table 15.4 shows age-standardized prevalence rates for hyperuricaemia in the populations studied. While the prevalence rates were similar for the two Polynesian groups (Funafuti and Western Samoa), the rates were significantly higher in the Micronesian inhabitants of Nauru. This difference may well be due to genetic factors. Similar prevalence rates for hyperuricaemia to those in our Polynesians have been reported in the Polynesian populations studied by Prior and his group (Prior *et al.*, 1966).

Further evidence that hyperuricaemia is genetically determined and unrelated to the extent of environmental change comes from studies in the American Pima Indians. This urbanized population has an extremely high prevalence of diabetes comparable with that of the Nauruans, but their mean serum uric acid concentrations are about half those of the Nauruans and much lower than those of American Caucasians. The prevalence of hyperuricaemia in Pima Indians aged 30 years and over is 3·3 per cent (O'Brien *et al.*, 1966).

The highest prevalence of hyperuricaemia found by Prior and his colleagues occurred among Pukapukan men (48·5 per cent) and women (49 per

Table 15.4   Age-standardized prevalence of hyperuricaemia in Funafuti, Western Samoa and Nauru islanders, aged 20 years and over

Population	Hyperuricaemia prevalence[1]		
	Male (%)	Female (%)	Combined sexes (%)
Funafuti	32·3	35·7	36·9
Western Samoa (rural)	43·5	32·0	37·6
Western Samoa (urban)	36·7	25·1	30·1
Nauru	63·6	59·2	61·3

[1] Diagnostic criteria: serum uric acid, males $\geqslant 0·42$ mmol/l (7·0 mg/dl); females $\geqslant 0·36$ mmol/l (6·0 mg/dl)

cent). These workers suggested that there was a strong genetic predisposition to hyperuricaemia because the extent of the problem in the three Polynesian groups studied (New Zealand Maoris, Rarotongans, and Pukapukans) was remarkably similar despite great differences in their environments. The high rates found among the Polynesians contrasted with a prevalence of hyperuricaemia among New Zealand Caucasians of 23 per cent in men and 16 per cent in women (Prior and Davidson, 1966).

Table 15.5 shows age-standardized prevalence rates for gout in these same populations. While there were no documented cases of gout in Funafutian subjects and only a few cases in Nauruan females, the prevalence rates were similar in rural and urban Samoans and Nauruan males. Overall, the relationship between increasing modernization and gout prevalence was not as dramatic as that noted earlier for diabetes and hypertension.

Prior and his co-workers noted a higher attack rate of gout among the more urbanized Polynesians whom they studied. They suggested that environmental factors might influence the precipitation of clinical gout in subjects with a genetic predisposition. Our findings in Tuvalu, Western Samoa, and Nauru support the contention that, while the hyperuricaemia has a genetic basis, clinical gout is probably caused by the dramatic environmental change from a traditional to Western lifestyle.

Cardiovascular epidemiology and risk factors in Funafuti, Western Samoa, and Nauru

Coronary heart disease

Reported prevalence rates for cardiovascular disease show a wide variation in different Pacific ethnic groups. As has been noted for diabetes, prevalence rates vary between different ethnic groups and within the same ethnic group depending on the degree of modernization (Prior and Evans, 1970).

Table 15.5   Age-standardized prevalence of gout in Funafuti, Western Samoa and Nauru islanders, aged 20 years and over

| Population | Gout prevalence[1] | | |
	Male (%)	Female (%)	Combined sexes (%)
Funafuti	0	0	0
Western Samoa (rural)	6·2	2·3	4·2
Western Samoa (urban)	7·2	3·9	5·3
Nauru	6·9	0·4	3·5

[1] Diagnostic criteria: a history of typical podagra affecting joints of great toe or foot (Prior *et al.* 1966)

Table 15.6   Coronary risk factors[1] among Funafuti, Western Samoa and Nauru islanders, aged 20 years and over, with one or more coronary risk factors

| Population | One or more risk factors | | |
	Male (%)	Female (%)	Combined sexes (%)
Funafuti	37	56	46
Western Samoa (rural)	40	46	43
Western Samoa (urban)	60	70	66
Nauru	91	86	88

[1] Risk factors:
1. Body mass index $\geqslant 30$
2. Diastolic BP $\geqslant 95$ mmHg or systolic BP $\geqslant 160$ mmHg
3. Serum cholesterol $\geqslant 6·8$ mmol/l (260 mg/dl)
4. Serum triglycerides $\geqslant 1·8$ mmol/l (160 mg/dl)
5. Smoking $\geqslant 20$ cigarettes/day
6. Diabetes

While coronary heart disease is still rare in Funafuti, Western Samoa, and Nauru, Table 15.6 indicates high risk factor status ranging from 43 per cent of rural Western Samoans to 88 per cent of Nauruans with one or more cardiac risk factor. Again, the trend shows a rise in risk status with increasing westernization.

It is possible that, as the development of the pathological process of atherosclerosis may take 15–20 years, the full brunt of the morbidity and mortality from coronary heart disease may not be seen in these populations for several decades.

Cerebrovascular disease

Table 15.7 shows prevalence rates for strokes in the Western Samoan rural and urban populations. Of the 13 cases of documented stroke, there were only two rural subjects—the other 11 people were all from the urban sample. Ten of the 13 subjects were hypertensives. It seems likely that the high prevalence of stroke is related to the high prevalence of documented hypertension in Western Samoa.

Appendicitis

There is some evidence that appendicitis rates are increasing in the populations we have studied. Unfortunately, documentation of this is difficult because of the poor medical records available in most of the islands. During our Funafuti survey in 1976, pre-World War II surgical records were examined at the Funafuti hospital and no instances of appendicectomy were recorded. In the 30 years post-war, increasing numbers of appendicectomies were performed. In our own survey 5·8 per cent of the subjects 20 years and over had had their appendix removed. In the Western Samoans studied, 1·7 per cent of rural subjects and 5·7 per cent of urban subjects had had an appendicectomy.

From this limited information, it does appear that there has been an increase in appendicitis in these populations and, even today, rural Western Samoans have a lower prevalence of appendicitis than their urban counterparts. The rural dwellers are still eating significant quantities of their traditional fruits and vegetables which do have a high fibre content, whereas their urban counterparts tend towards a Western-style diet.

Conclusion

Our studies in these three Pacific populations add weight to the mounting evidence that the adoption of a Western lifestyle by developing communities is associated with a dramatic increase in the incidence and prevalence of certain chronic non-communicable diseases.

While changing environmental habits clearly play a role, it is difficult to ignore the fact that some of these populations may have a genetic susceptibility to some of these diseases and that the environmental changes unmask the disease state. Diabetes mellitus seems to provide a model situation to illustrate this (Zimmet, 1979). Diabetes is rare in Melanesians even after urbanization. However, certain American Indian tribes, also Polynesians and Micronesians show prevalence rates up to 20 times higher than Caucasians after undergoing the modernization process.

Table 15.7   Age-adjusted prevalence of stroke in Western Samoa rural and urban populations

Population	Stroke prevalence		
	Male (%)	Female (%)	Combined sexes (%)
Western Samoa (rural)	0·3	0·3	0·3
Western Samoa (urban)	2·5	0·7	1·5

Why, then, has the hereditary tendency to diabetes, which is potentially lethal, survived the process of natural selection? After all, it appears to have survived through centuries in certain Pacific populations such as Polynesians and Micronesians. Its survival can only be explained by the fact that it must have conferred some survival advantage at certain times in the past.

Neel has proposed that people with an hereditary tendency to diabetes were better able to store food as fat when food was abundant—the thrifty genotype hypothesis (Neel, 1962).

The Polynesians and Micronesians have been subjected to long periods of food deprivation—during their long canoe voyages and later on the isolated Pacific atolls where they finally settled. Famines, high environmental temperatures, hurricanes, and tidal waves were frequent occurrences. Those with a predisposition to diabetes may have been better equipped for survival than the people without it, as the latter could not store food to withstand the long canoe voyages and famine periods. It is probable that this hereditary factor was significant in terms of modulation and stabilization of population density in response to varying food availability. As such, the predisposition to diabetes has been maintained selectively in those communities where high temperatures and widely fluctuating food availability have been present during major evolutionary periods. Wise has produced laboratory evidence that the thrifty genotype hypothesis may operate in this manner in diabetes (Wise, 1977) and he has suggested that this is the reason for the high prevalence of diabetes in the Australian Aboriginal (Wise *et al.*, 1976).

At the present time with westernization and plentiful food supplies, this possible survival factor becomes useless and, in fact, deterimental and the disease diabetes manifests.

It does appear that there is a certain degree of inevitability about these diseases occurring and that only a return to traditional lifestyle can prevent their occurrence and escalation.

The epidemiologist, having defined the extent of these diseases in developing populations, is faced with the fact that most of the morbidity and mortality from these diseases is due to their complications. In Nauru, a significant proportion of the diabetic population now exhibit diabetic retinopathy, cataracts, diabetic nephropathy and neuropathy, and peripheral vascular

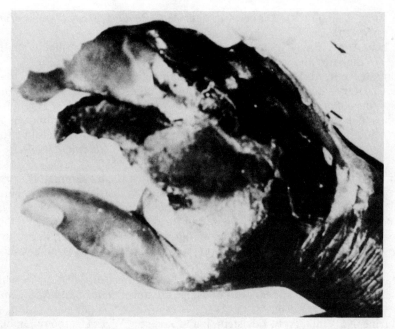

Fig. 15.6   Limb gangrene—a complication of diabetes that is becoming increasingly common in the islands

disease (Zimmet, 1979). Limb gangrene and infection is becoming increasingly common (Fig. 15.6) due to a combination of microangiopathy, neuropathy, and macro-vascular disease.

The full impact and severity of these chronic degenerative diseases in terms of the overall health of Pacific populations, as well as the serious morbidity and mortality of their complications, have yet to be fully manifested. These diseases are appearing in earlier age groups than in most westernized countries. As a result 30–40 per cent of the workforce in certain developing countries may have one or several of these chronic diseases which could render them disabled and unable to work. This fact alone could have serious implications on the economy in terms of productivity and an inevitable increase in cost of health care.

References

Beaglehole, R., Salmond, C. E. and Prior, I. A. M. (1975). A familial study of blood pressure in Polynesians. *International Journal of Epidemiology*, **4**, 217–220

Bennett, P. H., Rushforth, N. B., Miller, M. and Lecompte, P. M. (1976). Epidemiological studies of diabetes in the Pima Indians. *Recent Progress in Hormone Research*, **32**, 333–371

Cassidy, J. T. (1967). Diabetes in Fiji. *New Zealand Medical Journal,* **66,** 167–172

Cohen, A. M., Bavly, S. and Poznanski, R. (1961). Change of diet in relation to diabetes and ischaemic heart disease. *Lancet,* **ii,** 1399–1401

Hankin, J., Reed, D., Labarthe, D., Nichaman, A. and Stallones, R. (1970). Dietary and disease patterns among Micronesians. *The American Journal of Clinical Nutrition,* **23,** 346–357

Johnson, B. C., Epstein, F. H. and Kjelsberg, M. O. (1965). Distributions and familial studies of blood pressure and serum cholesterol levels in a total community. Tecumseh, Michigan. *Journal of Chronic Diseases,* **18,** 147–160

Kirk, R. L., Theophilus, J., Whitehouse, S., Court, J. and Zimmet, P. (1979). Genetic susceptibility to diabetes mellitus: the distribution of Properdin factor B (Bf) and Glyoxalase (Glo) phenotypes. *Diabetes,* **28,** 949–951

Koestler, A. (1976). *The Call Girls.* Pan Books, London and Sydney

Leading Article (1977). The epidemiological transition. *Lancet,* **ii,** 670–671

Lowenstein, F. W. (1961). Blood pressure in relation to age and sex in the tropics and sub-tropics. *Lancet,* **i,** 389–392

Maddocks, I. and Rovin, L. (1965). A New Guinea population in which blood pressure appears to fall as age advances. *Papua and New Guinea Journal of Medicine,* **8,** 17–21

Marine, N., Vinik, A. I., Edelstein, I. and Jackson, W. P. U. (1969). Diabetes hyperglycaemia and glycosuria among Indians, Malays and Africans (Bantu) in Cape Town, South Africa. *Diabetes,* **18,** 840–857

Mouratoff, G. J., Carroll, N. V. and Scott, E. M. (1967). Diabetes mellitis in Eskimos. *Journal of the American Medical Association,* **199,** 107–112

Neel, J. V. (1962). Diabetes mellitus: a thrifty genotype rendered deterimental by 'progress'? *American Journal of Human Genetics,* **14,** 353–362

Nerup, J. (1978). HLA studies in diabetes mellitis. *Advances in Metabolic Disorders,* **9,** 263–275. Editors R. Levine and R. Luft. Academic Press, New York

O'Brien, W. M., Burch, T. A. and Bunim, J. J. (1966). Genetics of hyperuricaemia in Blackfeet and Pima Indians. *Annals of Rheumatic Disorders,* **25,** 117–119

Prior, I. A. M. (1974). Cardiovascular epidemiology in New Zealand and the Pacific. *New Zealand Medical Journal,* **80,** 245–252

Prior, I. A. M. and Davidson, F. (1966). The epidemiology of diabetes in Polynesians and Europeans in New Zealand and the Pacific. *New Zealand Medical Journal,* **65,** 375–383

Prior, I. A. M. and Evans, J. G. (1970). Current developments in the Pacific. *Atherosclerosis: Proceedings of the Second International Symposium,* 335–342. Editor R. J. Jones. Springer-Verlag, New York, Heidelberg, Berlin

Prior, I. A. M., Rose, B. S., Harvey, H. P. B. and Davidson, F. (1966). Hyperuricaemia, gout and diabetic abnormality in Polynesian people. *Lancet,* **i,** 333–338

Reid, J. M., Fullmer, S. D., Pettigrew, K. D., Burch, T. A., Bennett, P. H.,

Miller, M. and Whedon, G. D. (1971). Nutrient intake of Pima Indian women: relationships to diabetes mellitis and gall bladder disease. *American Journal of Clinical Nutrition*, **24**, 1281–1289

Ringrose, H. and Zimmet, P. (1979). Nutrient intakes in an urbanized Micronesian population with a high diabetes prevalence. *American Journal of Clinical Nutrition*, **32**, 1334–1341

Sinnet, P. F. and Whyte, H. M. (1978). Lifestyle, health and disease: A comparison between Papua New Guinea and Australia. *Medical Journal of Australia*, **1**, 1–5

Stanhope, J. M. and Prior, I. A. M. (1976). The Tokelau Island migrant study: Prevalence of various conditions before migration. *International Journal of Epidemiology*, **5**, 259–266

Welborn, T. A., Curnow, D. H., Wearne, J. T., Cullen, K. J., McCall, M. G. and Stenhouse, N. S. (1968). Diabetes detected by blood sugar measurement after a glucose load: Report from the Busselton Survey, 1966. *Medical Journal of Australia*, **2**, 778–783

West, K. M. (1974). Diabetes in American Indians and other native populations of the New World. *Diabetes*, **23**, 841–855

West, K. M. and Kalbfleisch, J. M. (1970). Diabetes in Central America. *Diabetes*, **19**, 656–663

Wicking, J., Ringrose, H., Whitehouse, S. and Zimmet, P. (1980). Nutrient intake in a partly westernized isolated Polynesian population: The Funafuti survey. *Diabetes Care* (in press)

Wise, P. H. (1977). Significance of anomalous thermoregulation in the pre-diabetic spinymouse (Acomys Cahirinus): Oxygen consumption and temperature regulation. *Australian Journal of Experimental Biological Medical Science*, **55**, 463–473

Wise, P. H., Edwards, F. M., Craig, R. J., Evans, B., Murchland, J. B., Sutherland, B. and Thomas, D. W. (1976). Diabetes and associated variables in the South Australian Aboriginal. *Australian and New Zealand Journal of Medicine*, **6**, 191–196

Zimmet, P. (1978). Diabetes in Pacific populations—a price for Westernization. *Proceedings of 6th Asia and Oceania Congress of Endocrinology*, 256–265. Editor J. S. Cheah, Singapore

Zimmet, P. (1979). Epidemiology of diabetes and its macrovascular manifestations in Pacific populations: The medical effects of social progress. *Diabetes Care*, **2**, 144–153

Zimmet, P., Arblaster, M. and Thoma, K. (1978a). The effect of westernization on native populations. Studies on a Micronesian community with a high diabetes prevalence. *Australian and New Zealand Journal of Medicine*, **8**, 141–146

Zimmet, P., Seluka, A., Collins, J., Currie, P., Wicking, J. and Deboer, W. (1977a). Diabetes mellitus in an urbanized isolated Polynesian population. The Funafuti survey. *Diabetes*, **26**, 1101–1108

Zimmet, P. and Taft, P. (1978). The high prevalence of diabetes mellitus in Nauru, a Central Pacific island. *Advances in Metabolic Disorders*, **9**, 225–240. Editors R. Levine and R. Luft. Academic Press, New York

Zimmet, P., Taft, P., Guinea, A., Guthrie, W. and Thoma, K. (1977b). The high prevalence of diabetes mellitis on a Central Pacific island. *Diabetologia,* **13,** 111–115

Zimmet, P. and Whitehouse, S. (1978). Bimodality in fasting and two-hour glucose tolerance distributions in a Micronesian population. *Diabetes,* **27,** 793–800

Zimmet, P., Whitehouse, S., Jackson, L. and Thoma, K. (1978b). High prevalence of hyperuricaemia and gout in an urbanized Micronesian population. *British Medical Journal,* **1,** 1237–1239

Part V

Migrants and mixed ethnic groups

16

New Zealand Maori and Pacific Polynesians

Ian Prior and Clifford Tasman-Jones

Introduction

'He moana pukepuke e ekengia e te waka'

'Mountainous sea can be negotiated by the canoe.'
(Difficult problems can be solved by determination and effort.)

A Maori proverb.

Polynesian populations living in different parts of the Pacific provide a wide range of contrasts in their health and disease patterns. The rate of change is increasing in the Pacific, as in many other parts of the world, and there are a number of variables influencing the changes that take place. These include the varying physical environments, the extent of resources, the ways these are used, and a variety of factors which influence exposure of these populations to a Western style of living and to affluence. Some groups are living in an essentially traditional and subsistence economy, but even here some experience effects of 'subsistence affluence' that provide them with excess energy (calories) leading to obesity despite very little in the way of monetary resources. In contrast, other groups have more limited resources and are at much greater risk from hurricanes and periodic food shortages. The opportunities to develop obesity and its sequelae are much more limited in these groups. Polynesians are one of the distinct Pacific ethnic groups. They inhabit the 'Polynesian Triangle' which extends from Hawaii in the north, to Easter Island in the east and New Zealand in the south (see Fig. 15.1). The principal Polynesian populations are found in Hawaii, French Polynesia, Cook Islands, Western Samoa, American Samoa, Tonga, Niue, Tuvalu, Tokelau and New Zealand. Their combined populations total around 0·8 million, and historically they have functioned as separate communities. The vast areas of the Pacific Ocean which they span and the considerable variation in their resources have contributed to acceptance of migration from the earliest times until the present.

227

Migration and European contact

'He taru tawhiti'

'A weed from afar.'
A modern saying. In his natural state the Maori was prone to few diseases, but after the coming of the European he fell victim to tuberculosis, measles, and many other complaints which were brought to him from overseas.

Migrations of Maori from central Polynesia to New Zealand took place more than one thousand years ago. The explorers and settlers of New Zealand in the early part of the nineteenth century found well established Maori tribes of vigorous, apparently healthy people. Disastrous consequences of the European invasion included epidemics of measles, tuberculosis, syphilis and typhoid fever resulting in a decline of the Maori population from 250 000 in the early 1800s to 41 100 by the 1890s. By 1900 they were regarded as a declining and disappearing race.

The emergence of Maori leaders such as Te Rangi Hiroa (Peter Buck), Maui Pomare, and Apirana Ngata was an important milestone, as these men, and others, encouraged greater acceptance of the advantages of hygiene and sanitation, improved housing and a greater will to accept Western medicine. This awakening was a critical factor in the social and health history of the Maori in New Zealand. Much has happened since that time. Greatly decreased infant mortality rates have played an important part in the steady increase in Maori population. By 1945, the Maori population had reached 98 000, of whom around 25 per cent were urban dwellers. The rural to urban migration that has taken place since then has led to many changes in Maori society with some loss of tribal and community ties as more and more live in towns and cities. By the mid-1970s, 75 per cent of Maoris were urban dwellers and the total Maori population was 275 000 out of a total New Zealand population of 3 138 800.

The Maori have maintained a higher risk status for infectious diseases, as compared to European New Zealanders,[1] but have also shown a much greater predisposition to Western diseases such as hypertension, coronary heart disease, diabetes and carcinoma of the lung. It is the emergence of these conditions and the critical part they are playing in present-day Maori health that provide opportunities for examining their natural history and the factors which contribute to their development. It is on the basis of this knowledge that effective prevention programmes will need to be developed and evaluated. The part played by diet and in particular, the fibre content of the diet, is one of the important questions being examined in this book. Some reference will therefore be made to dietary data and to those areas where the New Zealand data appears to support, or not to support, certain of the hypotheses that are currently being examined and tested in many parts of the world and reported in this book. In this chapter the clinical picture of bowel disorders will be examined, in particular the evidence that the New Zealand Maori are at low risk from diverticular disease and carcinoma of the colon, in contrast to the

[1] The large majority of non-Maori New Zealanders are of European stock and will be called Europeans in this chapter.

New Zealand European. The high risk status of the New Zealand Maori for coronary heart disease and hypertension, and in particular the Maori females, will also be discussed. The results will be examined in the light of prevention programmes and future research. Diabetes, hyperuricaemia and gout constitute important components of the Maori metabolic maladies and must be considered if a clear picture is to be put forward of their major problems and potential for prevention (Prior *et al.*, 1964). Data will be presented showing a change in the use of tobacco as Polynesians move into more affluent societies and it is clear that these will contribute to disease patterns and must be examined as part of the picture of the emergence of Western diseases. Alcohol use also increases considerably but will not be dealt with in this chapter.

Coronary heart disease in New Zealand Maori

'He ta kakaho e kitea, he ta ngakau e kore e kitea'

'A bend in the stalk can be seen, but not a bend in the heart.'

National mortality statistics for a number of years have indicated that New Zealand Maori have high coronary heart disease (CHD) death rates. The rates in the Maori women are, in fact, higher than women in any other country assuming that basic mortality data are comparable and accurate. The age-adjusted rates in Maori and European men were in a similar range from 1955 to 1969, increasing from 500 per 100 000 to 700 per 100 000; since that time the Maori rates have increased to 800 per 100 000 while European rates have declined slightly to 600 per 100 000 in 1976. The age-adjusted rates have been higher in the Maori women than in European women throughout the period 1955–77. In 1974, the Maori women rates were 560 per 100 000 compared to 260 per 100 000 in European women. The age-standardized rates for men and women have been calculated by the direct method using the world population of Segi. A comparison of age-specific rates per 100 000 by race and sex is set out for certain age groups for the years 1960, 1965, 1970 and 1975 in Table 16.1.

Prevalence

Epidemiological surveys were first carried out among three New Zealand Maori samples in 1962 and 1963 and results of these studies have been reported (Prior, 1962; 1974). Further studies of these samples confirmed a high prevalence of CHD in Maori women and Maori men compared with a sample of Europeans. These studies suggested, however, that the high prevalence of CHD, in Maori women in particular, would not have been predicted from a knowledge of their risk-factor status although Maori women were heavier, smoked more, and had higher uric acids, than their European counterparts and the latter had higher cholesterol levels (Prior, 1974; Beaglehole *et al.*, 1975b). Data from the second round of Maori studies carried out in 1968 and 1969 were used to examine again the prevalence of CHD and its relationship to several standard risk factors. Comparisons were

Table 16.1   European and Maori deaths from coronary heart disease (CHD), age-specific rates per 100 000

Age (years)	35–44	45–54	55–64	65–74	35–44	45–54	55–64	65–74
Date	European Males				European Females			
1960	52	248	751	1548	9	59	221	694
1965	62	278	855	1729	9	41	279	837
1970	73	269	679	1905	14	63	261	862
1975	62	283	814	1714	16	50	239	775
	Maori Males				Maori Females			
1960	44	352	650	1440	57	223	862	1053
1965	47	300	928	1775	—[1]	243	816	1240
1970	128	372	1077	2156	39	178	585	1373
1975	89	369	811	1845	40	127	686	1089

[1] No cases

Table 16.2   Maori and European age-standardized CHD prevalence rates (%)

Maori		European	
Female	Male	Female	Male
$16 \cdot 1 \left(\dfrac{38}{246}\right)$ [1]	$7 \cdot 3 \left(\dfrac{17}{236}\right)$	$11 \cdot 5 \left(\dfrac{19}{151}\right)$	$6 \cdot 5 \left(\dfrac{8}{125}\right)$

[1] Observed number of cases and population at risk in parentheses

made with Europeans from the Carterton survey (Beaglehole *et al.*, 1978b). Cases of CHD were defined on the basis of the examining physician's assessment of angina pectoris and/or the presence of major ECG Q wave abnormalities (Minnesota Code 1:1 or 1:2). The association of CHD and risk factors under study were analysed by multiple cross tubulations. The results have been presented for persons aged 35–74 in the form of age-standardized prevalence rates of CHD by risk-factor level. The age-standardized prevalence rates of CHD by race and sex are set out in Table 16.2.

The age-standardized prevalence rates of CHD at three levels of systolic blood pressure are shown in Table 16.3. In both Maori males and Europeans of both sexes, the prevalence increased with increasing blood pressure, but not in Maori females. Smoking was associated with an increased risk of CHD only in European females. The age-standardized prevalence rates of CHD by uric acid level are shown in Table 16.4.

Table 16.3 Age-standardized CHD prevalence rates (%) and systolic blood pressure by race and sex, ages 35–74 years

		Systolic BP (mmHg)		
		<140	140–159	>160
Maori	Female	$17 \cdot 4 \left(\dfrac{19}{134}\right)$[1]	$12 \cdot 7 \left(\dfrac{6}{45}\right)$	$15 \cdot 6 \left(\dfrac{13}{67}\right)$
	Male	$5 \cdot 5 \left(\dfrac{7}{140}\right)$	$5 \cdot 9 \left(\dfrac{7}{40}\right)$	$12 \cdot 4 \left(\dfrac{7}{44}\right)$
European	Female	$2 \cdot 1 \left(\dfrac{1}{63}\right)$	$14 \cdot 4 \left(\dfrac{7}{40}\right)$	$16 \cdot 0 \left(\dfrac{11}{48}\right)$
	Male	$5 \cdot 8 \left(\dfrac{3}{60}\right)$	$2 \cdot 7 \left(\dfrac{1}{35}\right)$	$11 \cdot 7 \left(\dfrac{4}{30}\right)$

[1] Observed number of cases and population at risk in parentheses

Table 16.4 Age-standardized CHD prevalence rates (%) by serum uric acid by race and sex: ages 35–74 years

		Serum uric acid (mmol/l) (mg/dl)		
		<0·35 <6·0	0·35–0·41 6·0–7·0	>0·41 >7·0
Maori	Female	$13 \cdot 3 \left(\dfrac{13}{111}\right)$[1]	$16 \cdot 9 \left(\dfrac{9}{54}\right)$	$20 \cdot 7 \left(\dfrac{12}{50}\right)$
	Male	$1 \cdot 8 \left(\dfrac{1}{56}\right)$	$6 \cdot 8 \left(\dfrac{4}{61}\right)$	$10 \cdot 8 \left(\dfrac{10}{89}\right)$
European	Female	$8 \cdot 9 \left(\dfrac{12}{126}\right)$	$20 \cdot 7 \left(\dfrac{5}{19}\right)$	$37 \cdot 0 \left(\dfrac{2}{6}\right)$
	Male	$1 \cdot 8 \left(\dfrac{1}{58}\right)$	$8 \cdot 0 \left(\dfrac{3}{38}\right)$	$14 \cdot 1 \left(\dfrac{4}{29}\right)$

[1] Observed number of cases and population at risk in parentheses

Conversion: SI to traditional units uric acid 0·1 mmol/l ≈ 1·68 mg/dl

The prevalence rate increased with serum uric acid level in all four race/sex groups. No clear relationship was found between cholesterol and triglyceride levels and CHD in these subjects, except in European females. The Maori women stand out as the group with the highest prevalence of CHD. The unusual finding was that only one of the risk factors studied, uric acid, appeared important in Maori women. Cases include subjects with angina and a smaller number with major ECG Q waves as evidence of infarction and this must be taken into account. This is part of the problem of the relatively small sample sizes. Other epidemiological studies have demonstrated a marked difference in the sex ratios of various manifestations of CHD. In particular, the incidence of myocardial infarction was about five times greater in males in Framingham, while incidence of angina was similar in the two sexes (Kannel *et al.*, 1961). The New Zealand data suggest that a higher case fatality among men compared with women could be important in contributing to the higher prevalence rate of CHD in Maori women. The unusual finding was that the Maori female excess CHD prevalence was more notable because for all risk factors studied they were in the lowest category; this raised some unusual possibilities. One possibility was that CHD was produced by different factors to those operating in the three other groups. An alternative could be that there are two syndromes operating, those cases of CHD occurring largely in the absence of risk factors which are mainly responsible for the Maori female excess and those occurring in the presence of risk factors. A higher fatality rate occurring in those with risk factors than in those without, could also lead to a failure of relationship between risk factor and CHD being shown in a prevalence study. The picture that emerged from this study made it important that longitudinal studies be continued before intervention studies could be developed.

Incidence

The prevalence study performed in 1968–69 was followed up by a further examination in 1974, 5·3 years later. The incidence and case mortality of CHD have been reported (Beaglehole *et al.*, 1978b) and will be reviewed. Incidence cases were those who were classed as negative at the 1968–69 examination and who died from, or had evidence of, CHD in the 1974 examination. The study population, death rates and participation rates are set out in Table 16.5.

The association between CHD risk factors was examined by both univariate and multivariate analyses. Indirect age-adjusted incidence rates are presented by risk-factor level. Stepwise discriminate function analysis was used to define the best set of variables to predict new cases. Among the 493 Maori, aged 35–74 years, 40 new cases of CHD occurred. Twenty-one developed angina, 5 developed major Q wave changes, 8 suffered myocardial infarction and 6 sustained a sudden death. The five-year age-adjusted incidence rates were 9·4 per cent in men and 12·3 per cent in women. There was no significant sex difference in incidence rates in contrast to the female preponderance found in the prevalence surveys. The annual incidence rate of CHD was therefore 1·8 per cent for Maori men and 2·3 per cent for Maori women. These rates in the women are very high by world standards; compared with Framingham, 0·5 per cent per year for women aged 30–62 years. The strong relationship between increasing systolic blood pressure and increasing

Table 16.5 Study population CHD death rates and participation rates from 1968/69 to 1974, New Zealand Maori study

Age (years)	1968/69 Population Men (No.)	Women (No.)	1968/69–1974 Deaths Men (No.)	(%)	Women (No.)	(%)	1974 Re-examined Men (No.)	(%)[1]	Women (No.)	(%)[1]
35–44	78	87	2	2·6	8	9·2	73	96·1	73	92·4
45–54	70	79	4	5·7	3	3·8	65	98·5	73	96·1
55–64	68	53	24	35·3	12	22·6	42	95·5	41	100·0
65–74	23	35	7	30·4	17	48·6	16	100·0	18	100·0
Total	239	254	37	15·5	40	15·7	196	97·0	205	95·8

[1] Per cent of survivors

incidence of CHD is shown in Table 16.6. The incidence rises more than three-fold from the lowest to the highest blood pressure level.

Table 16.6   Age-adjusted 5-year Maori CHD incidence rates (%) by systolic blood pressure and by sex

Systolic pressure mmHg	<140	140–159	≥160
Females	$6 \cdot 1 \left(\frac{5}{103}\right)^1$	$15 \cdot 2 \left(\frac{6}{34}\right)$	$19 \cdot 3 \left(\frac{11}{43}\right)$
Males	$6 \cdot 3 \left(\frac{7}{117}\right)$	$4 \cdot 7 \left(\frac{2}{43}\right)$	$24 \cdot 2 \left(\frac{9}{29}\right)$

[1] Observed number of cases and population at risk in parentheses

Other risk factors examined by risk factor categories included serum cholesterol, serum uric acid, serum triglycerides, smoking habits and body mass index (BMI = weight/height^2). None of these, however, showed a significant relationship between risk factor level and age-adjusted incidence of CHD. Examining risk factors as continuous variables showed that in males, age, systolic blood pressure and their squares and product each provided significant discrimination between incident cases and non-cases. In females, systolic blood pressure and age, their squares and products, ECG, and products of age with BMI, serum uric acid and triglycerides, each provide significant discrimination. In the multivariate analyses, age and systolic blood pressure in both sexes, BMI in males and serum triglycerides and electrocardiographic left ventricular hypertrophy in females provide the best prediction but still only identifies half of the new cases occurring.

Case mortality
In the five-year period, a total of 77 individuals in the sample died. Twenty-one had been classified as having CHD in the 1968–69 prevalence examination. The prognostic significance of CHD has been related to the original CHD status. The risk of death increases with age and, in the absence of CHD, the age-adjusted five-year death rates were 13 per cent in males and 14·1 per cent in females. In those with CHD, the rates were 40·1 per cent in males and 20·8 per cent in females. The difference is significant ($\chi_1^2 = 5 \cdot 04$, $P < 0 \cdot 025$). The lack of association of CHD with serum cholesterol and smoking habits is contrary to a number of other studies. For technical reasons, cholesterol results were available for only two of the three Maori samples and thus included only in the initial analyses of risk factor level. It has not been shown to be a risk factor, however, in the prevalence surveys. There are some unusual patterns in Maori lipids that may contribute to their high risk status (see below). Smoking is common in Maori men and women and the lack of association with CHD may be surprising. In this sample, 14 per cent were

Table 16.7 Smoking among Maori by age and sex in 1974

Sex	Age (years)	Non-smokers		Ex-smokers		Smokers — Cigarettes smoked per day						(No.)
						<10		10–19		>20		
		(No.)	(%)	(No.)	(%)	(No.)	(%)	(No.)	(%)	(No.)	(%)	
Male	15–19											0
	20–24	7	16·7	4	9·5	16	38·1	9	21·4	6	14·3	42
	25–34	9	15·8	8	14·0	9	15·8	10	17·5	21	36·8	57
	35–44	25	24·3	13	12·6	20	19·4	19	18·4	26	25·2	103
	45–54	10	16·4	15	24·6	16	26·2	7	11·5	13	21·3	61
	55–64	15	27·3	21	38·2	7	12·7	5	9·1	7	12·7	55
	65–74	8	26·7	11	36·7	5	16·7	1	3·3	5	16·7	30
	75+	5	50·0	3	30·0	2	20·0	0	0·0	0	0·0	10
	total	79		75		75		51		78		358
Female	15–19											0
	20–24	3	10·0	4	13·3	6	20·0	14	46·7	3	10·0	30
	25–34	9	11·4	8	10·1	21	26·6	19	24·1	22	27·8	79
	35–44	26	26·5	11	11·2	17	17·3	22	22·4	22	22·4	98
	45–54	15	19·5	17	22·1	16	20·8	12	15·6	17	22·1	77
	55–64	32	45·7	12	17·1	15	21·4	6	8·6	5	7·1	70
	65–74	13	54·2	4	16·7	2	8·3	3	12·5	2	8·3	24
	75–94	2	22·2	5	55·6	1	11·1	1	11·1	0	0·0	9
	total	100		61		78		77		71		387

Note: smokers with an unknown amount coded as non-smokers

smoking more than 20 cigarettes per day. The overall distribution of smoking from the round of Maori studies in 1974 is set out in Table 16.7. There is some evidence that smoking is more related to sudden death than other manifestations of CHD and that this may have masked the relationship since all CHD manifestations have been pooled in the present study. The overall findings in relationship to the standard risk factors of hypertension, elevated cholesterol and smoking, place the New Zealand Maori and their predisposition to CHD in a somewhat different category from reported studies in many Western societies. The part being played by hypertension in predicting CHD does provide the basis for intervention programmes and effective treatment of this disorder must be given high priority.

Lipid patterns in New Zealand Maori

The first Maori surveys carried out in 1962–63 showed serum cholesterol levels in both Maori men and women that were notably lower than in a survey of European New Zealanders carried out in 1964 (Prior, 1974). A survey of adolescents aged 12–16 years in Rotorua in 1972 confirmed the same trend (Stanhope *et al.*, 1975). The third round of Maori adult examinations was carried out in 1974 and high density lipoprotein cholesterol (HDLC) levels were measured in addition to low density lipoprotein cholesterol (LDLC) and triglycerides (Beaglehole *et al.*, 1979). Participation was 93 per cent of survivors. The evidence from many sources that HDLC functions as an independent risk factor, inversely related to the occurrence of CHD, has reinforced the need to explore the part played by HDLC in New Zealand Maori, both men and women. The distribution of total cholesterol, HDLC, LDLC and triglycerides are set out in Table 16.8 for Maori men and Table 16.9 for Maori women. Serum cholesterol for men and women are not significantly different (5·92 ± 0·058 mmol/l or 228·6 mg/dl for men; 5·82 ± 0·060 mmol/l or 224·8 mg/dl for women). The serum HDLC levels were unrelated to age and there were no overall differences in mean HDLC levels between men and women (1·08 ± 0·02 mmol/l or 41·7 mg/dl in men and 1·06 ± 0·01 mmol/l or 40·9 mg/dl in women). Serum LDLC increased with age in females but not in males. The overall means were not different in the two sexes (4·02 ± 0·07 mmol/l or 155·2 mg/dl for men and 4·12 ± 0·06 mmol/l or 159 mg/dl for women). The distribution of triglycerides was skewed so that median values are presented. Overall median triglycerides were significantly higher in men (1·76 mmol/l) than in women (1·31 mmol/l). In the Maori study BMI is positively correlated with serum triglycerides and negatively correlated with HDLC in both men and women. Diabetes also positively correlated with triglycerides in both sexes. In Maori men there was a positive relationship between current alcohol drinking and HDLC but not in women. Both sexes showed a negative relationship between drinking and LDLC. Again the findings confirm that serum cholesterol levels are lower in New Zealand Maori than in European New Zealanders studied in Carterton (Evans and Prior, 1969) and in Milton when lipids were measured

Table 16.8 Distribution of serum lipids in Maori men by age

Age (years)	Total cholesterol (mmol/l)			High density lipoprotein cholesterol (mmol/l)			Low density lipoprotein cholesterol (mmol/l)			Triglycerides (mmol/l)		
	(mean)	(s.e. mean)	(no.)	(mean)	(s.e. mean)	(no.)	(mean)	(s.e. mean)	(no.)	(median)	(s.e. median)[1]	(no.)
20–24	5·559	0·158	41	1·04	0·04	36	3·84	0·16	36	1·382	0·313	41
25–34	5·787	0·138	55	1·13	0·05	37	3·82	0·19	37	1·920	0·363	55
35–44	6·013	0·099	95	1·08	0·03	76	4·04	0·11	76	1·902	0·243	97
45–54	5·986	0·127	60	1·09	0·04	45	4·06	0·15	45	1·745	0·563	60
55–64	6·150	0·171	55	1·13	0·04	43	4·24	0·19	43	1·830	0·267	55
65–74	5·780	0·241	27	1·01	0·04	23	4·01	0·24	23	1·580	0·185	27
75+	6·054	0·397	8	1·00	0·06	5	4·15	0·60	5	1·579	0·236	8
Total	5·922	0·058	341	1·08	0·02	265	4·02	0·07	265	1·763	0·148	343

Conversion: SI to traditional units cholesterol 1 mmol/l ≈ 39 mg/dl

[1] Approximate standard error of the median = 1·253 × s.e. mean

Table 16.9   Distribution of serum lipids in Maori women by age

Age (years)	Total cholesterol (mmol/l)			High density lipoprotein cholesterol (mmol/l)			Low density lipoprotein cholesterol (mmol/l)			Triglycerides (mmol/l)		
	(mean)	(s.e. mean)	(no.)	(mean)	(s.e. mean)	(no.)	(mean)	(s.e. mean)	(no.)	(median)	(s.e. median)[1]	(no.)
20–24	5·289	0·209	27	1·03	0·05	27	3·72	0·22	27	1·042	0·114	27
25–34	5·356	0·111	64	1·01	0·03	62	3·71	0·12	62	1·310	0·086	65
35–44	5·669	0·096	91	1·04	0·03	85	4·06	0·10	85	1·230	0·179	91
45–54	5·812	0·138	72	1·11	0·04	67	4·02	0·14	67	1·417	0·103	73
55–64	6·502	0·150	65	1·07	0·04	61	4·73	0·15	60	1·492	0·117	66
65–74	6·310	0·183	21	1·09	0·05	19	4·51	0·22	19	1·400	0·262	21
75–84	6·358	0·598	8	1·04	0·07	7	4·70	0·61	7	1·925	0·426	8
Total	5·822	0·060	348	1·06	0·01	328	4·12	0·06	327	1·310	0·063	351

Conversion: SI to traditional units cholesterol 1 mmol/l ≈ 39 mg/dl
[1] Approximate standard error of the median = 1·253 × s.e. mean

as part of a community cardiovascular study (Nye *et al.*, 1977). Triglycerides are higher in both Maori males and females than those reported in Europeans in New Zealand.

The HDLC levels are low in both men and women compared with blacks and whites in North Carolina (Castelle *et al.*, 1977). The usual sex difference, with women having higher levels than men, is not apparent in the New Zealand Maori data. This may be a contributing factor to the high risk status of Maori women. The Framingham study and others have shown a negative relationship with relative weight, measures of glucose intolerance and HDLC (Gordon *et al.*, 1977) and this was shown for body mass, but not for diabetes in Maori in this study. Lipid differences between Maori and Europeans in New Zealand have also been shown in adolescents, with lower HDLC and higher triglycerides in Maori compared with Europeans (Stanhope *et al.*, 1977).

It is clear that there are a wide range of environmental factors which play a part in setting the level of lipids in individuals and in groups and it is the summation and interaction of these that are observed. The habitual diet of New Zealand is high in fat with around 40 per cent of energy from this source, high in cholesterol (500–600 mg per day) and high in sucrose and carbohydrate. (Prior and Davidson, 1966). These earlier findings have been confirmed in 1977 by a National Diet Survey initiated by the National Heart Foundation of New Zealand. (See Table 16.11). There are no data available nor clear hypothesis that can explain Maori–European lipid differences on the basis of diet. Existing data would suggest that overall saturated fat intake could be somewhat higher in the Maori than in Europeans and so one could expect higher levels of LDLC in Maori, but these are not in fact seen. The higher rates of obesity and diabetes in the Maori could clearly contribute to the triglyceride levels and to the overall lower levels of HDLC—a clear association, however, was not shown in the analyses reported here. The high risk status of the New Zealand Maori for CHD has now been clearly established. The need for prevention programmes on the basis of identification of subjects with hypertension must now be tested as the most effective and likely measure that could be introduced. There is still inadequate information about the pathogenesis of atheroma and the pattern of risk factors should be explored further. This need not preclude intervention studies involving the earlier identification of obese subjects, early diabetes and testing ways and means of lessening or preventing the smoking habit. This represents a major challenge to those involved in the health service in New Zealand.

Polynesian diets and gastrointestinal disorders

'E hoa ma! Ina te ora o te tangata'

'Oh friends! Here indeed is the health of mankind.'
A statement made to a visitor when food is set before him.

Epidemiological studies have drawn attention to the marked differences in the incidence of non-infective bowel disease occurring between developed

Western societies and underdeveloped third world countries. These variations in incidence of certain diseases suggest that dietary factors are important in their aetiology. There are many bowel diseases such as appendicitis, gallbladder disease, diverticular disease, irritable bowel disease, cancer of the stomach, cancer of the colon and haemorrhoids which appear to have dietary factors in the aetiology. In the Polynesian Triangle there are many small but well defined communities, but the physical resources have not been available for accurate determination of disease distributions. Such communities, because of their distinctness, should provide ideal study areas providing the organizational, logistic and other problems can be met.

Gallstone disease occurs in the Maori and is the common cause for cholecystectomy in both Europeans and Maori in New Zealand. In those 45 years and over, deaths related to gallstones are about five times greater among the Maori than Europeans. No national statistics are currently available to indicate the incidence of gallstone disease or the variation in pattern of disease in these racial groups. If the frequency with which cholecystectomy is done is a reliable measure of this disorder cholelithiasis is very uncommon in Tonga and Western Samoa.

Inflammatory bowel diseases including ulcerative colitis are very uncommon in the Maori but common in the New Zealand European population. Wigley and MacLaurin (1962) showed that in a group of patients with ulcerative colitis there were no Maori represented. Subsequent hospital experience would support this, and the few patients with ulcerative colitis have mixed Maori–white ancestry. Crohn's ileitis on the other hand has been seen in New Zealand in a number of Polynesian people of pure or nearly pure extraction. Peptic ulcer occurs frequently in the New Zealand Maori and from the age of 45 and over is appreciably more common than in Europeans. It is the single most important cause of digestive disease deaths in Maori over 65 years of age. In Western Samoa peptic ulcer disease occurs with even greater frequency. The occurrence in Western Samoa is irregular and suggests that there are local aetiological factors which may be operating. An increased consumption of taro has been suggested as one factor which may contribute to the peptic ulcer pattern of Samoans. Further the type of ulcer appears to be different in that there is a high frequency of stenosing duodenal ulcer (MacLaurin et al., 1979a, b).

Diverticular disease occurs in both Maori and Pacific islanders living in New Zealand, but with a frequency which is less than would be expected. The sex ratio also is different. In New Zealanders of European descent the male to female ratio is approximately two to three, in the Polynesians with diverticular disease it appears to be equal.

The Maori population form about 8 per cent of New Zealand's population but the age distribution of the Maori population is different from that of the European. For the years 0–4, 12·3 per cent are Maori, whereas for 65 and over only 1·9 per cent are Maori. The significant change in the population disposition, with a marked urban drift, which is more pronounced for the Maori than the Europeans, has been referred to. At present over 80 per cent of the total New Zealand population and 75 per cent of the Maori population are urban dwellers. These differences in population structure are of importance when considering malignant disease. Up to the age of 15 there is no difference in death rates from cancer in Maori and Europeans, but after 15 the Maori death rates are higher than the European death rates, and between the ages of 15 and 25 are 75 per cent higher. The standardized rates of cancer of the alimentary tract are set out in Table 16.10. Cancer of the stomach, cancer of the liver, and pancreatic cancer show a much higher incidence in the Maori compared with the Europeans. For cancer of the oesophagus the standardized rates are equal between the two races. This trend is, however, very significantly reversed for cancer of the large bowel and cancer of the rectum where the Maori rates are notably lower.

Table 16.10 Cancer in different gastrointestinal sites. Standardized rates/100 000 of population in Maori and European

Site	Maori	European
Stomach	33·4	10·5
Liver	5·1	1·4
Pancreas	13·4	6·5
Oesophagus	3·6	3·6
Colon	9·3	26·0
Rectum	7·8	13·0

Current theories on the causation of cancer of the bowel are that it is most likely to be related to dietary factors (Kelsey, 1978). The dietary factors considered most frequently are high fat, high proteins and low fibre. It is suggested that, because one or more of these factors operate, there is an alteration in the bacterial breakdown of bile salts which leads to the formation of a carcinogen responsible for causing cancer. Only preliminary work has been done to indicate differences in diet which may be important in the aetiology of bowel cancer in the Maori and European in New Zealand. Little accurate scientific information is available on the changing patterns of the diet in New Zealand, on the variations in diet between urban and rural Maori, and of the detailed composition of Maori diets and particularly the dietary fibre content. Seafoods such as shellfish, sea urchins and a wide variety of fish are held in high regard by the Maori and where available will form an important part of the diet. Pork and eel are popular as is the sweet potato and a wild thistle.

With increasing ubranization the Maori is adopting a more Western style of diet. In spite of increasing use of westernized foods the Maori will favour fatty foods and traditional seafoods if available. The National Heart Foundation of New Zealand has recently carried out a national dietary survey in New Zealand (Table 16.11; Birbeck, 1979). In the age range 20–50 male

Europeans get approximately 43·5 per cent of their dietary energy from carbohydrate, 42·5 per cent from fat and 14 per cent from protein, while the Maori male gets 39 per cent of his energy from carbohydrate, 46 per cent from fat and 15 per cent from protein. A similar pattern is shown for females, for the European 41·5 per cent of the energy comes from carbohydrate, 44 per cent from fat and 14·5 per cent from protein and in the Maori 39 per cent from carbohydrate, 46 per cent from fat, 15 per cent from protein.

The higher dietary intake of fat relative to carbohydrate and protein is the consistent difference between the Maori and European shown in this survey of diet in New Zealand at the present time. The energy intake in the

Table 16.11   Sources of energy (%) in European and Maori diets of males and females aged 20–50 years. Data is based on 50th centile from National Heart Foundation Dietary Survey, 1978

	Carbohydrate	Fat	Protein
European males	43·5	42·5	14
Maori males	39	46	15
European females	41·5	44	14·5
Maori females	39	46	15

Maori diet is, however, somewhat higher than in the European diet. It has been previously shown that populations in whom undernutrition is common rarely develop cancer of the bowel or diverticular disease of the colon. While cancer in general is more common in the Maori than in the European, cancer of the colon and rectum is at a significantly lower level. Epidemiological evidence from the Maori would suggest that the high fat intake is unlikely to be a major factor in the incidence of large bowel cancer. Protein intakes between the Maori and European are similar and again would be unlikely to account for the relative differences between the racial groups. Data on the difference in the fibre intake of these population groups is only now being obtained (Pomare *et al.*, 1980). Until further information is available it must remain uncertain as to whether the differences in cancer are related to specific differences in dietary fat composition or to differences in dietary fibre intake or to differences unrelated to the diet but related to genetic and other socio-economic factors.

Dietary fibre in Tokelau and New Zealand diets

Collection of dietary data in Tokelau and New Zealand has been an important part of the Tokelau Island Migrant Study. In 1976, samples of certain island foods were obtained and subsequently analysed by the Chemistry Division of the Department of Scientific and Industrial Research NZ for fibre content (Drs. G. L. Disk and N. A. Moore, personal communication, 1980). The

Table 16.12   Dietary fibre and starch in some Tokelauan Island foods (g/100 g)

Total	Dietary fibre	Constituents			
		Non-cellulosic polysaccharides	Cellulose	Lignin	Starch
Pulaka	4·54	2·28	1·96	0·31	39·11
Breadfruit	3·52	1·61	1·83	0·09	11·11
Coconuts					
Matatalua (soft flesh)	1·42	0·93	0·32	0·17	0·67
Sua (drinking nut)	1·26	0·76	0·32	0·19	0·53
Agalele (firm flesh)	2·83	1·24	1·59	0·02	2·36
Popo (hard flesh, mature nut)	2·84	1·15	0·97	0·72	2·11

foods included coconuts at differing stages of maturity, breadfruit and pulaka, an edible arum. Foods were not cooked and results expressed as g/100 g (net weight) are set out in Table 16.12.

The very extensive and varied use of coconuts in the Tokelau diet had been demonstrated in 1968–71 and was again shown during the 1976 dietary survey (Drs. W. Harding and F. Davidson, personal communication, 1980). This provides a high fat intake, a large proportion in the form of short chain saturated fatty acids. The dietary fibre intake in Tokelau resident men ranged from 14·1 g/24 hours in those aged 75 and over to 19·4 g/24 hours in those aged 45–54 years. The overall mean in 95 men studied was 16·5 g/24 hours or 8·0 g/1000 calories. The intake in Tokelau resident women ranged from 13·5 g in those aged 20–24 to 16·8 g in those aged 65–74 years. The overall mean in 161 women was 14·9 g/24 hours or 9·9 g/1000 calories. The diet pattern in New Zealand is different in many ways, particularly in the availability of coconut, taro and other traditional foods. An estimate of dietary fibre intake in New Zealand has been made based on household dietary data collected from Tokelauan families in New Zealand. Food tables have been used to estimate the dietary fibre content of cereals, vegetables, fruit coconut and other foods in their diet. The mean dietary fibre intake was 12·8 g/24 hours or 5·7 g/1000 calories, made up from cereals 2·7 g, vegetables 6·1 g, fruit 2·3 g, coconut 0·4 g and miscellaneous 0·2 g.

While diets are different in Tokelau and the Tokelauans in New Zealand, these results do not indicate that fibre intake in the islands is much higher in Tokelau. The New Zealand pattern may well alter as the migrants spend longer in New Zealand and documentation of the dietary pattern is an important part of the ongoing study.

Bowel transit time studies in Tokelau and in New Zealand

Using the single stool analysis technique (Cummings and Wiggins, 1976), bowel transit times were carried out among 44 adults aged 30–59 years in Fakaofo in Tokelau, during the 1976 survey. The procedure was explained at a village meeting and excellent cooperation was achieved. Further explanations were given when the markers were given out to each individual together with the special container for collection of faeces on the fourth day. The absence of x-ray facilities meant that the markers had to be counted by sieving the faeces. This involved the use of large amounts of sea water and some fortitude, but proved satisfactory. Collections in New Zealand were made on a random sample of 40 Tokelau adults aged 30–59 years living in the Wellington area, who had been resident in New Zealand for five years or more. The median bowel transit times in Fakaofo were 32·5 hours while those of Tokelauans in New Zealand were 36·7 hours. The difference was small, but statistically significant ($P < 0.029$). These times are shorter than those reported in Western groups. Recent studies in other New Zealand and Pacific groups (Drs. E. W. Pomare, N. H. Stace, C. A. Fisher, S. Peters and L. Thomas, personal communication, 1980) have given times in New Zealand Europeans of 53·15 ± 23·7 hours, in New Zealand Maori of 53·2 ± 24·8 hours and in Tongans living in New Zealand 41·4 ± 16·7 hours. The gradient of transit times demonstrated between the groups that the change towards longer times is a relatively slow process following migration and dietary change. Certainly no differences exist between New Zealand Europeans and New Zealand Maori that could help explain the notably lower cancer of the colon rate in Maori compared with the European.

Future research into gastrointestinal disorders in the Pacific

Standardized rates of diseases are difficult to obtain, with the multiple and relatively small Polynesian groups and with their variable pattern of dietary intake, social environment and geographic circumstances. Considerable progress has, however, been made in recent years aided by the efforts of the South Pacific Commission and the Western Pacific Region of WHO. An opportunity certainly exists for study of a few of the more common disorders where more accurate and detailed disease indices could be correlated with specific dietary and environmental factors. With the larger Maori group in New Zealand concentrated studies are likely to be more productive. Studies to estimate the dietary fibre composition of diets in New Zealand foods will be of significant value. Of particular importance in New Zealand is the contrasting incidence of malignancy of the bowel and comprehensive dietary surveys are now indicated as part of such investigations. The high incidence of stomach and pancreatic cancers in the Maori compared to Europeans is worthy of specific study in relation to the differences in fat intake of the two ethnic groups.

Comparative studies of Polynesians in the Pacific

'Te taepaepatonga o te rangi'

'The place where the sky hangs down to the horizon.'
The expression refers to great distances and open spaces.

Surveys of Polynesians living in different environments and in societies varying from traditional to urban or modern provide a range of opportunities for testing certain specific hypotheses relating to health and disease. Migrations from outer islands or villages into towns, such as Nuku'alofa in Tonga, Apia in Western Samoa and Avarua in Rarotonga, are associated with many problems of urbanization, as well as some advantages. Housing is often inadequate and job opportunities limited. There is less reliance on traditional sources and supplies of food and greater use of processed foods. The modern migration of Pacific islanders to New Zealand represents a considerable change in physical, social and cultural environment, particularly for those from small traditional atoll societies such as Tokelau. In 1946 there were 1600 Pacific islanders in New Zealand. By 1977 they had increased to 60 000 and have become important contributors to the cultural diversity of New Zealand. The migrants have come from Western Samoa, Cook Islands, Niue, Tonga, Tokelau and Fiji. Migration to New Zealand is easier for subjects from Cook Islands, Niue and Tokelau since these groups have New Zealand citizenship. Quota systems operate for groups such as Samoans where the upper limit is 1500/year. The health consequences of migration, both harmful and advantageous, are influenced by the pattern of health prior to migration, by the response to the new environment, and the social and living patterns adopted. There are few studies reported in which migrants have been examined prior to migration, so that the characteristics of those who were to migrate can be compared with the non-migrants (sedentes), and where both groups are then followed in a prospective way.

The Tokelau Island Migrant Study (TIMS) has provided this opportunity and the general outline of the study will be set out later in this chapter (Prior *et al.*, 1974).

Blood pressure patterns in the Pacific Polynesians

The considerable gradient that can be shown among Pacific Polynesian populations highlights the fact that an increase in blood pressure with age is not inevitable. Such populations offer an unusual opportunity to seek out environmental and other factors playing a part in this process. They stand out as small traditional societies, often where resources are limited and where weight does not increase with age.

Studies in 1964 in Pukapuka in the Northern Cook Island group confirmed previous work in 1953 showing that they were a low blood pressure group (Murphy, 1955; Prior *et al.*, 1968). The Cook Island Maori in Rarotonga showed a considerable increase in blood pressure with age and were notably heavier and taller. Allowing for weight, the Rarotongans still had higher pressures than the Pukapukans. There was a much lower dietary salt intake in Pukapuka compared with Rarotonga. This was confirmed by 24-hour urine sodium outputs and dietary assessment, with intake around 50 mEq (3 g NaCl) in Pukapuka and 120 mEq (7·5 g NaCl) in Rarotonga (Prior *et al.*, 1968). Comparison of systolic and diastolic pressures and weights in males and females in Pukapuka and Rarotonga are set out in Fig. 16.1 and Fig. 16.2. Data available from the New Zealand Maori, Carterton European, Rarotonga, Pukapuka and Tokelau 1968 surveys have been analysed and the age-standardized rates are set out in Table 16.13. This confirms that Tokelau rates are at somewhat higher levels than Pukapuka but considerably lower than the other groups.

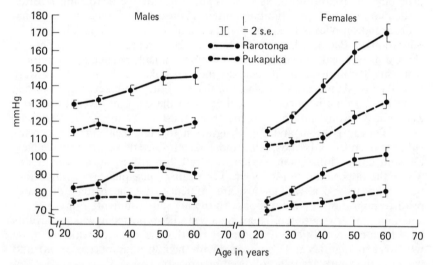

Fig. 16.1   Mean systolic and diastolic blood pressure in Rarotonga and Pukapuka by age for males and females

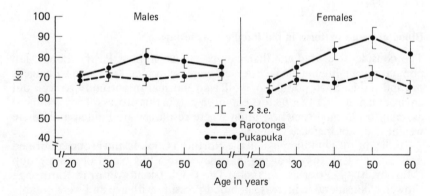

Fig. 16.2   Mean weights in Rarotonga and Pukapuka by age for males and females

Table 16.13 Age-standardized rates/1000 of definite hypertension[1] in four Polynesian and one New Zealand (NZ) European sample

	Males	Females
NZ Maori	288	318
NZ European	266	225
Rarotonga	343	366
Tokelau	80	151
Pukapuka	47	82

[1] BP 160 mmHg or more and/or diastolic 95 mmHg or more

Tokelau Island Migrant Study

Tokelau consists of three small atolls 480 km north of Western Samoa. In 1966 the total population consisted of just under 2000. A small compact Polynesian traditional atoll society, they have been a New Zealand dependency since 1925. In 1948 Tokelauans were granted New Zealand citizenship. A hurricane took place in early 1966 which drew the attention of the New Zealand government to the somewhat overcrowded conditions and limited opportunities for development. A programme was established aiming at resettling around 1000 inhabitants in New Zealand over a five-year period. The support of the New Zealand government and the Medical Research Council of New Zealand was obtained by the Wellington Hospital Epidemiology Unit for the establishment of a longitudinal study of the social and health consequences of migration of Tokelau islanders from Tokelau to New Zealand (Prior *et al.*, 1974). Baseline surveys in Tokelau were carried out in 1968 and 1971. A WHO sponsored meeting in Wellington, New Zealand, in 1970 on cardiovascular epidemiology in the Pacific, strengthened the protocol and planning for the study. It was recommended at this meeting that the Tokelau study should include children and that the register of Tokelauans in New Zealand should include all residents and not only those migrating with government assistance (Prior, 1976). This was implemented with a complete survey of Tokelauan adults and children in New Zealand in the period 1972–74, and again in 1975–77. In 1976, a return visit to Tokelau was made when adults and children on the three atolls were examined. The total study population comprises 3600 subjects and in 1976 there were 1600 in Tokelau and the remainder in New Zealand.

Basic hypothesis regarding blood pressure

There are two sets of hypotheses relating to why blood pressure increases with age in some populations and not in others that are being tested in the Tokelau study (Prior, *et al.*, 1974; Cassel, 1974). One holds that physical factors are important, including diet and the associated body weight, salt intake, exercise and the burden of parasites or chronic diseases such as tuberculosis. The other holds that much of the phenomenon can be accounted for by psychosocial factors; low pressures occurring in societies with coherent value systems which are showing little change. Migration to societies with different value systems leads to situations in which previously socially sanctioned patterns of behaviour, that the subject had learned in early life, can no longer be used to express normal behavioural urges and this in turn creates repeated autonomic system arousal that could influence blood pressure levels. It has been found that a pattern of social interaction predominantly with Tokelauans at work, at home and during leisure was associated with lower blood pressures than one of interaction predominantly with non-Tokelauans. The contribution of social interaction to the variance of blood pressure was, however, small compared with the contribution of weight (Beaglehole et al., 1977).

Blood pressure in Tokelauans

Blood pressure before migration

The analysis of the 1968 data showed that young adult male premigrants were taller and heavier and had slightly higher blood pressures than sedentes (Prior et al., 1974). It is suggested that younger and more athletic males were active initiators of migration while females and older males migrated in response to decisions made by the younger males.

The pooled data from the 1968 survey confirmed that Tokelauans had higher blood pressures than atoll-dwelling Pukupukans in the Northern Cook Islands, but notably lower than New Zealand Maori. Weights and cholesterol levels were higher in Tokelauans than in Pukapukans and approached the levels found in the New Zealand Maori.

Blood pressures in Tokelau and New Zealand

The major cross-sectional survey carried out in New Zealand in the period 1972–74 provided data on blood pressure, weight, lipid and other variables which can be compared with patterns found in Tokelau in 1971. The New Zealand subjects had been in New Zealand for varying periods, some came straight from Tokelau to New Zealand, 'one-step migrants', while others had spent periods of one year or more in Western Samoa, 'two-step migrants'. The mean systolic blood pressure by age is set out in Fig. 16.3 for males and females, while the mean weight by age is set out in Fig. 16.4 for males and females. Blood pressures, both systolic and diastolic, are higher in Tokelauans living in New Zealand than in Tokelau. Changes in weight are also occurring with those in New Zealand being heavier, in most age classes, than those in Tokelau.

Comparison of early morning urinary sodium concentrations in Tokelau and in New Zealand show higher mean values in New Zealand in all age groups, consistent with greater salt use in New Zealand.

The extent to which psychosocial and cultural factors related to migration could be contributing to the blood pressure pattern has been examined and

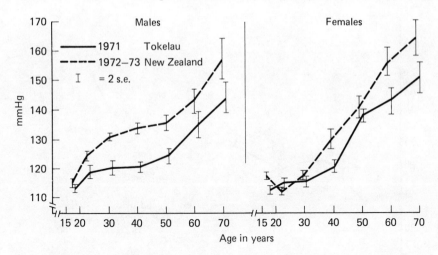

Fig. 16.3 Mean systolic blood pressures in males and females in Tokelau 1971 and migrants in New Zealand in 1972–73

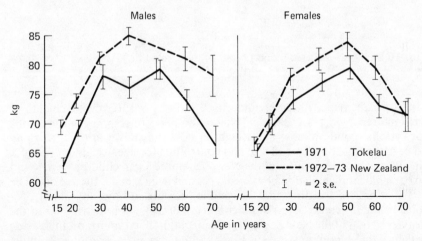

Fig. 16.4 Mean weights in males and females in Tokelau 1971 and migrants in New Zealand 1972–73

already referred to. There was a small but definite contribution to blood pressure related to the pattern of social interaction.

Blood pressure patterns in children
In 1975 Tokelauan children aged 2–14 years were examined in New Zealand with the blood pressures being recorded by one observer (Beaglehole *et al.*, 1978a). Among 856 children a 95 per cent response rate was obtained, with 550 (64 per cent) born in New Zealand and the rest born in the Pacific Islands.

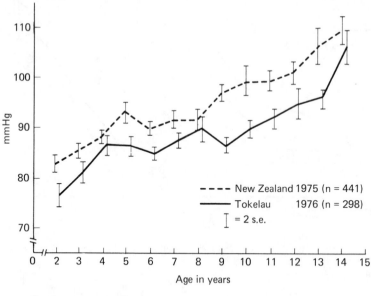

[*]Average of two readings
adjusted for cuff size

Fig. 16.5   Mean systolic blood pressures in Tokelau boys in two
environments in Tokelau 1976 and New Zealand 1975

In 1976, the same observer undertook blood pressure measurements of
571 children aged 2–14 years in Tokelau (96 per cent response). The results
for systolic blood pressure and weight in boys are shown in Figs. 16.5 and
16.6. After adjusting for cuff size and controlling for age, weight and height,
the systolic blood pressures of the New Zealand resident children were found
to be significantly higher in boys of all ages and in girls under the age of 8. The
fact that half of the difference in systolic pressure in boys and about one-
third of the difference in girls under 8 years of age can be attributed to the
heavier weight of the New Zealand resident children, is important. Increasing
evidence that blood pressure levels in children may predict adult levels must
be considered. Weight control in childhood might play a part in preventing
hypertension in later life (Beaglehole *et al.*, 1979).

The analysis of longitudinal changes of blood pressure and weight in
Tokelau migrant children has shown that major changes of blood pressure
and weight occurred following migration to New Zealand in Tokelau boys,
who were aged 5–9 when seen in Tokelau (Beaglehole *et al.*, 1978a). The
older age group 10–14 showed no greater increase in weight in New Zealand
than in Tokelau and no significant differences in blood pressures. The
development of the longitudinal adult file has allowed comparisons to be
made in those examined in Tokelau in 1968 or 1971 and then followed
through and examined in either Tokelau in 1976 or in New Zealand 1975–77.

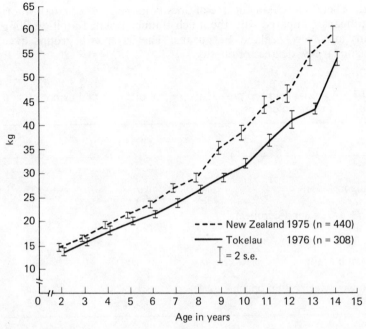

Fig. 16.6 Mean weights in Tokelau boys in two environments in Tokelau in 1976 and in New Zealand in 1975

The rates of increase in blood pressure, both systolic and diastolic, are greater in the adult migrants in New Zealand than in those living in Tokelau. Weight increases are also greater in the migrants.

Diabetes in Polynesians

'Papaku a ringaringa, hohonu a korokoro'

'The hand is shallow, but the throat is deep.'
Said of a lazy person with a gluttonous appetite.

Studies in the period 1962–64 showed a considerable variation in the prevalence of diabetes (Prior *et al.*, 1966). The highest prevalence was in New Zealand Maori while the lowest was in Pukapuka Polynesians and Carterton New Zealand Europeans. Rarotongans had an intermediate prevalence. In these surveys, glucose tolerance tests were carried out in subjects with glycosuria 0·10 per cent, or more, in non-fasting casual urines. Diabetic abnormality was assigned on the basis of a fasting blood sugar of 120 mg/dl, or more, and/or a two hours level of 130 mg/dl or greater. Known diabetics were accepted after checking of criteria. The age-standardized prevalence rates of diabetes and obesity (relative weight ⩾ 120 per cent) are set out in

Table 16.14. There is a striking degree of obesity in the New Zealand Maori and Rarotongans compared with the much thinner isolated atoll-dwelling Pukapukans and New Zealand Europeans. The latter two groups have essentially similar low degrees of obesity.

Table 16.14   Age-standardized prevalence (%) of diabetes and extent of obesity in different Pacific groups

	Diabetic	Obese
Males		
New Zealand Maori	8·7	37
Rarotongan	5·5	21
Carterton New Zealand European	1·5	7
Pukapukan	0·4	7
Females		
New Zealand Maori	6·9	59
Rarotongan	4·3	65
Carterton New Zealand European	3·1	24
Pukapukan	1·6	22

Energy, carbohydrate and sucrose intake

There is ample evidence from many sources that an increase in sucrose intake is one of the major dietary changes that occur as populations move from traditional to modern living patterns. The part which a change from a diet of high complex carbohydrate intake with low sucrose intake, to one of more refined carbohydrates with higher sucrose intake, plays in the development of diabetes and other disorders has been the basis of considerable enquiry and requires examination in a variety of populations. The contrasting environments of the different groups studied in this 1962–64 period and the types of food available have allowed a critical look at the inter-relationships between the intake of energy, carbohydrate and sucrose. The Pukapukan diet consisting of traditional atoll foods such as fish and coconut, taro, rice and flour, contrasts strongly with the Western-style diet of the New Zealand Maori and Carterton Europeans. Pukapukans had the lowest energy intake, Maori the highest, with Carterton Europeans and Rarotongans intermediate. The percentage of energy intake from carbohydrate was 44 per cent in the New Zealand Maori, 47 per cent in Carterton Europeans, 50 per cent in Pukapukans and 60 per cent in Rarotongans. The mean daily sucrose intake and percentage of energy from sucrose was 17 g, 4 per cent in Pukapuka; 73 g, 13 per cent in Carterton Europeans; 73 g, 11 per cent in New Zealand Maori; and 33 g, 7 per cent in Rarotongans. This data does not lend support to the hypothesis that sucrose intake in itself is important in the development of diabetes.

Diabetes in New Zealand Maori and Tokelauans, 1968–77 period

Examination of the pattern of diabetes in New Zealand Maori and Tokelauans living in New Zealand and in Tokelau, provides a further opportunity to examine groups living in different environments and with differing degrees of Westernization. (Prior *et al.*, 1978). From 1968 on, 100 g oral glucose loads were given to all adults after an overnight fast, with blood samples being taken at 1-hour intervals for plasma glucose determination. In these analyses, definite diabetics were those subjects whose 1-hour plasma glucose level was 250 mg/dl and over, or those subjects previously diagnosed by acceptable criteria. A comparison of age-specific prevalence rates in New Zealand Maori examined in 1974 with those found in Tokelau in 1976 and in Tokelauans seen in New Zealand during 1975–77 is set out in Table 16.15. The prevalence rates were higher in females than males in both Maori and Tokelauans. The Maori prevalences were higher than in Tokelauans. A comparison of age-specific rates show little difference between those males in Tokelau and those in New Zealand, while females show higher rates in New Zealand than in Tokelau.

The trends that have occurred since 1968 and 1971 in Tokelau and in New Zealand since the 1972–74 round of examinations are set out in Table 16.16 as the age-standardized prevalence of definite diabetes in subjects aged 24 and over. The results in the 1968–69 and 1974 Maori surveys are also included. The increase in diabetes prevalence in Tokelau since 1968 and 1971 in both males and females may relate to weight increases that were shown to have taken place in Tokelau in the 1976 survey. The similar trends in age-specific diabetes prevalences for men and women in Tokelau in 1976 and in New Zealand in 1975–77 suggest that body mass or obesity is the common factor rather than specific diet items, such as energy from carbohydrates and sucrose. The short duration of exposure of Tokelauans to the different diet and exercise pattern in New Zealand compared with the lifetime involvement of the New Zealand Maori could explain why New Zealand Tokelauan prevalence is not higher than observed. An examination of the prevalence of diabetes in Maori and Tokelauans in relationship to body mass provides further confirmation of the part played by body mass in both groups. The age-adjusted rates of definite diabetes category by tertiles of BMI are set out in Table 16.17.

In the New Zealand Maori the diabetes prevalence increases with body mass in both males and females. The rate of 14·8 per cent in the highest male tertile is significantly higher than those in the lower tertiles ($P < 0.001$). Among females, the prevalence increases significantly between the lower and medium tertiles. ($P < 0.001$.)

In the two Tokelau groups, the trend increased with body mass, but the only significant differences were found in females in the islands ($P < 0.049$).

The Maori males in the highest tertiles are clearly higher than the two Tokelau groups ($P < 0.001$) but rates in the highest tertiles in the females were not significantly different.

Table 16.15   Age- and sex-specific prevalence of definite diabetes[1] in Tokelauans (in Tokelau and in New Zealand) and New Zealand Maoris

| Age (years) | Tokelauans | | | | | | New Zealand Maoris (1974) | | |
| | Tokelau (1976) | | | New Zealand (1975–77) | | | | | |
	Examined (no.)	Definite diabetes (no.)	Definite diabetes (%)	Examined (no.)	Definite diabetes (no.)	Definite diabetes (%)	Examined (no.)	Definite diabetes (no.)	Definite diabetes (%)
Males									
25–34	35	0	—	165	3	1·8	42	3	7·1
35–44	46	1	2·2	103	8	7·8	90	6	6·6
45–54	50	2	4·0	71	4	5·6	59	8	13·6
55–64	33	2	6·0	35	1	2·9	51	13	25·5
65–74	27	3	11·1	15	2	13·3	27	8	29·6
Total	191	8	4·2	389	18	4·6	269	38	14·1
Females									
25–34	70	1	1·4	136	4	2·9	62	4	6·4
35–44	80	4	5·1	76	6	7·9	87	9	10·3
45–54	61	6	9·8	57	12	21·0	72	19	26·3
55–64	41	12	29·3	25	8	32·0	64	19	29·7
65–74	29	2	6·9	19	4	21·1	20	5	25·0
Total	281	25	8·9	313	34	10·9	305	56	18·4

[1] Definite diabetes: 1 hour plasma glucose ⩾ 250 mg/dl or known diabetes (criteria examined and accepted)

Table 16.16 Age-standardized[1] prevalence (per hundred) of definite diabetes,[2] by sex, at two points in time in Tokelauans (in Tokelau and in New Zealand) and New Zealand Maoris, aged 24 and over

	Tokelauans				New Zealand Maoris	
	in Tokelau		in New Zealand			
	1968–71	1976	1972–74	1975–77	1968–69	1974
Male	1·0	3·7	5·6	5·4	10·7	12·4
Female	3·3	8·6	8·0	13·6	11·1	16·4

[1] Indirect standardization using pooled groups as reference population
[2] See definition footnote Table 16.15

Table 16.17 Age-standardized prevalence of definite diabetes[1] (%) in Polynesians by sex and tertiles of Body Mass Index (W/H²) (ages 35–74)

Males	Body Mass Index		
	Low (⩽2·45)	Medium (2·46–2·77)	High (⩾2·78)
Maori (New Zealand)	3·9	4·1	14·8
Tokelauans (New Zealand)	1·9	4·3	6·3
Tokelauans (Islands)	2·1	1·5	3·6

Females	Body Mass Index		
	Low (⩽2·59	Medium (2·60–3·03)	High (⩾3·04)
Maori (New Zealand)	3·1	11·3	12·8
Tokelauans (New Zealand)	2·9	6·7	8·5
Tokelauans (Islands)	2·5	4·3	9·1

[1] See definition footnote Table 16.15

Varicose veins in Polynesians

'Ka mahi te waewae, i toia i, te ata hapara'
'How beautiful are the legs moistened in the dawn.'

There is a marked geographical variation in the prevalence of varicose veins
in different parts of the world including the Pacific (Stanhope, 1975). A
variety of factors have been proposed as contributing to the high prevalence
in the Western world. These include a diet high in refined carbohydrate and
low in fibre (Cleave and Campbell, 1969; Burkitt, 1972), chair sitting
(Alexander, 1972), effect of prolonged standing and constricting garments
and genetic susceptibility. Other factors have been put forward as having a
direct association with varicose veins, including weight and parity (Mekky
et al., 1969), height (Stewart *et al.*, 1955) and heavyweight lifting (Weddel,
1969). Systematic examination for varicose veins has been included in the
epidemiological studies carried out in New Zealand and the Pacific and the
results have been reviewed (Beaglehole *et al.*, 1975a). The study populations
consisted of New Zealand Europeans studied in Carterton (Prior *et al.*, 1970)
and Polynesians living in contrasting environments, already referred to, New
Zealand Maori, Cook islanders in Rarotonga and the atoll of Pukapuka and
atoll-dwelling Tokelau Islanders.

Details of the samples and participation rates and methods have been
reported previously (Beaglehole *et al.*, 1975a). This report dealt with males
and non-pregnant females aged 15–64 years. There was a striking variation
in the age-standardized prevalence rates of varicose veins in the five samples
set out in Table 16.18. The atoll-dwelling Pukapukans and Tokelauans had
the lowest prevalence, Rarotongans were intermediate and the New Zealand
Maori and Europeans had the highest rates. In the New Zealand samples,
the Maori male rates were significantly higher than Europeans ($P < 0.01$),
while there was no significant difference in the females. Age was a risk factor
in the New Zealand and Rarotonga samples, while female sex and parity
were risk factors in the New Zealand samples, both Maori and European.

Parity
The age-standardized prevalence rates of varicose veins in relationship to
parity are set out in Table 16.19. The small numbers of cases of varicose veins
in the Pukapukans and Tokelauans prevented examination of these relationships. This indicated, however, that parity could not have been a factor
responsible for the differing prevalence rates.

Height
A relationship with height was found in the New Zealand European Maori
and Rarotonga males but only in the Maori females. The prevalence rates
percentage of varicose veins by height is shown for males in Table 16.20.

Weight
Weight showed a relationship to varicose vein prevalence in the New

Table 16.18 Age-standardized prevalence rates (%) of varicose veins in South Pacific samples of males and females 15–64 years

	New Zealand		Cook Islands		Tokelau Island
	Maori	European	Rarotonga	Pukapuka	
Males	$33\cdot4\left(\dfrac{129}{366}\right)^{1}$	$19\cdot6\left(\dfrac{39}{173}\right)$	$15\cdot6\left(\dfrac{34}{219}\right)$	$2\cdot1\left(\dfrac{4}{199}\right)$	$2\cdot9\left(\dfrac{9}{347}\right)$
Females	$43\cdot6\left(\dfrac{166}{355}\right)$	$37\cdot8\left(\dfrac{77}{183}\right)$	$14\cdot9\left(\dfrac{29}{198}\right)$	$4\cdot0\left(\dfrac{7}{178}\right)$	$0\cdot8\left(\dfrac{3}{439}\right)$

[1] Number of cases and population at risk in parentheses

Table 16.19 Age-standardized prevalence rates (%) of varicose veins by parity in South Pacific samples of females 15–64 years

Parity	0	1–2	3–4	5–8	>8
Maori	$22 \cdot 3 \left(\frac{11}{63}\right)$ [1]	$38 \cdot 6 \left(\frac{26}{63}\right)$	$46 \cdot 3 \left(\frac{25}{51}\right)$	$51 \cdot 3 \left(\frac{53}{87}\right)$	$49 \cdot 2 \left(\frac{51}{79}\right)$
European	$13 \cdot 1 \left(\frac{3}{26}\right)$	$30 \cdot 7 \left(\frac{22}{66}\right)$	$44 \cdot 4 \left(\frac{35}{62}\right)$	$46 \cdot 9 \left(\frac{17}{29}\right)$	$-\left(\frac{0}{0}\right)$
Rarotonga	$27 \cdot 4 \left(\frac{5}{16}\right)$	$10 \cdot 9 \left(\frac{4}{48}\right)$	$12 \cdot 7 \left(\frac{3}{35}\right)$	$15 \cdot 0 \left(\frac{8}{47}\right)$	$13 \cdot 9 \left(\frac{7}{37}\right)$

[1] Number of cases and population at risk in parentheses

Table 16.20 Age-standardized prevalence rates (%) of varicose veins by height (cm) in South Pacific samples of males 15–64 years

Height (cm)	<165	165–169	170–174	>175
Maori	$28 \cdot 6 \left(\frac{21}{68}\right)$ [1]	$30 \cdot 7 \left(\frac{36}{110}\right)$	$33 \cdot 2 \left(\frac{38}{111}\right)$	$42 \cdot 1 \left(\frac{34}{77}\right)$
European	$6 \cdot 0 \left(\frac{1}{13}\right)$	$14 \cdot 3 \left(\frac{7}{40}\right)$	$21 \cdot 4 \left(\frac{12}{51}\right)$	$24 \cdot 4 \left(\frac{19}{69}\right)$
Rarotonga	$7 \cdot 9 \left(\frac{2}{29}\right)$	$17 \cdot 0 \left(\frac{7}{38}\right)$	$13 \cdot 2 \left(\frac{11}{82}\right)$	$21 \cdot 2 \left(\frac{14}{68}\right)$

[1] Number of cases and population at risk in parentheses

Zealand European and Maori samples, both male and female but not in Rarotongans. The differing weight pattern of the groups was such that weight cannot be invoked as a factor contributing to the striking variation in prevalence of varicose veins in Polynesians.

The positive associations documented in the New Zealand European and Maori survey were in accordance with results reported by other workers. The Rarotongans represented an intermediate picture where age was the only significant relationship. The gradient observed followed the pattern of contact with the Western world and it is here that the answers to the question may lie. Atoll dwellers have had the least contact, Rarotongans an intermediate degree of contact, and the New Zealand samples the most contact and direct involvement in Western industralized lifestyle. The data from these studies certainly rules out genetic susceptibility as the primary cause for varicose veins and must invoke the importance of environmental factors.

Table 16.21 Age-standardized prevalence rates (%) of varicose veins by weight (kg) in South Pacific samples of males and females 15–64 years

Weight		<60	60–69	70–79	>80
Males	Maori	$16 \cdot 6 \left(\frac{2}{18}\right)^{1}$	$32 \cdot 3 \left(\frac{17}{66}\right)$	$29 \cdot 3 \left(\frac{31}{100}\right)$	$36 \cdot 7 \left(\frac{79}{182}\right)$
	European	$6 \cdot 2 \left(\frac{1}{15}\right)$	$21 \cdot 8 \left(\frac{14}{56}\right)$	$16 \cdot 1 \left(\frac{10}{58}\right)$	$24 \cdot 6 \left(\frac{14}{44}\right)$
	Rarotonga	$11 \cdot 9 \left(\frac{2}{19}\right)$	$12 \cdot 9 \left(\frac{7}{59}\right)$	$20 \cdot 0 \left(\frac{14}{74}\right)$	$14 \cdot 6 \left(\frac{11}{65}\right)$
Females	Maori	$36 \cdot 4 \left(\frac{22}{74}\right)$	$43 \cdot 8 \left(\frac{42}{94}\right)$	$46 \cdot 7 \left(\frac{39}{73}\right)$	$45 \cdot 0 \left(\frac{63}{116}\right)$
	European	$32 \cdot 0 \left(\frac{30}{88}\right)$	$36 \cdot 0 \left(\frac{23}{55}\right)$	$45 \cdot 4 \left(\frac{11}{19}\right)$	$45 \cdot 5 \left(\frac{13}{21}\right)$
	Rarotonga	$12 \cdot 9 \left(\frac{4}{36}\right)$	$12 \cdot 8 \left(\frac{4}{45}\right)$	$15 \cdot 0 \left(\frac{7}{48}\right)$	$17 \cdot 6 \left(\frac{14}{64}\right)$

[1] Number of cases and population at risk in parentheses

Reference has already been made to the traditional atoll diet of Pukapukans and Tokelauans and to the extent of energy from carbohydrate and sucrose being used in the different groups. The atoll dwellers, with reliance on coconut, fish, starchy roots, breadfruit, flour and rice, are on very different diets from these in Rarotonga where traditional foods are being replaced by flour, rice, canned meat and fish and much higher use of sucrose.

Smoking and smoking disorders in the Pacific

The pattern of tobacco use in the Pacific shows a wide and interesting distribution in different populations. The type and amount of tobacco used is influenced by the stage of westernization, the cash income, by the societal constraints, particularly the influence of the church on what women should or should not do. In many of the more traditional subsistence economies the tobacco used is Derby plug, a coarse type of compressed leaf from which small amounts are cut and smoked in a dried leaf of a pandanas tree. The strong church influence in such societies tends to frown on tobacco use by women, but not by men. The smoking rates are high in men, reaching 80 per cent in Tokelau, but the mean number of cigarettes smoked per day is low, four per day.

In societies with greater per capita income, cigarettes are either rolled, using tobacco and cigarette papers, or tailor-made. The use of tailor-made cigarettes is limited for the most part to the higher income group such as doctors, school teachers and those in the public service in such societies. The contrast with New Zealand Maori is very considerable where smoking by both men and women has been very common, and where few constraints have ever influenced the pattern. The long period of tobacco availability and the wide acceptance by the New Zealand Maori are important contributing factors to their high rate of morbidity and mortality from lung cancer, chronic obstructive airways diseases, bronchitis and coronary artery disease, that is, the smoking diseases. It is certainly a highly significant fact that the New Zealand Maori female death rate from coronary artery disease and lung cancer is the highest in the world.

Studies have been carried out among secondary school students in New Zealand that indicate the extent of the problem in both Maoris and Europeans (Stanhope, 1978). Among students reporting half or more Maori ancestry, this prevalence was 57 per cent in boys and 65 per cent in girls, compared with rates of 26 per cent and 20 per cent in European boys and girls respectively. Elder siblings, peers and parental attitudes were seen as important factors in determining smoking habits in these groups. The differences demonstrated in a survey among different adult groups in the Pacific for different categories are set out in Table 16.22 for men and Table 16.23 for women. The period when the data was collected is also set out. The much higher rate in New Zealand Maori males and females has been confirmed in the National Census of 1976 where questions were asked about smoking status and the number of cigarettes per day. This has been linked with

Table 16.22 Smoking rates (%) in males in four Polynesian and one New Zealand European sample

	Non-	Ex-	Smoking	Light	Medium	Heavy
Pukapuka 1964	22	4	74	25	60	15
Rarotonga 1964	23	9	68	16	57	27
Tokelau 1976	31	7	62	99	1	—
Tokelau NZ 1975–77	31	14	55	35	42	23
NZ Maori 1974	22	21	57	37	25	38
NZ European 1964	20	24	55	11	37	52

Table 16.23 Smoking rates (%) in females in four Polynesian and one New Zealand European sample

	Non-	Ex-	Smoking	Light	Medium	Heavy
Pukapuka 1964	56	4	40	84	12	4
Rarotonga 1964	68	1	31	63	31	6
Tokelau 1976	65	12	23	99	1	—
Tokelau NZ 1975–77	58	11	31	73	20	7
NZ Maori 1974	26	16	61	37	33	30
Carterton European 1964	61	9	29	22	50	28

ethnicity and has produced valuable data concerning the extent of smoking in New Zealand. This illustrates the value that can accrue from simple health-related questions at the time of national census collections. The distribution of smoking practice from the National Census is set out in Table 16.24.

The health and disease problems of the tobacco-related disorders present important areas of potential prevention. The inadequacies of our present methods of health education in the Western world make it important that methods of intervention be developed for the emerging countries that are worked out with the indigenous people and adapted to their societies.

Table 16.24 Smoking practice of ethnic groups in New Zealand, percentage distribution of males and females in the New Zealand population according to smoking status (1976 Census data)

	Male			Female		
Group	Never smoked	Used to smoke	Smoke regularly	Never smoked	Used to smoke	Smoke regularly
Maori	31	13	56	30	11	59
Pacific islander	44	10	46	69	7	24
All others	39	23	38	58	12	30

Migrants are at greater risk in their new societies and data from the Tokelauan study in fact show a small decline in the number of male smokers, but they smoke more than in Tokelau, a median of 14 per day. More migrant Tokelau women are smoking and they are clearly following the pattern coming forward in European young women in New Zealand and other parts of the world.

Primordial[1] prevention—a new concept

An expert committee of the World Health Organization has recently put forward the case for the prevention of the development of high cardiovascular risk in those traditional, isolated and developing third world countries where these disorders at present are only minor problems (WHO Report, 1978). They have put forward the concept of primordial prevention, and make the case for intensive research into ways and means of lessening the steady progression which is emerging in many groups as they take on the Western pattern of living, diet and society. The contrast between some of the Pacific Polynesian populations and the fully developed atheroma-prone hypertensive, diabetic and obese New Zealand Maori highlights the problem and provides some clues as to how the problem should be tackled. The concept of primordial prevention is central to the theme of this book and the summation of experience described in the different chapters may act as a catalyst for sustained serious research and work in this area. Certainly the detailed data on coronary disease in the New Zealand Maori produced from the cross-sectional and longitudinal surveys carried out between 1962 and 1974 have added to knowledge of the natural history and correlates of the disorder in the Maori. The part played by hypertension and the lack of predictive power of cholesterol levels and smoking pose a number of questions and illustrate that coronary artery disease may have a different mix of predisposing factors in

[1]Existing from the beginning (*Chambers Twentieth Century Dictionary*).

different populations. The rate of development and emergence of the varied consequences of movement into Western living and eating habits is well illustrated from the Pacific data. The New Zealand Maori have the full picture, but still with total cholesterol levels that are lower than in New Zealand Europeans. Their low HDLC levels in both males and females, adults and adolescents and lowish LDLC levels clearly separate them from what is seen in New Zealand Europeans. Higher triglycerides, higher diabetes, obesity, hyperuricaemia and gout are other concomitants that add to their risk status. The low risk status on most of these counts of the Pakapukans and the intermediate status of Tokelauans offer clear examples of the 'emergence' effect. They give clues also to directions for prevention. The changes occurring in the Tokelauan migrants to New Zealand, both adult and children, indicate the all-pervading influence of migration into a Western environment. Weight, blood pressure and diabetes increase and social patterns alter. However, those who remain in a Tokelau environment and network maintain lower blood pressures and so derive some protection compared with those who move more clearly into a European environment and personal relationships.

The process of change following migration is being observed and the time for interventions is drawing close. Knowledge of how to intervene, how to measure the process and the outcomes will require new approaches. The involvement of the Tokelau community will be a keystone to any progress that is made. Lessons will be learnt from the major efforts of community health education that have shown considerable success in North Karelia in Eastern Finland (Puska, 1973; 1977) and the Stanford Heart Disease Prevention Programme (Farquhar *et al.*, 1977). In both of these studies significant changes in coronary risk factors, blood pressure control and diet were achieved by well-planned and sustained health education programmes. Major involvement of the communities was a key part of these. The application of these intensive methods would need considerable modification for use in developing societies in a state of rapid change and with limited resources, where new values are replacing old, where emphasis is now being placed on the nuclear family, individual betterment and decreased acceptance of responsibilities to extended family and to the community. There is talk in the Pacific of 'The Pacific Way', an approach which embodies many of these long-held and valuable characteristics together with a real sense of cooperation and calm in the approach to life and its activities. Changes are taking place as more and more of the Pacific countries become independent and have to make their way in a changing world. Urbanization and migration are the major components of the changes taking place. Westernization is a central part in this process and the conflicts and advantages involved influence health and disease status. Knowledge of these relationships and a willingness to collect information concerning the way they produce their effects must be given high priority if the otherwise relentless progress towards a high risk atherogenic cardiovascular and metabolic status is to be avoided or lessened. The Western world has been overtaken by its plagues and ills and they are many and pervasive. Knowledge, understanding, application and legislation and a greater awareness of the need for personal responsibility for health will all be needed if progress is to be made by those countries who still have the opportunity to do so.

Can the scientists now work with the politicians, health service personnel and people of those many countries at 'serious risk' and make primordial prevention a reality? If it is not done in the next few years it will be too late.

'Mauri tu, Mauri ora, mauri noho, mauri mate,'

'He who stands, lives, who sleeps dies.'

Mauri is the life principle of a man. Nowadays most use it to signify that one must work and be alert in a European world if he wishes to succeed. What costs does this carry?

Acknowledgements

The authors wish to acknowledge the help received from many sources in preparation of this chapter. The Epidemiology Unit, Wellington Hospital, receives and gratefully acknowledges support from the Medical Research Council of New Zealand, the Cardiovascular Disease Unit of WHO and the Wellington Hospital Board. The participation of the many Pacific people in the studies is particularly acknowledged.

References

Alexander, C. J. (1972). Chair sitting and varicose veins. *Lancet*, **i**, 822–823

Beaglehole, R., Eyles, Elaine, Salmond Clare, E. and Prior, Ian (1978a). Blood pressure in Tokelauan children in two contrasting environments. *American Journal of Epidemiology*, **108**, 283–288

Beaglehole, R., Prior, I. A. M., Salmond Clare, E. and Eyles, Elaine (1978b). Coronary heart disease in Maoris: incidence and case mortality. *New Zealand Medical Journal*, **88**, 138–141

Beaglehole, R., Prior, I. A. M., Salmond Clare, E. and Davidson, Flora (1975a). Varicose veins in the South Pacific. *International Journal of Epidemiology*, **4**, 295–299

Beaglehole, R., Prior, I. A. M. and Salmond Clare, E. (1975b). Prevalence of coronary heart disease in New Zealand Maoris and Pakehas. *New Zealand Medical Journal*, **82**, 119–122

Beaglehole, R., Prior, I. A. M., Eyles, E. and Sampson, V. (1979). High density lipoprotein cholesterol and other serum lipids in New Zealand Maoris. *New Zealand Medical Journal*, **90**, 139–142

Beaglehole, R., Salmond Clare, E., Hooper, Antony, Huntsman, Judith, Stanhope, J., Cassel, John C. and Prior, I. A. M. (1977). Blood pressure and social interaction in Tokelau migrants in New Zealand. *Journal of Chronic Diseases*, **30**, 803–812

Birkbeck, J. A. (1979). New Zealanders and their diet. *A Report to the National Heart Foundation of New Zealand on the National Diet Survey 1977*. Department of Nutrition, University of Otago, Dunedin, New Zealand

Burkitt, D. P. (1972). Varicose veins, deep vein thrombosis, and haemorrhoids: epidemiology and suggested aetiology. *British Medical Journal*, 2, 556–561

Cassel, J. (1974). Hypertension and cardiovascular disease in migrants: a potential source of clues? *International Journal of Epidemiology*, 3, 204–206

Castelle, W. P., Cooper, G. R., Doyle, J. T., Garcia-Palmieri, M., Gordon, T., Hames, C., Hulley, S. B., Kagan, A., Kuchmak, M., McGee, D. and Vicic, W. J. (1977). Distribution of triglyceride and total LDL and HDL cholesterol in several populations: a cooperative lipoprotein phenotyping study. *Journal of Chronic Diseases*, 30, 147–169

Cleave, T. L. and Campbell, G. D. (1969). *Diabetes, Coronary Thrombosis and the Saccharine Disease*, 78–83. John Wright, Bristol

Cummings, J. H. and Wiggins, J. S., (1976). Transit through the gut measured by analysis of a single stool. *Gut*, 1, 219–223

Evans, J. G. and Prior, I. A. M. (1969). The Carterton study: 4. Serum cholesterol levels of a sample of New Zealand European adults. *New Zealand Medical Journal*, 69, 346–350

Farquhar, J. W., Maccoby, N., Wood, P. D., Alexander, J. K., Breitrose, H., Brown, B. W. Jr., Haskell, W. L., McAlister, A. L., Meyer, A. J., Nash, J. D. and Stern, M. P. (1977). Community education for cardiovascular health. *Lancet*, i, 1192–1195

Gordon, T., Castelle, W. P., Hjortland, M. C., Kannel, W. B. and Dawber, T. R. (1977). High density lipoprotein as a protective factor against coronary heart disease. The Framingham Study. *American Journal of Medicine*, 62, 707–714

Kannel, W. B., Dawber, T. R., Kagan, A., Revotski, W. and Stokes, J. (1961). Factors of risk in the development of coronary heart disease—six year follow up experience. The Framingham Study. *Annals of Internal Medicine*, 55, 33–50

Kelsey, J. L. (1978). A review of research on effects of fiber intake in human nutrition. *American Journal of Clinical Nutrition*, 31, 142–159

MacLaurin, B. P., Wardell, T. E. M. and Faaiuau, S. T. (1979a). Environmental aspects of peptic ulcer disease in Western Samoa. *New Zealand Medical Journal*, 89, 376–378

MacLaurin, B. P., Wardell, T. E. M., Faaiuau, S. T. and McKinnon, M. (1979b). Geographic distribution of peptic ulcer disease in Western Samoa. *New Zealand Medical Journal*, 89, 341–344

Mekky, S., Schilling, R. S. F. and Walford, J. (1969). Varicose veins in women cotton workers. An epidemiological study in England and Egypt. *British Medical Journal*, 2, 591–595

Murphy, W. (1955). Some observations on blood pressure in the humid tropics. *New Zealand Medical Journal*, 54, 64–73

Nye, E. R., Sutherland, W. H. F., Larking, P. W. and Spears, G. F. S. (1977). Blood lipids and lipo-proteins in a rural New Zealand population. *Australian and New Zealand Journal of Medicine*, **7**, 134–137

Prior, I. A. M. (1962). A health survey in a rural Maori community. With particular emphasis on cardiovascular, nutritional and metabolic findings. *New Zealand Medical Journal*, **61**, 333–348

Prior, I. A. M. (1974). Cardiovascular epidemiology in New Zealand and the Pacific. *New Zealand Medical Journal*, **80**, 245–252

Prior, I. A. M. (1976). *Population Studies in New Zealanders and in South Pacific Populations. Cardiovascular Epidemiology in the Pacific.* World Health Organization Report

Prior, I. A. M., Beaglehole, R., Davidson, Flora and Salmond Clare, E. (1978). The relationship of diabetes, blood lipids and uric acid levels in Polynesians. *Advances in Metabolic Disorders*, **9**, 241–261. Editors P. H. Bennet and M. Miller. Academic Press Inc., New York

Prior, I. A. M. and Davidson, F. (1966). The epidemiology of diabetes in Polynesians and Europeans in New Zealand and the Pacific. *New Zealand Medical Journal*, **65**, 375–383

Prior, I. A. M., Evans, J. G., Harvey, H. P. B., Davidson, F. and Lindsey, M. (1968). Sodium intake and blood pressure in two Polynesian populations. *New England Journal of Medicine*, **279**, 515–520

Prior, I. A. M., Evans, J. G., Morrison, R. B. I. and Rose, B. S. (1970). The Carterton study: 6. Patterns of vascular, respiratory, rheumatic and related abnormalities in a sample of New Zealand European adults. *New Zealand Medical Journal* **72**, 169–177

Prior, I. A. M., Rose, B. S. and Davidson, F. (1964). Metabolic maladies in New Zealand Maoris. *British Medical Journal*, **1**, 1065–1069

Prior, I. A. M., Stanhope, J. M., Evans, J. G. and Salmond Clare, E. (1974). The Tokelau Island Migrant Study. *International Journal of Epidemiology*, **3**, 225–232

Puska, P. (1973). The North Karelia project. An attempt at the community prevention of cardiovascular disease. *World Health Organisation Chronicle*, **27**, 55

Puska, P. (1977). Heart attacks fell sturdiest of Finns. *New York Times*, p. 24. September 19

Stanhope, J. M. (1975). Varicose veins in a population of lowland New Guinea. *International Journal of Epidemiology*, **4**, 221–225

Stanhope, J. M. (1978). Social patterns of adolescent cigarette smoking in a rural community. *New Zealand Medical Journal*, **87**, 343–348

Stanhope, J. M., Prior, I. A. M. and Malcolm, J. B. (1975). Coronary risk factors in New Zealand Maori and European adolescents: the Rotorua Lakes Study 2. *New Zealand Medical Journal*, **82**, 336–339

Stanhope, J. M., Sampson, Vivienne M. and Clarkson, Patricia M. (1977). High density lipoprotein cholesterol and other serum lipids in a New Zealand biracial adolescent sample: the Wairoa College survey. *Lancet*, **i**, 968–970

Stewart, A. M., Webb, H. W. and Hewitt, D. (1955). Social medicine studies on civilian medical records. II Physical and occupational characteristics of men with varicose conditions. *British Journal of Preventive and Social Medicine,* **9,** 26–32

Weddell, J. M. (1969). Varicose veins pilot survey 1966. *British Journal of Preventive and Social Medicine,* **23,** 179–186

Wigley, R. D. and MacLaurin, B. P. (1962). A study of ulcerative colitis in New Zealand showing a low incidence in Maoris. *British Medical Journal,* **ii,** 228–231

World Health Organisation (1978). *Report of WHO Consultation on Primordial Prevention of Cardiovascular Diseases in Developing Countries.* CUD/791. WHO, Geneva

17

Israeli Migrants

Baruch Modan

Ethnic and population groups

Israel, with a total population of approximately 3·6 million, comprises a
wide variety of ethnic groups, originating from every corner of the globe.
This heterogeneous mixture, which undergoes a rapid amalgamation process,
due to a common environment and a dynamic society, provides an optimal
milieu for the study of differential disease distribution, and of the effect of
migration on disease patterns.

Not infrequently, disease characteristics in Israel are compared between
two main population categories—Ashkenazi ('German' in literal translation)
and Sephardic ('Spanish'). The first category is used as a synonym for Jews
of European extraction and encompasses migrants from Europe, the
Americas, South Africa, Australia and New Zealand. The second category is
usually, but wrongly, used as a synonym for those originating from the
Middle East and North Africa, who are also referred to as 'Oriental' or
'Eastern'. Although there are no 'Ashkenazi' constituents among the latter,
the true 'Sephardi', who are descendants of migrants sent into exile from
Spain and Portugal in the fifteenth century, include migrants and native-born
originating from Bulgaria, Greece, Italy, Turkey, Yugoslavia and to a lesser
extent from North Africa.

In fact, we should consider five major population groups as follows.

European and American
This category constitutes the largest ethnic group, and totals now about
800 000 individuals. These have migrated from Russia and Poland since the
end of the nineteenth century through the 1920s, followed by waves of
migration from Germany and Poland in the 1930s, and Rumania, Bulgaria
and Poland in the late 1940s and 1950s. The major influx in recent years has
been from Russia, and South and North America. Persons born in Australia,
New Zealand and South Africa are usually considered as part of this group
because of basically similar parentage.

Some recent immigrants from France and Spain are, in fact, of North
African extraction.

North African

The vast majority of these individuals, currently amounting to 340 000, have arrived in Israel between 1948 and 1970, primarily from Morocco, Algiers, Tunisia, Libya, and to a lesser extent from Egypt. In 1948 they constituted only 2 per cent of the total foreign-born Jewish population in the country as compared to 24 per cent today.

There are no Israeli migrants from Central Africa.

Middle Eastern

Currently, this group amounts to 300 000 individuals. They also constituted a minority prior to the establishment of the State of Israel—12 per cent of the foreign-born—but gained strength during the 1948–54 period by migrants coming from Yemen, Iraq, Turkey and in more recent years from Iran. Others came from Syria, the Lebanon, India and Afghanistan. They resemble the North African group in most of their socioeconomic characteristics, and despite their different genetic background are frequently grouped with the latter for demographic purposes.

There are practically no migrants from Eastern and South Eastern Asia, with the exception of a small Russian community, coming from China, who are grouped for demographic purposes with the European-born.

Israeli-born Jews

This is a very heterogeneous group, reflecting the migration patterns since the end of the last century. Today, they comprise close to 55 per cent of the total Jewish population in Israel, with an outstanding age distribution— about 88 per cent are younger than 30, while less than one per cent are above 60. Forty-seven per cent of the Israeli natives are of Asian and North African parentage, and 31 per cent are of European extraction. There is a negative correlation between age and the proportion of the non-Europeans among the natives, since the non-Europeans arrived in Israel relatively recently, and because they have more children per family than the European-born.

Non-Jews

Within the 1967 borderlines, there are close to 600 000 non-Jews, the vast majority of whom are Moslem and Christian Arabs, and Druz. Most, but not all, of these are Israeli-born. They are concentrated primarily in the Northern and East–Central parts of the country, and have a relatively larger proportion of rural residents.

Hospitalization referrals and data accuracy are lower in this population segment and thus comparison of disease patterns with the Jewish subgroups is ambiguous.

Population characteristics

This review will be limited to the Jewish population. Emphasis will be made on those disorders that are at present of prime attention in the Western world.

Comparisons will be focused at variation in disease patterns between the two major migrant groups, (a) European–American ('Western'), (b) North African and Middle Eastern ('Eastern') that differ in their genetic, cultural and socioeconomic and environmental backgrounds.

From a genetic viewpoint, there is no pure 'Jewish' group. The nucleus of the 'Western' Jews were descendants of the Diaspora taken into exile by the Romans in the first century. Genetic heterogeneity started as far back as then, because of the ancient Roman custom of intermarrying slaves from different nationalities. This admixture has been strongly augmented during the eighth century when a large Russian tribe—the Kazars—converted to Judaism, and subsequently, by continuous forceful mixture of the neighbouring populations.

The equivalent 'Eastern' Diaspora dates to the destruction of the First Temple in 586 BC and subsequent, voluntary, out-migration to the East, South and West of Old Judea, during the following five centuries. Cross-breeding, due to a variety of reasons, though less thoroughly documented than among the 'Western', also occurred.

The best illustration of the genetic polymorphism is provided by the prevalence of G6PD deficiency, first described by Sheba *et al.* (1962) over 20 years ago. The enzyme deficiency ranges from less than one per cent in those of European extraction to over 50 per cent among those originating in Kurdistan. Similar observations with regard to other genetic traits were made by Bonneh *et al.* (1979) and Adam (1973).

Coming from diametrically opposed cultures, the two populations vary markedly in their socioeconomic backgrounds and in life habits. The Europeans, as a group, have achieved a relatively higher educational and economic status as compared to the Middle Asian and North African. They tend to reside in better urban areas, have smaller families, and a relatively lower dwelling density.

Due to the integration process of the Israeli society and the small geographical size of the country, the variability in life patterns is rapidly disappearing. Uncovering the potential relationship of this social change to disease patterns, while it lasts, provides an intriguing challenge to the epidemiologist.

Disease patterns

The optimal method to determine a disease pattern in a given population group is to define the incidence of the disease at given time periods, and to make comparisons with other populations. Temporal and spatial changes in disease distribution over time may yield aetiological clues. This approach is dependent on four factors:

1. availability and validity of data sources;
2. continuous updating and data monitoring;
3. cost of data accrual;
4. disease severity.

In contrast to infectious diseases, the prolonged latency in chronic conditions presents a particular burden in the evaluation of environmental factors in a migrant population, due to the inability to determine whether the disease process started in the country of origin, or was acquired in the country of residence; unless the factors are related to life habits that have not been abandoned in the second country.

Genetic disorders

Hundreds of years of isolation of small Jewish communities, with frequent consanguinous marriages, have contributed to a high frequency of certain genetic disorders in certain Jewish populations. These genetic diseases are prevalent either in the European or in the non-European groups; never in both.

At least six rare metabolic disorders tend to appear more frequently among Jews of Eastern European origin, than among any other ethnic group in the world. Foremost of these is Tay–Sachs disease, which occurs in one out of 4000 Ashkenazi births, both in Israel and in the USA, as compared with 1 : 500 000 among non-Jews in the USA. Other conditions that follow a similar pattern are Neimann–Pick's and Gaucher's diseases, Riley–Day's (familial disautonomia) and Bloom's syndromes and pentosuria.

Several other inborn errors of metabolism are highly prevalent among selected non-European subgroups. The most prominent of these is haemolytic anaemia due to glucose-6-phosphate dehydrogenase deficiency (G6PD), which reaches a frequency of 58 per cent in Jews coming from Kurdistan, 25 per cent in the rest of Iraqi Jews, and only 0·5 per cent among the Europeans (Sheba *et al.*, 1962). Thalassaemia is also found primarily in Iraqi Jews. Dubin–Johnson's disease, a chronic liver syndrome, is concentrated among Iranian migrants, who have the world's highest incidence of this condition. Phenylketonuria occurs primarily in Jews originating from Yemen and is practically non-existent in Ashkenazis. Familial Mediterranean fever (FMF), a disorder manifested by repetitive inflammatory attacks of abdominal, pleural and joint pains, as well as by amyloidosis, is prevalent primarily among North Africans, notably those coming from Libya. Ataxia-telangiectasia is more prevalent among the Moroccan-born.

The increasing number of inter-ethnic marriages in Israel, coupled with a decrease in consanguinity, should lead to a dilution of the gene pools and to a decline in the overt frequency of these deleterious conditions.

Diseases of a potential environmental background

In general terms, diseases known to be more prevalent in Western society, and/or among individuals of higher socioeconomic status in developed countries, are relatively more prevalent in the European segment of the Israeli population. The most prominent examples are cardiovascular disorders and cancer. These are also the conditions most extensively investigated.

Cardiovascular disorders

Ischaemic heart disease

One of the first observations on the differential incidence of non-infectious diseases in Israel was made by Dreyfuss (1953), who emphasized an extremely low rate of myocardial infarction among Yemenites. The observation was subsequently expanded to the broader category of 'Eastern' Jews and confirmed through death certificates by Kallner and Blondheim (1956), and later by morbidity studies by Toor *et al.* (1960), Medalie *et al.* (1973) and others. The studies have consistently demonstrated a higher incidence of the various manifestations of ischaemic heart disease in the European- and American-born, low rate in the Yemenites, and intermediate among those coming from the rest of Asia and North Africa. The Yemenites, originating from the southern tip of the Arabian Peninsula, also have the lowest rates for a series of other 'Western-type' diseases.

Incidence rates of ischaemic heart disease are high among the first generation Israeli-born of all ethnic groups; while those of non-European parentage are rapidly approaching the rate of the foreign-born Europeans. One interesting aspect is the finding that incidence of myocardial infarction in Israeli-born males is similar to that of the European-born, while in females it is closer to the rate of the Asian–African-born (Shani *et al.,* 1975). A similar observation was noted only in colon cancer (Mass and Modan, 1969), and may suggest common aetiology. This topic will be elaborated later.

Recently, there has been an indication of an overall decline in the mortality from ischaemic heart disease, which is compatible with similar observations in the USA. However, since this conclusion is not based on morbidity data, it is plausible that the decline reflects a decrease in case–fatality ratio. The latter could be ascribed to earlier hospitalization, introduction of coronary care units, mobile care teams and/or improved drug therapy, rather than reflect a true decrease of disease incidence.

Hypertension

While the inter-ethnic differences in arteriosclerotic heart disease seem clear-cut, the patterns of related disorders, such as diabetes and hypertension, are less certain. Current data (Modan *et al.,* 1979) suggest a slightly higher prevalence of hypertension in the North African and a low one among the Yemenites. This finding is consistent with a higher incidence of end-stage kidney disease (Modan *et al.,* 1975b) and of mortality from stroke in the North African-born. However, no distinction is usually made between primary and secondary hypertension.

Diabetes

Earlier reports by Cohen (1961) indicated a low incidence of diabetes in the

Yemenites, while more recent studies (Medalie *et al.*, 1974; Modan, M., Modan, B. and Spitz, I., unpublished data) demonstrate a relatively higher incidence in the Yemenites, a relatively high incidence in the Middle Eastern and North African, and a lower incidence in the Europeans. The different results can be explained by varying methodology, for instance, fasting blood glucose, versus urinary samples, or glucose tolerance test; also, by lack of consideration of related variables such as weight or height. In any case, there is hardly any basis to support a single aetiological structure for the three disorders—ischaemic heart disease, hypertension and diabetes—which are, quite often, nosologically grouped.

Cancer

Patterns of cancer incidence in Israel show strong parallelism with findings in the Western world (Modan, 1974). Thus, by and large, cancer sites that occur more frequently among the white US population, are more prevalent among the European-born Israeli, while those that occur more frequently among US blacks are relatively more prevalent among the non-Europeans.

Cancer sites occurring more frequently among the European-born are colon and rectum (Mass and Modan, 1969), breast (Shani *et al.*, 1966), ovary (Schenker *et al.*, 1968), uterine corpus (Sharon *et al.*, 1977), brain tumours (Cohen and Modan, 1968), chronic lymphatic leukaemia (Waterhouse *et al.*, 1976), malignant melanoma (Movshovitz and Modan, 1973) and gall-bladder in females (Hart *et al.*, 1972). On the other hand, cancer of the uterine cervix (Sharon *et al.*, 1977) and the nasopharynx (Turgman *et al.*, 1977) occur more frequently among the North African- and to a certain extent among the Asian-born. Cancer of the oesophagus is more prevalent among Jews coming from Iran and Yemen (Shani and Modan, 1975), hepatic cancer among Yemenites (Costin and Steinitz, 1971) and cancer of the larynx among immigrants coming from Bulgaria, Greece and Turkey (Shiloh, S. and Modan, B., unpublished data). Cancer of the stomach (Tulchinsky and Modan, 1967) and lung (Modan, 1978) are also higher in the European-born, contrary to the expected pattern of a lower risk in higher socioeconomic groups.

Since there is little common genetic background for the Israeli and American subgroups, it seems that the similarities observed may be associated with inter-ethnic differences in socioeconomic status. These findings corroborate previously made observations regarding the role of environmental factors in carcinogenesis.

An alternative hypothesis would be a similarity in certain biochemical parameters such as, for instance, glucose-6-phosphate dehydrogenase deficiency, which is also more prevalent in US blacks (Sheba *et al.*, 1962; Beaconsfield *et al.*, 1965). Although this explanation cannot be ruled out, it does not seem likely in view of the very similar cancer pattern among the North African- and Asian-born groups in Israel, despite the marked difference in the frequency of the enzyme deficiency.

Thus, we are faced with three different types of neoplasia in the population:

1. sites associated with high socioeconomic status—particularly breast, ovary, endometrium, brain and the large bowel;
2. those more prevalent in the lower socioeconomic groups, such as the uterine cervix or the nasopharynx; and
3. sites that might be attributed either to endogenous factors, or alternatively, to environmental factors that operate to a similar extent in all socioeconomic levels, e.g. the thyroid.

The fact that more recent data from the USA based on the 1969 cancer survey (Cutler *et al.*, 1974) demonstrate an increase of cancer incidence among the blacks, strengthens this hypothesis; i.e. with upgrading of socioeconomic standards, differences in cancer incidence tend to disappear.

The two leading sites of cancer in Israel (excluding skin) are lung and stomach in males and breast and stomach in females. This is true for all ethnic categories except for the North African-born females, where cancer of the uterine cervix assumes second place.

Cervical cancer

This has frequently been singled out as a rare malignancy among Jewish women (Kessler, 1974). This apparent rarity has been construed to indicate the protective role of circumcision. Recently it has been demonstrated that the low incidence is limited to Jews of European origin, and that incidence is actually high in those originating from Morocco (Sharon *et al.*, 1977) in comparison to rates among non-Jewish populations outside Israel. The 'protective' role of circumcision has also been challenged on the basis of lack of observations of an increased risk in case-controlled studies in the USA (Terris *et al.*, 1967), as well as by the fact that the disease is prevalent in circumcised non-Jewish populations such as those of Iran and Turkey (Laurent *et al.*, 1969).

It seems now that the low risk of the disease in the European-born Israeli females, as well as among Jewish women in the USA and Europe, is related to factors associated with sexual behaviour, and possibly the availability of a reservoir of a viral agent such as herpes type II. Higher antibody titres to this virus were found in Israeli women of all ethnic groups with cervical cancer, as compared to respective controls (Menczer *et al.*, 1975). The viral hypothesis is also consistent with the closed community life led by Diaspora Jews throughout the years.

The higher rate of this neoplasm in the Moroccan-born is limited to squamous cell carcinoma, while in the adenocarcinoma variety there are practically no differences (Menczer *et al.*, 1978). Consequently, in the other Israeli groups, the proportion of cervical adenocarcinoma is relatively higher than elsewhere in the world, reaching a value of close to 10 per cent. This may indicate different aetiology, but attempts to delineate a different aetiology have thus far been unsuccessful (Menczer *et al.*: in Press 1981).

On the other hand, the long-term observation on the rarity of cancer of the penis among Jews has not yet been refuted (Waterhouse *et al.*, 1976), and there is a strong possibility that in this case circumcision may actually play a preventive role. The disease is practically non-existent in Israel, among Jews and Arabs alike.

Cancer of other female organs

These present a mirror image to cervical cancer. The patterns of cancer of the breast, the ovary and the uterine corpus show a marked similarity (Modan, 1974) in their age patterns, and all three are significantly more common in European-born women. Of particular importance is the repeatedly described pattern of breast cancer in Western society (de Waard, 1969), i.e. the presence of Clemenses hook (Lilienfeld, 1956) around the menopause. In contrast, in the non-Europeans, the incidence curve tends to form a plateau around the menopause in a form which is intermediate between the one of Central Europe and that of Japan (Fig. 17.1). The ongoing westernization of the 'Eastern' population segment in Israel is clearly reflected in the fact that both the rate and the disease pattern in the first generation of the native-born Israeli women of non-European extraction, is starting to approximate those of the Europeans.

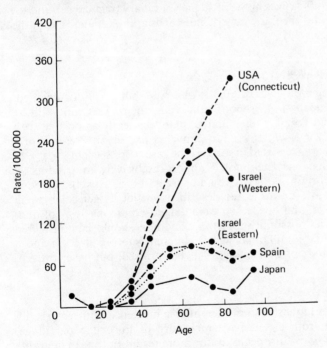

Fig. 17.1 Breast cancer age-specific rates in Israeli women, Western (European-born) and Eastern (not European-born) compared with USA and Japan

Hormonal studies conducted in a sample of healthy post-menopausal women of various ethnic groups, revealed an inverse correlation between the rate of oestriol excretion and breast cancer in each of the groups (Gross *et al.*, 1977). This finding is consistent with the observations of MacMahon *et al.* (1971) and Cole and MacMahon (1970) on differential hormonal patterns in high and low risk American and Japanese women; though their interpretation was related to the ratio $E_3/E_1 + E_2$ rather than to oestriol *per se*.

Three other cancer categories deserve special mentioning, whereby differential incidence patterns may bear an aetiological significance.

Gallbladder cancer

This cancer is relatively more frequent among 'Western' than among 'Eastern' women, but not among the men (Hart *et al.*, 1972); this is in line with the incidence pattern of cholelithiasis. By the same token the male: female ratio is $1:4\cdot5$, similar to the one observed in cholelithiasis. This may indicate a causal relationship between these two conditions (Hart *et al.*, 1971). The presence of gallstones in the vast majority of patients with gallbladder cancer—up to 80 per cent in both sexes—as well as the prolonged period of previous abdominal complaints support this notion. In contrast, there are no ethnic differences in the incidence of biliary tract cancer, the sex ratio is only $1:1\cdot6$, and the frequency of gallstones approximates that of the general population.

Small intestinal lymphoma

This most interesting entity was originally observed, but never documented, by Brandstetter (Modan *et al.*, 1969; Shani *et al.*, 1969). This entity affects primary children and young adults, and is quite frequently associated with malabsorption (Seltzer *et al.*, 1979; Rappaport *et al.*, 1972). Presence of a light chain molecule was reported in some of the cases (Brouet *et al.*, 1977). In Israel, this syndrome has been noted almost exclusively in patients of African and Asian origin, both native and foreign-born, as well as among Arabs. Similarly, most of the cases described outside Israel, such as in France, North Africa, and in Mexico were diagnosed among Jews of non-European origin. The possibility that this condition should be considered analogous to Burkitt's lymphoma, with a different site predilection and a possibly different mode of transmission has been raised, but never proven.

Malignant melanoma

This cancer shows the highest ethnic differential in incidence, with a markedly decreasing gradient from the native Israeli-born of European parentage, through the veteran-born Europeans, to the more recent European migrants and finally to the non-Europeans. This is compatible with the hypothesis that sunlight exposure plays a major role in the aetiology of this disease (Movshovitz and Modan, 1973), particularly among fair-skinned individuals, while the low risk among the non-Europeans indicates the presence of a protective mechanism offered by a darkly pigmented skin. This hypothesis is supported by the higher disease incidence among females, which is limited to sites originating on the extremities, and lack of site predilection in other parts of the body.

Time trends

Comparison of incidence trends over time may be indicative of environmental influence. At present, only preliminary data are available to evaluate this effect and they could reflect only rapidly occurring changes. For all cancer sites combined, there is a trend for an increased incidence, which is evident in both sexes and in all ethnic groups. However, such a generalization may be misleading, since, in fact, this is a combined effect of a clear trend of increase in those sites that are related to high socioeconomic standards, such as colorectal, breast, gallbladder and uterine corpus (as well as—though for different reasons—malignant melanoma) accompanied by a decrease in the sites related to lower socioeconomic standards, e.g. stomach and cervix.

With the exception of gallbladder cancer, where the increased incidence is similar in all ethnic groups, possibly due to better awareness, and brain tumours where there is practically no increase, the increase in the other, so-called Western types of cancer is mostly evident in the low risk non-European groups, indicating, once again, the strong effect of westernization.

Yet, the dramatic increase in the incidence in malignant melanoma among the European and Israeli-born—between two- and three-fold over a 10-year period—should be ascribed to sunlight.

Most interesting, from the viewpoint of aetiological inference, are the secular trends in cervical cancer. There is a significant decrease in the high risk North African, in the middle risk Middle Eastern, and in the low risk Europeans, beyond age 60, but a significant increase in the Israeli-born. The pattern probably reflects the diversification of sexual relations in the Israeli society. The North African female, originating from a community with a high reservoir of a transmissible agent, is now exposed to a decreasing proportion of high risk (North African) partners, while the Israeli-born is being exposed to an increasing proportion of high risk (North African) partners. The lack of change in the post-menopausal European-born women reflects the net effect of an overall decrease in cervical cancer, due to improved socioeconomic standards, coupled with an increased exposure to high risk partners.

The effect of length of residence in Israel on cancer incidence, which may reflect the role of change in environment, culture and daily life habits, has only partly been studied. Yet, there are (Tulchinsky and Modan, 1967; Royston and Modan, 1968) certain indications to support findings obtained in other countries (Buell and Dunn, 1965) that cancer among migrants tends to assume an intermediate position between the range in the country of origin and their host country. The changes are too early to be explained by an increasing frequency of inter-ethnic marriage.

Aetiological considerations

Evaluation of differential incidence of a disease is valuable in pointing out patterns of dynamic changes and in suggesting clues towards aetiology. By now, it should be clear that the Israeli population carries a load of distinct genetic backgrounds, and a multitude of imported environmental factors, augmented by rapidly occurring changes in life habits.

Potential environmental factors that might be instrumental in explaining both the differential incidence and the changing disease patterns are listed below:

Diet	Drugs
Smoking	Stress
Drinking	Hygiene
Water content	Occupation
Air pollution	Fertility
Radiation	Other life habits

It is intriguing to look for a common denominator that could explain the variation in disease patterns and would enable a comprehensive model. Unfortunately, since most chronic diseases are multifactorial, one cannot isolate a single aetiological cause. We have, therefore, to assume that a variety of factors strongly related to socioeconomic status, such as diet, smoking, occupation, sexual attitudes, and/or exposure to environmental hazards, lead to a conglomerate effect. The importance of sun exposure and sexual habits has already been discussed. A third factor, therapeutic radiation in childhood, has been shown to lead to a transient increase in thyroid cancer in a cohort of North African and Middle Eastern-born individuals (Ron and Modan, 1980).

Diet

One of the most prominent components that should be examined in this context is diet. This will be developed somewhat more in detail and taken as a model.

Nutritional habits constitute one of the most obvious differential population parameters. They constitute a daily life habit, which is strongly adhered to, despite migration, but it is also a parameter that is rapidly adaptable in a new environment. Current epidemiological inference with regard to the role of diet in disease aetiology is based mainly on two types of observations: correlations between disease incidence and consumption patterns, and case control studies. The most consistently cited correlations are between Western-type diseases and the consumption of high fat or low fibre food items (Drasar and Irving, 1973; Howell, 1974; Wynder, 1975).

Changes in disease risk with migration have provided some additional leads. One good example for a process of this kind has been demonstrated in a study of Hawaiian Japanese, a population undergoing displacement from low to high risk colon cancer, and of ischaemic heart disease, where a transition pattern from Japanese to Western-style diet (Hankin *et al.*, 1975) has simultaneously occurred. Similar observations were made with regard to breast cancer (Dunn, 1975). A more general observation refers to the fact that colon cancer is rare in developing countries, where fibre consumption is abundant (Burkitt, 1975). The above observations are, however, hampered by the fact that food consumption patterns are highly correlated with one another and with a variety of life habits that differ markedly in industrial and developing societies.

At attempt to identify a specific dietary factor is also difficult, due to the long latent period in cardiovascular and neoplastic conditions, and hence the difficulty to determine the point in time when a dietary component was influential.

One of the intriguing recent epidemiological observations has been the strong correlation between the incidence patterns of arteriosclerotic heart disease (Rose *et al.*, 1974; Howell, 1975) and cancer of the colon and the breast. The reason for this odd triad is unclear. Sugar consumption has been suggested as the most important food item to undergo a change in the Yemenite diet upon immigration to Israel (Cohen *et al.*, 1961), but there are no supportive data to relate it as such to the other non-cardiovascular 'Western'-type diseases, and thus provide a common denominator. We are, therefore, left with the perennial choice of high fats versus low fibre (Modan and Lubin, 1980), a difficult choice between two almost inseparable items, which is being more specifically discussed in other chapters of this book.

High fat diet has been claimed as a common denominator for all three diseases. On the other hand, a 20-year prospective study conducted by Morris and his associates (Morris *et al.*, 1977) revealed that fibre rather than fat was the only food group of influence in the development of subsequent coronary events. This is compatible with the lowering effect of fibre on blood lipids (Ershoff, 1974; Kritchevsky *et al.*, 1975; Eastwood and Mowbray, 1976; Palumbo *et al.*, 1978), and suggests similar pathways towards protection in each of the three disorders. We have been able to demonstrate an aetiological role of low fibre consumption in colon cancer aetiology (Modan *et al.*, 1975a). Dales *et al.* (1979) underlined the aetiological importance of high fat–low fibre diet. These observations constitute matching pieces of the jigsaw puzzle of epidemiological and experimental observation, pointing towards a protective role of fibre in at least some of the so-called 'Western diseases'.

The possibility that these two negatively correlated food components may act synergistically cannot be discarded. Descriptive data on low incidence of the above enumerated disorders in developing societies, or among Seventh Day Adventists, who conform to a vegetarian diet, results of case control dietary studies, and experimental laboratory evidence are compatible with both interpretations.

It has frequently been claimed that 'the fibre theory is too good to be true to lead us anywhere'. Yet, the fibre theory is too promising to be abandoned, since, if true, it implies a possibility of protection by adding a substance to the diet, which is far more acceptable to the public than deletion of a favourite item.

Though it is hard to foresee a unifying model that will explain the marked differences observed in disease patterns between 'Western' and 'Eastern' Israeli Jews, the dietary story, and particularly its fibre angle, has only been offered as a model. Further monitoring of the changing differences with relationship to time, process of integration and intermarriage will, it is hoped, provide additional clues. Comparison with other rapidly changing societies is more than desirable.

Acknowledgements

The invaluable help of Ms. Elaine Ron and Ms. Marion Zinn is more than appreciated.

References

Adam, A. (1973). Genetic diseases among Jews. *Israel Journal of Medical Sciences*, **9,** 1383–1392

Beaconsfield, P., Rainsbury, R. and Kalton, G. (1965). Glucose-6-phosphate dehydrogenase deficiency and the incidence of cancer. *Oncologia (Basel)*, **99,** 11–19

Bonneh, T. B., Ashbell, S. and Kennet, R. (1979). Genetic markers: benign and normal traits of Ashkenazi Jews. In: *Genetic Diseases Among Ashkenazi Jews*, 59–76. Editors R. M. Goodman and A. G. Motulsky. Raven Press, New York

Brouet, Y. C., Mason, D. Y., Danon, F., Preud'homme, J. L., Seligman, A., Reyes, F., Navab, F., Galian, Z., Rene, E. and Rambaud, J. C. (1977). Alpha chain disease. Evidence for common clonal origin of intestinal immunoblastic lymphoma and plasmacytic proliferation. *Lancet*, **i,** 861

Buell, P. and Dunn, J. E. (1965). Cancer mortality among Japanese Issei and Nisei of California. *Cancer*, **18,** 656–664

Burkitt, D. P. (1975). Large bowel cancer: an epidemiologic jigsaw puzzle. *Journal of the National Cancer Institute*, **54,** 3–6

Cohen, A. M. (1961). Prevalence of diabetes among different ethnic Jewish groups in Israel. *Metabolism*, **10,** 50–58

Cohen, A. M., Bavly, S. and Poznanski, R. (1961). Change of diet of Yemenite Jews in relation to diabetes and ischaemic heart disease. *Lancet*, **ii,** 1399–1401

Cohen, A. and Modan, B. (1968). Some epidemiologic aspects of brain tumors in Israel. *Cancer*, **22,** 1323–1328

Cole, P. and MacMahon, B. (1970). Urinary oestrogen profiles and aetiology of breast cancer. *Lancet*, **ii,** 153

Costin, C. and Steinitz, R. (1971). Primary liver carcinoma in Israel. *Israel Journal of Medical Sciences*, **7,** 1471–1474

Cutler, S. J., Scotto, J., Devesa, S. S. and Conelly, R. R. (1974). Third National cancer curvey—an overview of available information. *Journal of the National Cancer Institute*, **53,** 1565–1575

Dales, L. G., Friedman, G. D., Ury, H. K., Grossman, S. and Williams, S. R. (1979). Colorectal cancer and diet in Blacks. *American Journal of Epidemiology,* **109,** 132–144

de Waard, F. (1969). The epidemiology of breast cancer. Review and prospects. *International Journal of Cancer,* **4,** 577–586

Drasar, B. S. and Irving, D. (1973). Environmental factors and cancer of the colon and breast. *British Journal of Cancer,* **27,** 167–172

Dreyfuss, F. (1953). Incidence of myocardial infarction in various communities in Israel. *American Heart Journal,* **45,** 749–755

Dunn, J. E. Jr. (1975). Cancer epidemiology in populations of the United States—with emphasis on Hawaii and California—and Japan. *Cancer Research,* **35,** 3240–3245

Eastwood, M. and Mowbray, L. (1976). The binding of the components of mixed micelle to dietary fiber. *American Journal of Clinical Nutrition,* **29,** 1461–1467

Ershoff, B. H. (1974). Antitoxic effects of plant fiber. *American Journal of Clinical Nutrition,* **27,** 1395–1398

Gross, J., Modan, B., Bertini, B., Spira, O., de Waard, F., Thijssen, J. H. H., and Vestergrand, P. (1977). Relationship between steroid excretion pattern and breast cancer incidence in Israeli women of various origin. *Journal of the National Cancer Institute,* **59,** 7–11

Hankin, J. H., Nomura, A. and Rhoads, G. G. (1975). Dietary patterns among men of Japanese ancestry in Hawaii. *Cancer Research,* **35,** 3259–3264

Hart, J., Modan, B. and Shani, M. (1971). Cholelithiasis in the aetiology of gallbladder neoplasm. *Lancet,* **i,** 1151–1153

Hart, J., Shani, M. and Modan, B. (1972). Epidemiological aspects of gallbladder and biliary tract neoplasms. *American Journal of Public Health,* **62,** 36–39

Howell, M. A. (1974). Factor analysis of international cancer mortality data and per capita food consumption. *British Journal of Cancer,* **29,** 328–336

Howell, M. A. (1975). Diet as an etiological factor in the development of cancer of the colon and rectum. *Journal of Chronic Diseases,* **28,** 67–80

Kallner, G. and Blondheim, S. H. (1956). Incidence of diseases among the communities of Israel. *Harefuah,* **51,** 81–85

Kessler, I. (1974). Epidemiology of cervical cancer. *Journal of the National Cancer Institute,* **53,** 51–60

Kritchevsky, D., Tepper, S. A. and Story, J. A. (1975). Symposium: nutritional perspectives and atherosclerosis, non-nutritive fibre and lipid metabolism. *Journal of Food Science,* **40,** 8–11

Laurent, C., Leguerinais, J. and Maujol, L. (Eds.) (1969). *Le Cancer au Moyen-Orient* (II. Turquie et Liban). Paris, Monographie de L'Institut National D'Hygiène, No. 26

Lilienfeld, A. M. (1956). Relationship of cancer of female breast to artificial menopause and marital status. *Cancer,* **9,** 927–934

MacMahon, B., Cole, P. and Brown, J. B. (1971). Urine oestrogen profiles of Asian and North American women. *Lancet,* **ii,** 900–902

Mass, N. and Modan, B. (1969). Epidemiological aspects of neoplastic disorders in Israeli migrant populations. IV. Cancer of the colon and rectum. *Journal of the National Cancer Institute*, **42**, 529–536

Medalie, J. H., Kahn, H. A., Neufeld, H. N., Riss, E., Goldbourt, U., Perlstein, T. and Oron, D. (1973). Myocardial infarction over a five-year period. I. Prevalence, incidence and mortality experience. *Journal of Chronic Diseases*, **26**, 63–84

Medalie, J. H., Papier, C., Herman, J. B., Goldbourt, U., Tamir, S., Neufeld, H. N. and Riss, E. (1974). Diabetes mellitus among 10,000 adult men. I. Five Year Incidence and associated variables. *Israel Journal of Medical Sciences*, **10**, 681–697

Menczer, J., Leventon-Kriss, S., Modan, M., Oelsner, G. and Gerichter, C. B. (1975). Antibodies to Herpes simplex virus in Jewish women with cervical cancer and in healthy Jewish women of Israel. *Journal of the National Cancer Institute*, **55**, 3–6

Menczer, J., Modan B., Oelsner, G., Sharon, Z., Steinitz, R. and Sampson, S. (1978). Adenocarcinoma of the uterine cervix in Jewish women. A district epidemiological entity. *Cancer*, **41**, 2464–2467

Modan, B. (1974). Role of ethnic background in cancer development. *Israel Journal of Medical Sciences*, **10**, 1112–1116

Modan, B. (1978). Population distribution of cell type specific lung cancer. *Israel Journal of Medical Sciences*, **14**, 771–784

Modan, B., Barrell, V., Lubin, F., Modan, M., Greenberg, R. A. and Graham, S. (1975a). Low fiber intake as an etiological factor in cancer of the colon. *Journal of the National Cancer Institute*, **55**, 15–18

Modan, B., Boischis, H., Bott-Kanner, G., Barrell, V., Bar-Noach, N. and Eliahou, H. (1975b). An epidemiological study of renal failure. I. The need for maintenance haemodialysis. *American Journal of Epidemiology*, **101**, 276–280

Modan, B. and Lubin, F. (1980). Epidemiology of colon cancer. Fiber and fats, fallacies and facts. In: *Medical Aspects of Dietary Fiber*, 119–135. Editor G. A. Spiller. Plenum Publishing Corporation, New York

Modan, B., Shani, M., Goldman, B. and Modan, M. (1969). Nodal and extranodal malignant lymphoma in Israel. *British Journal of Haematology*, **16**, 53–59

Modan, M., Modan, B., Shani, M., Rabin, D. and Thurm, R. (1979). Nationwide study of hypertension in Israel. In: *Essential Hypertension*, 21–27. Editor R. H. Thurm. Year Book Publishers, Chicago and London

Morris, J. N., Marr, J. W. and Clayton, D. G. (1977). Diet and heart: a postscript. *British Medical Journal*, **2**, 1307–1314

Movshovitz, M. and Modan, B. (1973). Role of sun exposure in the etiology of malignant melanoma. Epidemiological inference. *Journal of the National Cancer Institute*, **51**, 777–779

Palumbo, P. J., Briones, E. R. and Nelson, R. A. (1978). High fiber diet in hyperlipemia: comparison with cholecystyramine treatment type 11a hyperlipoproteinemia. *Journal of the American Medical Association,* **240,** 223–227

Rappaport, H., Ramot, B., Hulu, N. and Park, J. K. (1972). The pathology of so-called Mediterranean abdominal lymphoma with malabsorption. *Cancer,* **29,** 1502–1511

Ron, E. and Modan, B. (1980). Benign and malignant thyroid neoplasms after child irradiation for tinea capitis. *Journal of the National Cancer Institute,* **65,** 7–11

Rose, G., Blackburn, H., Keys, A., Taylor, H. L., Kannel, W. B., Paul, O., Reid, D. D. and Stamler, J. (1974). Colon cancer and blood cholesterol. *Lancet,* **i,** 181–183

Royston, L. and Modan B. (1968). Comparative mortality of childhood leukaemia and lymphoma among the immigrants and native born in Israel. *Cancer,* **22.** 385–390

Schenker, J. C., Polishuk, W. Z. and Steinitz, R. (1968). An epidemiological study of carcinoma of ovary in Israel. *Israel Journal of Medical Sciences,* **4,** 820–826

Seltzer, G., Sherman, B., Callihan, T. and Schwartz, Y. (1979). Primary small intestinal lymphomas and heavy chain disease. *Israel Journal of Medical Sciences,* **15,** 111–123

Shani, M. and Modan, B. (1975). Esophageal cancer in Israel. *American Journal of Digestive Diseases,* **20,** 951–954

Shani, M., Modan, B., Goldman, B., Brandstetter, S. and Ramot, B. (1969). Primary gastrointestinal lymphoma. *Israel Journal of Medical Sciences,* **5,** 1173–1177

Shani, M., Modan, B., Steinitz, R. and Modan, M. (1966). The incidence of breast cancer in Jewish females in Israel. *Harefuah,* **71,** 337–338

Shani, M., Schor, S. S. and Modan, B. (1975). Some epidemiologic aspects of acute myocardial infarction in Israel. *Chest,* **68,** 214–221

Sharon, Z., Shani, M. and Modan, B. (1977). Clinico-epidemiologic study of uterine cancer. Comparative aspects of endometrial and cervical sites. *Obstetrics and Gynaecology,* **50,** 536–540

Sheba, C., Scheinberg, A., Ramot, B., Adam, A. and Ashkenazi, I. (1962). Epidemiologic surveys of deleterious genes in different population groups in Israel. *American Journal of Public Health,* **52,** 1101–1106

Terris, M., Wilson, F., Smith, H., Sprung, E. and Nelson, J. H. Jr. (1967). The relationship of coitus to carcinoma of the cervix. *American Journal of Public Health,* **57,** 890–897

Toor, M., Katchalsky, A., Agmon, J. and Allalouf, D. (1960). Atherosclerosis and related factors in immigrants to Israel. *Circulation,* **22,** 265–279

Tulchinsky, D. and Modan, B. (1967). Epidemiological aspects of cancer of the stomach in Israel. *Cancer,* **20,** 1311–1317

Turgman, J., Modan, B., Shilon, M., Rappaport, Y. and Shanon, E. (1977). Nasopharyngeal cancer in a total population: selected clinical and epidemiological aspects. *British Journal of Cancer,* **36,** 783–786

Waterhouse, J., Muir, C., Correa, P. and Powell, J. (1976). *Cancer Incidence in Five Continents*. Volume III. Lyon, International Agency for Research in Cancer

Wynder, E. L. (1975). The epidemiology of large bowel cancer. *Cancer Research*, **35**, 3388–3394

18

South African Black, Indian and Coloured populations

Alexander Walker

South Africa occupies about 1·5 million square kilometres (0·5 million square miles). Its populations include about 18·25 million Blacks, 0·75 million Indians, 2·5 million coloureds (Eur-African-Malay), and 4·5 million Whites.

The first three populations will be discussed regarding:

1. particulars of origin, numbers, location, occupations;
2. environmental factors: non-dietary and dietary;
3. vital statistics;
4. general characteristics;
5. diseases of deficiency and low privilege;
6. diseases of excess and westernization.

After their presentation, there will be a discussion.

Understandably, the information presented is by no means exhaustive. The changes in the biological and other variables described are primarily those which the writer, his associates and collaborators have been most involved in seeking to characterize and elucidate.

South African Blacks

Origin, numbers, locations, occupations

The black population (18·25 million) in South Africa resulted from migrations from central Africa from the seventeenth to nineteenth centuries. Chief tribal populations are Zulu and Xhosa, each of about 5 millions, and Tswana about 2 millions. Roughly 40 per cent of blacks are urban dwellers (in Soweto, Johannesburg, there are over 1 million; in Pretoria, 300 000; Durban, 250 000; Cape Town, 100 000). The remainder live in Homelands or on farms owned by Whites. In 1970, a third of economically active persons worked on farms, forests and fisheries. A third worked in production, transport and mines. Less than a tenth were employed in professional, administrative and sales occupations, although the proportion is now rapidly increasing.

Environmental factors

Non-dietary factors

Physical activity
Rural dwellers pursue physically active lives. Many children walk long distances to school. Pupils run races well (Walker *et al.*, 1972c). Traditionally, girls and women are more active than boys and men. In urban areas the situation tends to be reversed. Although activity is reduced, it is not as low as that among whites. In Soweto, one in seven families has a motor vehicle, a proportion higher than that found in some countries in Eastern Europe.

Smoking habits
In rural areas, from studies on series of high school pupils (16–18 years), roughly 25 per cent of males and 0–5 per cent of females smoked cigarettes. In town areas, proportions were about 35 and 10 per cent. Among middle-aged men in rural and urban areas, roughly 40 and 60 per cent, respectively, smoked. In a series of white high school boys and girls of 16–19 years, 33 and 25 per cent smoked; among middle-aged men and women, the figures were 40 and 33 per cent, respectively. The number of cigarettes smoked daily remains much higher with whites than with blacks.

Overcrowding
In rural areas, overcrowding, i.e. persons per dwelling (not dwellings per unit of area), is certainly a health hazard which promotes the spread of tuberculosis and other infectious diseases. In town areas, the same adverse situation prevails despite satisfactory spacing of dwellings.

Stress
There are all the anxieties usual to a developing population (especially in urban areas), e.g. competition for jobs, intertribal jealousies, traditional superstitions, increasing crime, etc.

Health services
In rural areas, accessibility to hospitals (largely mission hospitals) and clinics varies from region to region. Services, in the main, while good, could be improved. In urban areas, medical services are comparatively satisfactory. In Soweto, Baragwanath Hospital (2500 beds) treats about 100 000 in-patients and 300 000 out-patients annually. Witch doctors, with varying skills, remain popular.

Diet

Diet varies (Walker, 1966; Lubbe, 1971; Manning *et al.*, 1974; Waldmann, 1975; Wagstaff, 1976). Among dwellers in Homelands and on farms, the traditional diet with local modifications is still followed. Broadly, maize, mainly of high extraction rate, is still the staple, supplemented in parts with 'kaffir corn' (*Sorghum vulgare*), and wheat products (currently mostly brown bread because of its lower price). Additional foods include dried peas and beans, groundnuts, pumpkin, kaffir melon, tomatoes, onions, and other vegetables, fruits, and wild greens (*m'fino, morogo*). Consumption of fermented cereal products (*marewu*, 'kaffir beer') varies greatly. Meat is consumed irregularly, often twice a week or more, and milk usually in small quantities. Rural blacks buy varying, although increasing, amounts of sugar, tea, coffee, soft drinks, condensed milk, margarine, and tinned fish.

In towns, house servants eat much the same foods as their employers; yet maize-meal porridge remains popular. Some groups, e.g. gold and coal miners, are well catered for by industrial concerns. However, most urban Blacks buy their own food and eat a partially westernized diet. Bread and maize products, usually refined in character, are major sources of energy. Intakes of sugar, also milk and condensed milk, are increasing. Meat is eaten fairly regularly, sometimes one or more times a day. Municipally prepared 'kaffir beer' (3 per cent alcohol) made from maize and 'kaffir corn' is popular with men, and, to a lesser extent with women. Unfortunately, consumption of alcohol-containing drinks, home-made or purchased, from both legal and illegal sources, is high and increasing, as with other developing (and developed) populations. Seftel (1977) has listed alcoholic ills, several serious, encountered in Black patients in city hospitals.

For most older children and adults, the diet is probably adequate in energy (i.e. few go hungry) and gross protein, but low in animal protein and fat, high in carbohydrate and crude fibre (more especially in rural areas), low in calcium, usually or frequently high in iron, and borderline or low (with exceptions in some groups) in most vitamins. For blacks generally, carbohydrate supplies 65–80 per cent of energy, fat 10–25 per cent, and protein 10–12 per cent. In the study by Manning *et al.* (1974) on dietary patterns of Blacks in Cape Town, despite noting increasing taste for sophisticated town 'foods', the basic partiality for carbohydrate foods still prevailed.

Vital statistics

Birth rate
In country areas birth rate is high, about 35–50 per 1000 population, as in other African countries (Reis, 1978). In cities the figure is lower; in Soweto it is 35 per 1000. The figure is 19 for whites in Johannesburg.

Infantile mortality rate (IMR)
In rural areas, an IMR of 60–80 per 1000 live births is usual (Richardson, 1970). In urban centres, the rate is about 40–60. Among families of teachers and similarly placed workers, the figure is about 30–35. In other parts of Africa, the rate is usually higher, i.e. 100–200 (Reis, 1978). Among white populations, current IMR data are: South Africa, 18; Sweden, 18; UK, 16; USA, 19; USA Navajo Indians, 13·5; Poland, 24; Portugal, 45; all per 1000 live births. Historically, in 1840, in Limerick, admittedly an impoverished part of Ireland, the figure was 327.

Percentage mortality of children under 5 years
In rural and urban areas, proportions of 10–19 per cent, and 8–15 per cent, respectively, have been found. In some parts of Africa the figure is as high as 50 per cent (Morley, 1974; Reis, 1978). Among white populations, proportions are: South Africa, 2·5 per cent; Sweden, 1·9 per cent; UK, 2·0 per cent; Porgugal, 4·0 per cent. In Limerick, Ireland, in 1840, the proportion was 74 per cent. In Great Britain during the nineteenth century, in some 'workhouses' the figure reached 90 per cent.

Mortality of the young as a percentage of total mortality
In large centres, deaths of black infants account for 16–21 per cent of total deaths. The figure is 2–4 per cent for South African whites.

Total mortality rate
In big cities, the mortality rate is about 11 per 1000 of total population. This is about half the figure reported for many African populations (Reis, 1978). Precise data in rural areas are not available. For South African whites the figure is about 9 per 1000. The rate is very much affected by the population's age structure.

Cause of death
In large cities causes of death are roughly: violence, 5–13 per cent; perinatal diseases, 5–16 per cent; cancer, 6–8 per cent; 'strokes', 3–7 per cent; total heart disease, 7–8 per cent; tuberculosis, 4–5 per cent; pneumonia, 5–12 per cent. Corresponding data on local whites are: total heart disease, 30–32 per cent; cancer, 19–21 per cent; 'strokes', 7–10 per cent; pneumonia, 4–5 per cent; perinatal disease, 1–2 per cent; violence, 4–6 per cent.

Expectation of life at birth
Data for 1970 were: males, 51·2 years, females, 58·9 years. Expectations are 10 years greater, respectively, in black males and females in New York. In 1971, data for South African white males and females were 64·5 and 72·3 years, respectively. Data elsewhere are: UK, 69·2 and 75·6 years; Sweden, 71·9 and 76·4 years.

Expectation of life at middle-age
Of South African blacks aged 50 years or over in 1951, by 1971, 39·5 per cent had survived. The corresponding figure for USA blacks was 34·8 per cent. For whites in South Africa and the USA, proportions were lower, 32·7 and 37·4 per cent, respectively (Walker, 1974). Thus, entirely contrary to popular belief, middle-aged blacks compared with whites currently live longer. The more favourable situation in middle-aged blacks is due to their much lower mortality from degenerative diseases, particularly coronary heart disease and cancer.

Age structure
From limited surveys made in rural and urban areas, and from the 1970 Census data, the present general picture is that about 55 per cent of the population is under 20 years, and that 4 per cent are aged 65+ years. Data for whites are 32 and 10 per cent, respectively.

General characteristics

Rate of growth
More than half of prepuberty black children fall under the third percentile of weight for age of Harvard reference standards, although the huge majority have normal weight for height (Richardson, 1977; Walker and Walker, 1977a). It is strongly questioned whether shortfalls *per se* connote malnutrition, or are essentially prejudicial to health. By mid-adolescence, without dietary intervention, the proportion falls to about 10–20 per cent. Then, obesity in girls (using the index of triceps skinfold of 25 mm or more), but *not* boys, is present in up to a third of that population, and occurs far more commonly in black than in Indian, coloured, or white girls (for the latter the figure is about 10 per cent). The commonness of obesity in older black girls has been reported from other parts of Africa. The cause is not obvious, but may be partly genetic.

Skinfold measurements
From preschool to school-leaving age, mean triceps measurements in black, Indian and coloured *boys* are similar; all are lower than mean values for white *boys*. By mid-adolescence, as noted, in black girls mean values are far higher than in girls in the other ethnic groups.

General health of school children
School attendance records of black pupils, if anything, are superior to those of white pupils. Mortality rate of black pupils is not higher than that of white pupils (Walker *et al.*, 1978a).

Height at maturity
While there is a secular trend in rate of attainment of height, boys and girls when fully grown, even in good circumstances, are shorter than their white counterparts.

Menarche
Breast development begins in girls in the four ethnic groups at closely similar ages, but mean onset of menstruation occurs later in black girls (rural, 14·1 years, urban, 13·0 years; white girls, 12·9 years (Richardson and Pieters, 1977).

Lactation
Virtually all mothers in both rural and urban areas lactate well, usually for many months (Walker, 1978). Breast milk has satisfactory composition.

Laboratory biological values: haematology
In preschool children, but not school children, iron deficiency anaemia is common (Margo *et al.*, 1978). In a series of pregnant women (third trimester) in country and town areas, mean haemoglobin concentrations were less than 10 g/100 ml in 8 and 12 per cent, respectively. Mean haematocrit levels were 45 and 41 per cent. Elevated ESR is common; in some parts values for most are abnormally high, especially in pregnant women in schistosomal regions. Mean MCHC seldom is seriously less than 30. Mean whole blood clot lysis time (Fearnley technique) is significantly shorter than that of white groups (Walker, 1961).

Biochemical values
In serum protein electrophoretic fractions, in series of adolescents, mean albumin and gammaglobulin fractions were 49–54 per cent and 19–24 per cent, respectively. For the latter fraction, high proportions were commoner in schistosomal regions. Mean values for serum cholesterol and triglyceride in adolescent groups were 3·37–3·89 mmol/l (130–150 mg/dl) and 0·79–1·02 mmol/l (70–90 mg/dl), respectively. Means for serum high density lipoprotein concentrations were very high, 1·81–2·33 mmol/l (70–90 mg/dl); the constituent composes half or more of total cholesterol (Walker and Walker, 1978a). For adolescents, mean blood glucose values at fasting and 1 hour after glucose drink were low, 3·05–3·61 mmol/l (55–65 mg/dl), and 4·44–5·0 mmol/l (80–90 mg/dl), respectively. Mean serum uric acid concentrations in adolescent males and females were 0·29–0·25 mmol/l (4·8 and 4·2 mg/dl).

Diseases of nutritional deficiency and low privilege

Some information on disease patterns of blacks in rural and urban areas has been published (Edginton *et al.*, 1972; Seftel, 1977; Adams *et al.*, 1978; Scragg and Rubidge, 1978).

It is very much regretted that incidence and prevalence data on diseases of deficiency and of prosperity not only for black, but for Indian and coloured populations, are very far from adequate.

Marasmus and kwashiorkor
With rise in socioeconomic circumstances, these diseases are less common and severe than previously recorded. Almost a decade ago, in rural villages in Western Transvaal about 5 per cent of infants were reported to have been affected (Richardson, 1977). More recent studies have shown a lower figure. In cities, the disease remains a serious health problem.

Rickets
The disease occurs not infrequently in infants and very young children, especially in crowded urban areas, yet patients seldom are hospitalized. Rickets has not been a serious public health problem in African compared

with white populations in the past, where, in the UK a century ago it was almost the chief cause of death in infants. In New World populations, e.g. Jamaican blacks, rickets is rare. Interestingly, in the UK, while the disease is common in *Indian* immigrants (not only in infants but in preschool children and even in school attenders), it is rare in black immigrants from African and Caribbean countries (Hunt *et al.*, 1977).

Pellagra

Although less common and severe than in the past, pellagra is still a health problem in some rural areas. Hospitalization of child and adult patients is becoming infrequent. In a series of school pupils in Northern Transvaal, pellagrinous lesions, at four periods of examination, were detected in 0·5 per cent (du Plessis *et al.*, 1971). More recent studies indicate a lower figure. In urban centres, alcoholic pellagra is frequently seen in malnourished hard-drinking single black men (Seftel, 1977).

Scurvy

This disease is very seldom seen in infants or adults.

Beri-beri

Beri-beri heart disease occurs almost exclusively in men in big cities (mainly hostel dwellers) who are in poor nutritional state and addicted to alcohol (Seftel *et al.*, 1972).

Anaemia

Iron deficiency anaemia is not a serious problem among South African blacks (as it is occasionally among American blacks), largely because of the uptake of adventitious iron from food and beverage preparation vessels (Walker and Arvidsson, 1953). But since the use of such utensils is decreasing, prevalence of anaemia may be expected to rise, especially in pregnant women. Among the latter, megaloblastic anaemia occurs in about 2–5 per cent.

Infectious and parasitic diseases

Deficiency diseases, especially among the young, are aggravated by infections, and *vice versa*. Among very young Blacks, gastroenteritis remains a serious health problem, accounting for about a third of deaths (Spencer and Coster, 1969). In younger and older populations, helminthiasis presents little problem, save in certain areas; e.g. in parts of Natal where schistosomiasis, amoebiasis and ancylostomiasis are endemic. Tuberculosis remains a major health challenge, although less formidable than it was formerly. Total respiratory disease accounts for about 10 per cent of all classified deaths. As to venereal diseases, satisfactory epidemiological information is lacking since attendance at clinics is voluntary. Judging from data published for populations in large cities, frequency of infections due to gonorrhoea is four times that from syphilis. In Durban, in 1975, attack rates for venereal diseases per 100 population were Blacks, 6·04; Indians, 0·26; Coloureds, 0·25; Whites, 0·16. While rates fluctuate annually, that for blacks appears steady, whereas, in the three other populations mentioned, decreases are occurring.

Western diseases: diseases primarily of excessive consumption or of altered pattern of diet

Dental caries
Among rural and urban black senior pupils, DMF (decayed, missing, filled teeth) scores average 1·2 and 2·3 respectively, i.e. teeth remain excellent (Retief *et al.*, 1975), even, inexplicably, among high consumers of snacks. For white pupils DMF score is about 10.

Obesity
In rural areas in the past, while obesity certainly occurred, it was infrequent. Nowadays, especially in young and older women, it is common. In urban areas, obesity (defined as 20 per cent or more of ideal weight for height) affects roughly 10–20 per cent of middle-aged men, and 40–60 per cent of women. Some data for white men and women are about 35 and 30 per cent, respectively. A similar pattern of differences prevails in regard to black and white men and women in the USA.

Hypertension
School children have lower blood pressures than those of white school children (Walker and Walker, 1978b). In rural areas in the past, and in present-day rural and urban areas, proportions of black adults with diastolic pressures of 90 mmHg or more were about 5–15 per cent, and (currently) 15–25 per cent and 40–60 per cent, respectively (Walker, 1975). The corresponding proportion among urban white adults is about 30–35 per cent. Salt intake is variable but not excessive. High blood pressure clearly is a serious health problem among urban blacks (Seedat *et al.*, 1978a). Seftel (1977) believes it to be the main cause of non-violent death in Soweto. A rural–urban differential in blood pressure prevails in blacks in other parts of Africa.

Glucose tolerance abnormality and diabetes
Until the last decade diabetes was rare in rural areas. Now its frequency is increasing. In cities, in some segments the disease has almost the same frequency as in whites (Jackson, 1978). Remarkably, black diabetics very seldom die from coronary heart disease (Seftel, 1977).

Coronary heart disease
Among country dwellers, the disease is virtually unknown (Walker, 1975; Walker and Walker, 1978a). In urban areas, CHD remains rare (Seftel, 1978). In Johannesburg in 1977 there were 14 deaths from CHD at Baragwanath Hospital. This favourable situation obtains despite the presence of all risk factors, some to a major degree (e.g. hypertension), in a not insignificant proportion of the urban population. In a white population of the same size, age and sex structure as that of blacks in Soweto, calculations suggest that 1500–1750 CHD episodes or sudden deaths would be expected annually (Walker *et al.*, 1979).

Cardiomyopathies
These include, according to Seftel *et al.* (1972), beri-beri heart disease (just mentioned) and idiopathic cardiomyopathy. While the latter is attributed to alcohol excess, or to chronic malnutrition, or both, many aspects of its aetiology remain unclear. Cardiomyopathies are the commonest forms of heart diseases seen in urban blacks.

Cerebral vascular disease
Death from 'stroke' is by no means uncommon in rural areas. In cities, mortality is high and accounts for 8–10 per cent of non-violent deaths (Walker, 1975; Walker *et al.*, 1979).

Peripheral vascular disease
This disease, virtually unknown in rural areas, remains rare in cities, even among smokers.

Bowel diseases

Bowel behaviour
For children and adults, mean transit times (carmine method) are 8 and 18 hours—half or less than those of white populations. Defaecation frequency is twice that of whites. Mean weight of dry faeces voided *per diem*, 30–60 g, is 50–150 per cent greater than that of whites. Their percentage of unformed stools is double that of whites. Remarkably, the high majority of black children and adolescents readily pass a stool on request (Walker *et al.*, 1973a; Walker, 1976). Their faeces smell as offensively as those of whites.

Constipation
The taking of laxatives is common in both rural and urban population although not primarily for difficulty of bowel movement. Culturally, as with other populations, ancient and modern, primitive and sophisticated, purging is considered beneficial.

Haemorrhoids
While rare in country populations, haemorrhoids are becoming more common in urban dwellers. Frequency of operations for haemorrhoidectomy is about a fifth of that prevailing with whites (Walker and Segal, 1979).

Polyps
These are extremely rare even in urban dwellers (Bremner and Ackerman, 1970). Of great significance, in the few cases of colon cancer that occur among blacks (see later), according to Segal *et al.* (1980a) tumours rarely arise from polyps—in diametrical contrast to what prevails with white populations (Hill *et al.*, 1978).

Appendicitis
Even in city dwellers, acute appendicitis remains very uncommon—less than

10 per cent of that found in white populations. Evidence is forthcoming from Mine Hospitals (which cater for the needs of a quarter of a million mine labourers), Baragwanath Hospital (100–120 cases per annum), and appendicectomy prevalences in groups of adolescents (0·5–1·5 per cent). Interestingly, frequency does not appear to be significantly increasing (Walker *et al.*, 1973a).

Ulcerative colitis, irritable bowel syndrome, Crohn's disease
These diseases, while still extremely rare, are becoming very slightly more common in big cities (Giraud *et al.*, 1969; Segal and Hunt, 1975; Segal *et al.*, 1980b). Crohn's disease is not conspicuously linked with 'Westernization'.

Diverticular disease
While still very uncommon in urban areas, frequency is increasing. In 1974–75, 16 cases were seen at Baragwanath Hospital (Segal *et al.*, 1977).

Colon cancer
This disease, virtually unknown in country blacks, rarely occurs in city dwellers. At Baragwanath Hospital in 1977, there were 17 cases. Colon cancer in blacks has less than 10 per cent of the age-specific mortality prevailing in whites (Walker, 1976; Segal *et al.*, 1980a). Its occurrence is increasing very slowly or hardly at all (Robertson *et al.*, 1971).

Other conditions and diseases

Wearing spectacles
In series of pupils of 16–18 years, 2–3 per cent used spectacles, compared with 15–25 per cent in corresponding white populations. Poverty is not the explanation; black pupils (especially rural dwellers) have significantly superior visual acuity as based on performance using the Snellen chart.

Tonsillectomy
Frequency of operation in series of pupils of 16–18 years was about 3 per cent. In series of white pupils it was 35–45 per cent (at one school it was 75 per cent).

Hiatus hernia
While rare in rural populations, in 1977 15 cases were seen at Baragwanath Hospital (Segal *et al.*, 1980c).

Gallstones
Although absent in rural populations, 10 cases were seen in 1978 at Baragwanath Hospital.

Varicose veins
Arising from inter-ethnic studies made by Burkitt (1976), studies were made on series of hospital out-patients of 30–55 years in urban and rural areas. An

overall prevalence of 4 per cent was found; this is lower than the value, 8 per cent, reported in a similar study made on blacks in Tanzania (Richardson and Dixon, 1977). For whites, a corresponding figure of 18 per cent (for moderate to severe lesions) has been reported.

Renal calculi
These are extremely rare.

Osteoporosis
Although habitual calcium intake is low, 300–500 mg *per diem*, there are no adverse sequelae. Thus, cortical dimensions of metacarpal and humerus in series of black mothers with numerous pregnancies and long lactations indicated no significant depletion of calcium (Walker *et al.*, 1972b). South African observations are entirely at variance with the belief that high fibre diets seriously prejudice utilization of mineral salts (Walker and Walker, 1977b).

Cancer patterns
According to Robertson *et al.* (1971), Bradshaw and Harington (1975), and other workers, broadly, overall cancer mortality (age-specific) rate in blacks is about half that for whites. Rates for oesophagus (Rose, 1978), liver (both very high in certain parts) and cervix are much higher than those for whites. Cancers of the stomach, colon and rectum are rare, and apparently are not increasing significantly, as is duodenal ulcer (Robbs and Moshal, 1979). That of the breast is low and not increasing. Rates for lung and prostate cancers, while lower than those of whites, are increasing.

South African Indians
Origin, numbers, location, occupations

Emigrations of Indians to South Africa took place mainly before or soon after 1900, principally from south and south-east India, United Provinces, and around Bombay. Indians were brought in primarily as workers on sugar plantations. Their ethnic make-up, Dravidian and Aryan, has been described by Mistry (1965). About 70 per cent are Hindu, 20 per cent Moslem, and 10 per cent Christian. The huge majority live in cities or small towns. Of the 780 000 Indians, those living in Durban and Johannesburg number about 350 000 and 45 000, respectively. As to occupations, in 1970, of those economically active, 42 and 12 per cent of males and females were employed in professional, administrative and sales capacities.

Environmental factors
Non-dietary factors

Physical activity
Apart from workers on the land and labourers, level of activity is low, although probably not as low as that of Whites.

Smoking practices
Surveys indicate that among high school pupils of 16–18 years, about 20 per cent of males and 0–5 per cent of females smoke cigarettes. Among middle-aged men and women, proportions are about 40–55 per cent and 15–30 per cent, respectively.

Stress
Many Indians, socioeconomically, are poor, and hence exposed to the usual associated stresses.

Overcrowding
This is common in urban populations.

Health services
Those for Indians, mainly urban dwellers, while reasonably satisfactory, could be improved upon. Certainly services for blacks, Indians and coloureds are less adequate than those for whites, in the same manner that services for poorer whites are inferior to those for whites in affluent circumstances. Yet, for the less privileged populations mentioned, services are considerably superior to those available in the rest of Africa, in rural and in much of urban India.

Dietary factors

The diet varies (Walker, 1966; Booyens and de Waal, 1969). Moslems usually are non-vegetarian, and eat all common foods save pork. Some Hindus are vegetarian. Carbohydrate is supplied largely by rice, white bread, potatoes, and sugar. Fat is derived from *ghee* (produced by heating butter and removing the sediment by filtering through cloth) and to a lesser extent from vegetable oils. Milk, pulses, and cereals are chief sources of protein for Hindu vegetarians. Mutton, chicken, eggs, pulses and cereals are main sources of protein for Hindu non-vegetarians. Consumption of beef is forbidden by their religion. Additionally, spices, chillies, garlic, and other flavourings are ingredients in everyday dishes. As to intakes, in a group of Indian male students in Durban, mean intakes *per diem* were: energy value 8·6 MJ (2043 calories); protein, 64 g; fat, 67 g (Booyens and de Waal, 1969). Speaking generally, carbohydrate foods contribute about 55–65 per cent of energy, fat 25–30 per cent and protein 10–12 per cent.

Vital statistics

All data relate to Indians in Durban for 1976.

Birth rate
The rate was high, 29 per 1000.

Infant mortality rate
The rate was 32 per 1000 live births. As with similarly placed populations,

the figure is lower, 20–25, in families in higher socioeconomic circumstances. In India, a general figure of 100–110 has been reported (Konar, 1974).

Percentage mortality of children under 5 years
The figure was 8 per cent. In rural India, proportions of 10–30 per cent have been reported.

Mortality of infants as percentage of total mortality
The figure was 17 per cent.

Total mortality rate
The rate was 6·5 per 1000.

Causes of death
Chief causes listed were ischaemic heart disease, 13 per cent; perinatal disease, 10 per cent; pneumonia, 5 per cent; cerebral vascular disease, 5 per cent; tuberculosis, 1·5 per cent; violence, 8 per cent. This pattern is in gross contrast to that in rural India, where, in most parts, infections remain by far the primary cause of death.

Expectation of life
In 1971, for all Indians in South Africa, data were: males, 59·3 years; females, 63·9 years.

Survival at 50 years
Of those aged 50 or more years in 1950, by 1970, only 22·2 per cent had survived (Walker, 1974). This proportion is lower than that for whites, 32·7 per cent, and for blacks, 39·5 per cent; i.e. middle-aged Indians die far earlier than would be expected.

Age structure
55 per cent were under 20 years (compared with 32 per cent for whites); 3 per cent were aged 65+ years (compared with 10 per cent for whites).

General characteristics

Rate of growth
Interestingly, in South African Indian children, in contrast to the situation with black and white children, there is little difference in rates of growth of children from poor or from rich homes. Rates are slower than those of white children. Up to puberty, half to two-thirds of pupils lie under the third percentile of Harvard reference standards of weight for age, although the huge majority have normal weight for height. The proportion under the third percentile decreases considerably by adolescence, when obesity is still very uncommon in boys, and in girls is less frequent (7 per cent) than in white girls (10 per cent) (Walker and Walker, 1977a). Indian children, as a race, are more slender in body build than children of the other ethnic groups.

Skinfold measurements
Triceps skinfold values for Indian boys and girls are lower than those of groups of pupils in the other ethnic groups.

Menarche
Average time of onset is 13·1 years.

Height at maturity
Both boys and girls when fully grown remain shorter and lighter than their white counterparts; this is the case even in well-to-do Indian families, not only in India and South Africa, but also in the USA (Clarke, 1966).

Lactation
In India, more particularly in rural India, virtually all mothers lactate well for up to 2 years. Most South African Indian mothers initiate breast-feeding, although only about a third to a half are still feeding by 3–4 months (Walker, 1978). In the UK several reports have noted the small proportion (one study indicated only 8 per cent) of Indian mothers who attempted even to initiate breast-feeding (Jivani, 1978).

Laboratory biological values: haematology and biochemistry
In representative series of high school pupils of 16–18 years, mean haemoglobin levels of 10 g/dl or less were present in 0 and 8 per cent of boys and girls, respectively. ESR (Wintrobe method) were abnormally high in 41 and 72 per cent of boys and girls. Iron deficiency anaemia (see later) is very common in later life. Mean values for serum cholesterol and triglyceride were 4·61 and 0·78, and 4·81 and 0·77 mmol/l (177·9 and 68·8 mg, and 185·8 and 67·8 mg/dl). Uric acid values averaged 0·35 and 0·26 mmol/l (5·86 and 4·39 mg/dl). Mean serum gammaglobulin fractions (electrophoretic), 18·58 and 20·4 per cent, for boys and girls, were higher than those of white pupils, although not significantly so. Insufficient representative data on adults are available for citation.

Diseases of deficiency and low privilege

Marasmus and kwashiorkor
Reports are unanimous that these diseases very rarely occur in Indian infants (Scragg and Rubidge, 1978).

Rickets
Rickets appears to be neither common nor severe. The commonness of rickets in Indian immigrants (young and older children) to the UK has already been alluded to (Hunt *et al.*, 1977).

Pellagra, scurvy, beri-beri
These deficiency diseases are very rarely seen in Indian children or adults.

Anaemia

For reasons not apparent, iron deficiency anaemia is common in children (mainly in girls) and in adults, both in men and women (especially in pregnant women) (Mayet, 1976). Her data for fractions having values below 10 g/dl were not given, but in India, using this criterion, 40–80 per cent of pregnant women were anaemic (Chatterjea, 1969). Level of total iron intake does not appear to be low in Indians in Durban. The anaemia situation is thus less favourable in local Indians than in blacks.

Infections

Gastroenteritis occurs far less frequently in Indian than in black or coloured infants. Parasitic diseases of a tropical environment (amoebiasis, schisto-somiasis, ancylostomiasis) occur commonly, but are not major health hazards. Tuberculosis is far less of a public health problem in Indians than in blacks. Morbidity and mortality rates from respiratory diseases (other than tuber-culosis) are only slightly higher than those for the white population. In Indians, as to venereal disease (mainly gonorrhoea), attack rate per 100 000 (as reckoned solely from attendances at clinics) is little different from that of coloureds and whites, which are only 3–5 per cent of that of blacks.

Western diseases of excessive consumption and of altered pattern of diet

Dental caries

According to Retief *et al.* (1975), DMF scores of pupils of 16–17 years average 7·7 (urban blacks, 2·3; whites, 10·0).

Obesity

By middle-age, obesity is very common in men, 35–45 per cent, and especially so in women, 50–60 per cent.

Hypertension

Mean blood pressures in school children do not differ from those in the other ethnic groups (Walker *et al.*, 1978b). At 40–59 years, limited studies in the Transvaal indicate that 34 per cent of males and 32 per cent of females have a diastolic pressure of 90 mmHg or more. Very comprehensive studies on hypertension and disease in Indians in Durban have been made by Seedat *et al.* (1978b). They reported that 15 and 22 per cent of adult males and females, respectively, had a diastolic pressure of 95 mmHg or more, or a systolic pressure of 160 mmHg or more. These two series of data indicate higher prevalences of hypertension than such reported on Indians in India or on many white populations.

Glucose tolerance abnormality and diabetes

The diabetes situation in Indians is fascinating. Historically, Hippocrates did not mention the disease, yet it was recognized in India several hundred years BC. Currently, in India it is common in city dwellers, although much less so in rural populations (which constitute about 90 per cent of the total population). In that country, diabetes, as expected, occurs more often in higher income groups (professional workers, merchants, army officers, etc.) (Gupta *et al.*, 1978). As to South African Indians, their proneness to diabetes has been known for long; early knowledge is due principally to Campbell (1963). Prevalence is either approximately the same as, or, in some segments even greater than, that in whites (Jackson, 1978). In three country towns in the Transvaal, glucose tolerance abnormality was noted in over a quarter of Indians aged 50 years and over (Walker, 1966). In the diabetes survey made in Birmingham in 1966, the corresponding proportion was 11 per cent. In Cape Town, Jackson (1978) found an extremely high prevalence in Tamil Indians.

An important feature of local Indians is excessive insulinaemia following a glucose drink (Keller *et al.*, 1972). In Johannesburg, Indian children of 10–12 years were found to exhibit a significantly greater rise in mean serum insulin level following glucose drink, compared with that observed in black, coloured or white children; indeed, hyperinsulinaemia was detected in Indian children as young as 8 years (Walker *et al.*, 1972a).

Coronary heart disease
While coronary heart disease (CHD) was known to John Hunter, and later to Jenner, Heberden, Osler, and other great British physicians, its clinical description was not published until early in the present century (Herrick, 1912), when it evoked minimal interest. In remarkable contrast, in India, classifications of heart diseases were made by Charaka and Sushruta in the post-Vedic period which started about 800 BC, i.e. four centuries before the time of Hippocrates. One symptom described as 'a sense of constriction in the precordium, stitching pain and sensations of churning or bursting or rubbing' (Mukerjee, 1975).

In rural India, clinical CHD is rare, but it is common in centres of population. In South African Indians, while crude death rates from CHD are considerably lower than those of whites, age-specific data reveal a much smaller disparity (Walker *et al.*, 1979). Actually, in all countries to which Indians have migrated, their proneness to CHD has increased tremendously. In a study made in London, CHD incidence in the Indian moiety was *higher* than that in the white moiety; in startling contrast, incidence in Caribbean black immigrants was only a *tenth* of that in whites (Pedoe *et al.*, 1975).

In Indian patients peak mortality from CHD occurs early. In Western populations, whereas about two-thirds of deaths from CHD occur *after* 60 years, among Indian patients (both in India and South Africa) three-quarters or more of deaths occur *before* that age. In one study undertaken in India, peak period of mortality was 40–49 years; 11 per cent died under 40 years (Lal and Caroli, 1967). The corresponding proportion in Western populations is very much lower, about 1–2 per cent. 'Precocious' CHD is stated to be 'common in India'. A further unusual feature is that in India (and to a lesser extent in South Africa), serum cholesterol levels of CHD patients are relatively low. In one study in India, about half of the patients had cholesterol levels less than 4·2 mmol/l (162 mg/dl) (Parkash *et al.*, 1968). Thus, the same relatively low levels which have noxious significance to Indians, would be regarded as intensely desirable for whites, and would virtually guarantee to them freedom from severe atheroma and from CHD episodes.

Cerebral vascular disease
Mortality from this disease is common, accounting for 5 per cent of all deaths, being due largely to the commonness of hypertension (Seftel, 1977; Seedat, *et al.*, 1978b).

Peripheral vascular disease
This condition is rarely seen in women and seldom in men.

Bowel diseases

Bowel behaviour
Data on transit time, amount of faeces voided *per diem*, and stool consistency are meagre, due to reluctance of persons to undergo tests or supply information.

Constipation
This condition certainly occurs, but data on its commonness, also on laxative practices, are lacking.

Appendicitis
Frequency of operation noted in series of pupils aged 16–18 years is 2–3 per cent, i.e. far less than the frequency in white pupils of the same age, namely, 8–12 per cent.

Haemorrhoids
This condition is not uncommon; yet its frequency, also frequency of haemorrhoidectomy, appear less than such prevailing in white populations.

Polyps
No information is available.

Ulcerative colitis, irritable bowel syndrome, Crohn's disease, and diverticular disease
Judging by clinical experience at Coronation Hospital (about 800 beds), Johannesburg, where about 30 per cent of patients are Indian, all these diseases are considered to occur far less frequently in Indian than in white populations. A complicating factor is that not all Indians (45 000 in Johannesburg), when sick, go to Coronation Hospital; those with greater means attend private physicians.

Colon cancer
According to death certificates, crude mortality rate in Johannesburg Indians from 1963 to 1971 was only a fifth of that in the white population. This very low rate, occurring in the same context as high death rates from diabetes and coronary heart disease, is not explicable on the fibre-depletion hypothesis.

Other conditions and diseases

Wearing spectacles
In series of pupils of 16–18 years, 13–17 per cent wore spectacles (whites, average 19 per cent).

Tonsillectomies
Frequency of operation in series of pupils of 16–18 years was 16–21 per cent (whites, 35–45 per cent).

Duodenal ulcer
This disease, while less common than in whites, is increasing (Robbs and Moshal, 1979).

Hiatus hernia, gallstones, renal calculi
From clinical experience at Coronation Hospital, these diseases occur less frequently than in the white population. Satisfactory comparative data are lacking.

Varicose veins
While no frequency data are available, the impression is that varicose veins are less of a health problem than they are in whites.

Osteoporosis
No good data are available. Mean cortical dimensions of metacarpal in series of Indian school children at different age periods do not differ significantly from those of black, coloured, or white children (Walker *et al.*, 1973b).

Cancer patterns
According to Bradshaw and Harington (1975), during 1949–69 the most common cancer in Indian *men* was stomach cancer, although its occurrence decreased. Cancers of the colon and oesophagus also became less common. Decrease in the latter possibly stemmed from changes in betel-chewing habits. The gradual increases in lung and prostatic cancers might be sequelae of 'westernization'. The overall cancer risk remained the same over the period of observation and continued to be low. In Indian, as in coloured and white women, frequencies of cancers of the stomach and uterus decreased; yet rates for cervix and especially oesophagus rose. Since decreases exceeded increases, the overall cancer risk in women fell to a level as low as that

prevailing in Indian men. The rate for breast cancer rose only slightly; it remained less than half of that in white women.

Alcoholism
This problem is of far less public health significance than that prevailing with the black, coloured, or white populations.

South African coloured population

Origin, numbers, location, occupation

The coloured people originated from four stocks:

1. slaves brought from East India to the Cape in the early seventeenth and eighteenth centuries;
2. Hottentots;
3. Bushmen and
4. whites.

Populations 1 and 2 made the greatest contribution. Additionally, in recent times there has been admixture with the black population. The coloured people, evolving over a period of 250 years, while still being modified by outside influences, are relatively stabilized. Of the present 2·5 million, about 500 000 live in Cape Town and its environs, 100 000 in Johannesburg, and 50 000 in Durban. For many generations these people have lived in small relatively distinct residential areas scattered throughout South Africa, more especially in the Cape Peninsula. The coloured population, in the main, occupy inferior social and economic positions. In 1970, of those employed, only 12 and 15 per cent of males and females were employed in professional, administrative and sales occupations.

Environmental factors

Non-dietary factors

Physical activity
Most rural dwellers, mainly workers on farms and labourers, pursue physically active lives. In towns, apart from labourers and manual workers, the level of activity is low, although not as low as among whites.

Smoking
In series of urban high school pupils aged 16–18 years, roughly 20–30 per cent of males and 10–20 per cent of females smoked cigarettes. Among middle-aged men and women, 35–40 and 25–30 per cent, respectively, smoked.

Stress
The coloured population, in a relatively low socioeconomic position, contends with the usual associated worries and difficulties. The excessive consumption of alcoholic drinks, especially by males, constitutes a tremendous and widespread social and medical problem (see later).

Health services
While they are less adequate than would be desired, the services, broadly, are improving. In big cities, services may be regarded as reasonably satisfactory.

Dietary factors

Although recent studies have been made of the diet and health status of young children by Margo *et al.* (1976a, b), no corresponding recent investigations have been made on adults. Such information as is available indicates that the habitual diet, compared with that of whites, contains less animal protein and fat foods, but more of fibre-containing foods, primarily from cereal products, legumes and vegetables. Of total energy, carbohydrate supplies 55–65 per cent, fat 25–35 per cent, and protein 10–13 per cent.

Vital statistics

All data relate to coloureds in Cape Town in 1977.

Birth rate
The rate was 24 per 1000.

Infantile mortality rate
The rate was 26 per 1000 live births, a figure much lower than previously recorded. As with blacks and Indians, the rate is lower in the more privileged segment.

Percentage mortality of children under 5 years
Data for coloureds in Cape Town are not available. For those in Johannesburg, in 1973, 15 per cent died before their fifth birthday.

Mortality of infants as a percentage of total mortality
Deaths of infants up to 1 year accounted for 10 per cent of total deaths.

Total mortality rate
The rate was 6·2 per 1000.

Causes of death
Principal causes listed were cancer, 14 per cent; ischaemic heart disease, 12 per cent; cerebrovascular disease, 10 per cent; tuberculosis and pneumonia, each 4 per cent; violence, 9 per cent.

Expectation of life at birth
For the total coloured population in South Africa, in 1971 data were: males, 48·8 years, females, 56·1 years.

Expectation of life at middle-age
Of the coloured population aged 50 or more years in 1950, by 1970, the proportion surviving was 33·2 per cent.

Age structure
53 per cent of the population were under 20 years (as against 32 per cent for whites); 5 per cent were aged 65 + years (the figure was 10 per cent for whites).

General characteristics

Rate of growth
Of prepubertal school children, a third to a half lie under the third percentile of weight for age of Harvard reference standards. By mid-adolescence, the proportion is 10–15 per cent (Margo *et al.*, 1976a, b; Richardson, 1977).

Skinfold measurements
For series of boys, mean thickness of triceps invariably is less than that of white boys. For girls, mean value reaches, and, in some groups, slightly exceeds that of white girls.

Height at maturity
Mean heights of men and women are slightly lower than values for whites.

Lactation
Over 90 per cent of mothers initiate lactation. The proportion still breast-feeding at 3–4 months is roughly 50 per cent (Walker, 1978).

Laboratory biological values: haematology
Low haematological values are common in young preschool children, although not in school children (Margo *et al.*, 1977). Among adults, while there are no satisfactory comparative data, available information indicates anaemia to be less of a problem compared with that in Indian adults.

Biochemistry
Mean values for serum lipids in children and adults are intermediate between corresponding mean values for black and white populations (Truswell and Mann, 1972). Hyperglycaemia in older children and adults is commoner than in corresponding black, Indian and white populations, for reasons not apparent (Michael *et al.*, 1971).

Diseases of deficiency and low privilege

Marasmus and kwashiorkor
Frequencies of these diseases lie between those of blacks and Indians; they are much lower than they were 10–15 years ago.

Rickets
The disease still occurs, although few children are hospitalized. In the last few years the position has improved.

Pellagra
With rise in socioeconomic circumstances this disease is not the health problem that it was 10–20 years ago. Patients seldom are hospitalized.

Scurvy
This disease does occur but it is very uncommon.

Beri-beri
No cases have been reported, even in those with high alcohol consumption (see later).

Anaemia
Iron deficiency anaemia in young preschool children, but not school children, is common (Margo *et al.*, 1977). In adults, satisfactory data are not available.

Infections
Among the very young, gastroenteritis remains a health problem, although not as serious as it was previously. Helminthiasis presents no serious health hazard. Tuberculosis certainly still constitutes a challenge; yet again, there have been marked improvements compared with the past. As just noted, tuberculosis and pneumonia account for 9 per cent of all deaths. Concerning venereal diseases, they are common, although no satisfactory comparative data are available. Reports indicate a possible worsening of the position in coloureds in Cape Town, although not in those in Durban.

Western diseases: diseases of excessive consumption and altered pattern of diet

Dental caries
According to Retief *et al.* (1975), DMF scores of pupils of 16–17 years average 5·8; with urban blacks, 2·3; Indians, 7·7; whites, 10·0.

Obesity
At middle-age proportions found to be obese were, men, 35–45 per cent, women, 70–80 per cent.

Hypertension
Mean blood pressures of school children do not differ significantly from those in other ethnic groups (Walker *et al.*, 1978b). At 40–59 years, limited studies indicate that 25–30 per cent of males and 25–35 per cent of females have a diastolic pressure of 90 mmHg or more.

Diabetes
In studies on the Cape coloured community aged over 10 years (1385 persons), prevalence of known diabetes was 1·1 per cent, and of 'discovered diabetes', 6·1 per cent (Michael *et al.*, 1971). Prevalence of known diabetes was similar to that found in most white communities, also in blacks in Cape Town. 'Discovered diabetes', however, was very much commoner in coloureds than in whites or blacks. Data for the sexes differed little. Diabetes was rare in the young; none had symptoms, which in fact were extremely uncommon at all ages, even in persons with gross hyperglycaemia and fasting glycosuria. In many diabetics, glycosuria was absent; urine testing alone proved of little diagnostic help. A family history was given in 18 per cent. The coloured population is thus remarkably hyperglycaemic (for obscure reasons) which is rarely associated with symptoms; neither symptoms nor glycosuria can be relied upon to herald the presence of even biochemically severe diabetes.

Coronary heart disease
Crude and age-specific mortality rates from CHD in coloureds in Cape Town (1977) were a third, and slightly less than a half, of the respective figures for whites.

Cerebral vascular disease
Although crude mortality rates in coloureds in Cape Town were less than that of whites, age-specific rates were much the same.

Peripheral vascular disease
Mortality from this disease is low, and far less than that in whites.

Bowel diseases

Bowel behaviour
In children, transit time, defaecation frequency and consistency of faeces are intermediate between those of blacks and whites. No data are available on amount of faeces voided *per diem*.

Constipation
The condition certainly occurs among these people, but quantitative information is lacking. The taking of laxatives by adults appears less frequent than that found in a comparable white population.

Appendicitis
Frequency of the operation in pupils of 16–18 years is about 2·5 per cent, i.e. less than a quarter of the frequency in a comparable white population.

Diverticulitis
No prevalence data are available. The disease is believed to be uncommon.

Colon cancer
For coloureds in Johannesburg for the period 1963–71, mean crude annual mortality rate was 4·0 per 100000, a figure about a third of that for whites.

Other conditions and diseases

Wearing spectacles
In series of pupils of 16–18 years, 4–7 per cent wore spectacles (whites, average 19 per cent).

Tonsillectomies
Frequency of operation in series of pupils of 16–18 years was about 10 per cent (whites, 35–45 per cent).

Hiatus hernia, gallstones, and renal calculi
No prevalence data are available. The opinion is that they are less common than in the white population.

Varicose veins
In a series of out-patients aged 30–55 years attending hospital, prevalence was 10 per cent, i.e. higher than that of blacks, but lower than that of whites.

Osteoporosis
Mean cortical dimensions of metacarpal in series of coloured school children were, if anything, superior to those of white children (Walker *et al.*, 1973b). Prevalence of osteoporosis in adults is believed to be less than that in whites.

Cancer patterns
According to Bradshaw and Harington (1975), males have very high total cancer rates, especially respecting stomach, oesophagus, and, to a lesser extent, lung. Those for colon and rectum remain low. Females have lower total rates. Those for stomach and uterus have risen, although those for cervix and lung have fallen. While breast cancer frequency has increased, it remains a third of that for white females.

Alcoholism
As indicated by Gillis *et al.* (1973), alcoholism in this population is a very serious problem. A survey of a random sample of 500 persons in the Cape Peninsula revealed a very high rate of excessive drinking (4 per cent addictive drinkers, 3·2 per cent pre-addictive drinkers, 3·2 per cent heavy drinkers). The rate was particularly high among males leading to psychiatric disturbances, socioeconomic problems and physical ill health. Of drinkers, only a small proportion were social drinkers (33·9 per cent) compared with the figure reported for whites in South Africa (88·8 per cent). There were con-

siderably more male than female social drinkers (males: coloured, 43·3; Malays, 10·5; females: coloured 24·6 per cent; Malays, 6·3 per cent). Of all who drank (198), 73·7 per cent were social drinkers, 10·1 per cent addictive drinkers, 8·1 per cent pre-addictive, and 8·1 per cent heavy drinkers. These data are higher than those in most populations throughout the world. The excessive drinkers very largely imbibed wine.

Discussion

Summary of present health and ill health situations in black, Indian and coloured populations

A description has now been given of levels of health, disease, and biological variables in relation to the graded transitions of black, Indian and coloured populations from less privileged states to those more prosperous and westernized. The changes involved have been dietary and non-dietary, i.e. changes in physical activity, smoking practices and lifestyle.

Clearly there are differences in rates and in stages of transition in the three populations, for Western diseases are not emerging in a uniform profile nor with uniform consistency.

Among blacks, with urbanization and rise in socioeconomic state, reduced pronenesses to infection, but increased pronenesses to obesity, hypertension, diabetes and 'strokes' are such as would be expected. But their near immunity to coronary heart disease is not readily explicable, nor are the very low rises that have occurred in the emergence of gastrointestinal diseases, nor the low and little changing liability of women to breast cancer.

Among Indians, the enormous contrast in patterns of morbidity and mortality between those of rural Indians in India and the Indians in South Africa is remarkable. While causes of death of the former remain primarily infections, those of the latter are largely degenerative diseases. The intriguing situation is that expectation of life at 5 years of age appears to be much the same in both populations, despite the greater prosperity and far superior medical services available to South African Indians. Other fascinating aspects include: why, for millennia, have Indians been unusually prone to diabetes and coronary heart disease? Why, currently, are bowel diseases (e.g. appendicitis and colon cancer) much less common than would be expected? Why, indeed, do Indian adults die at much younger ages than can be accounted for?

The coloured population, with rise in prosperity, also evinces unexpected and unexplicable features, e.g. the high frequencies of non-specific diabetes and of certain types of cancer (e.g. oesophageal and stomach cancers).

Evidently, in emergence of increasing prevalences of Western diseases, there must be tremendous interplay between:

1. genetic factors whose role in the case of particular diseases must be extremely powerful; and
2. environmental factors, assuredly not all of which have been identified or are fully characterized.

What changes may be expected in the future?

There will be:

1. decreases, in the very young, in prevalences of nutritional deficiency diseases and of infections (especially gastroenteritis) leading to further falls in mortality rates of infants and young children;
2. more rapid growth in children;
3. falls in morbidity and mortality rates from tuberculosis and associated infections;
4. increases in prevalences of dental caries, obesity, hypertension, diabetes and circulation diseases (chiefly coronary heart disease and 'strokes');
5. increases in prevalences of bowel and other diseases of the gastro-intestinal tract;
6. decreases in prevalences of certain cancers (e.g. liver), but increases in others (e.g. lung, breast);
7. while expectation of life at *birth* will certainly improve, that at *middle-age* may change little (that of blacks will decrease).

The changes envisaged are much the same as those which have occurred in USA populations since the turn of the century (Burch, 1974). Such changes doubtless were also experienced by Western populations. Furthermore they have occurred with Indians who have migrated to various prosperous countries, and with Japanese who have migrated to Pacific Islands and California.

The changes predicted for the three South African populations will take place willy-nilly, for neither State nor society can significantly control nor modify them. In the case of blacks, were it possible, two pre-eminent desires would be, first to reduce morbidity and mortality in early childhood due to malnutrition and infections, and to do the same regarding tuberculosis and associated infections in later life. Second, it would be urgently desirable to *retain* their current pattern of diet (low intakes of animal fat and protein, high intakes of fibre-containing foods), and equally, to retain their higher level of physical activity and lower frequency of smoking, and, not least, their more phlegmatic approach to life. Obviously, the dietary features to be retained are analogous to those recommended in *Dietary Goals for the United States* (1977), which, although challenged by Harper (1978), have received strong support from others (Leading article, 1977a, b; Hegsted, 1978).

What are the chances of prevention, amelioration or regression of Western diseases?

Involuntary changes

When communities have made *involuntary* dietary changes, as has occurred occasionally in some countries during wartime, changes in disease pattern have in measure occurred (Saunders, 1944; Banks and Magee, 1945; Fleisch, 1946). The changes to the good (which in some respects are those hopefully predicted by protagonists for the adoption of *Dietary Goals*) included reductions in prevalences of dental caries, obesity, diabetes, atherosclerosis, constipation and appendicitis. These changes are the exact converse of those transpiring with most emerging populations (Burkitt and Trowell, 1975).

Voluntary changes

What is the situation when dietary and other changes are not imposed, but left to individual volition? Confucious wrote 'The essence of knowledge is, having acquired it, to apply it.' But even with unanimous support from recognized authorities, and with full cooperation from the media, it is very doubtful whether any serious reversion will occur to patterns of diets previously consumed but now recommended. Why not?—principally because of the conservative character of most people's dietary likes and dislikes, and because the changes recommended would detract from the diet's palatability. The likelihood of people being persuaded or frightened into making changes which involve a lessening of palatability is remote, because food occupies a far more central role in people's enjoyment of life than it is given credit for. Thus, historically, in the Sinai wilderness the Children of Israel, even at cost of returning to very rigorous slavery, cried, 'Oh, for a few bites of meat! Oh, that we had some of the delicious fish we enjoyed so much in Egypt, and the wonderful cucumbers and melons, leeks, onions, and garlic . . .' (Living Bible, 1971). One of the causes of the French Revolution was the scarcity of salt, because of the high tax; for salt was needed by the peasantry, not just to preserve food and make it palatable, but simply to mask the appalling taste of unfresh meat. In South Africa, there was tremendous euphoria after World War II when white bread replaced the standard wartime brown bread. A Leading article (1974) in *Lancet* declared that drastic reduction in serum lipids is likely to be 'rarely achieved except in small numbers of almost fanatically determined patients'. Meade (1975), writing of the USA 'prudent diet', stated that 'even the highly motivated often won't stick to it'. In a Leading Article (1976), The *British Medical Journal* commented, with nostalgia, 'no longer should we be urged from hoardings to "go to work on an egg" or to "drink another pinta . . ." '.

It has been emphasized *ad nauseum* that the seeds of degenerative diseases are sown by the time of adolescence when habits of eating, physical activity and smoking are formed, so that preventive measures must be started in youth. Lauer *et al.* (1975) noted marked hypercholesterolaemia in 3 per cent, obesity in 8 per cent and hypertension in 12 per cent of post-puberty pupils in Iowa. Yet entreaties to the young, as every parent knows, to modify their diet or manner of life to avoid future ill health or worse, are virtually unheeded. As William Hazlitt wrote, 'No young man believes he shall ever die.'

In South African populations, one item of evidence of partial reversion to the diet and lifestyle of the past concerns middle-aged and elderly blacks who have returned from towns and cities to villages of origin—either of their own or those of their parents. In two regions, small groups of such persons, who had returned at least a year prior to observations, have been studied, also groups of villagers who had not migrated or who had migrated only for short periods, and of course groups of urban dwellers. The tests undertaken included measurements of weight, blood pressure, serum lipids, and blood sugar at fasting and 1 hour after glucose load. For all the variables, mean values for the groups of returned persons lay approximately midway between mean values for villagers and for city dwellers. This certainly indicates that changes in dietary and non-dietary factors, in the directions recommended, ready evoke changes in biological variables—to the good.

Adoption of *Dietary Goals* and like recommendations may be inevitable

The view is hazarded that, in the long run, changes in dietary pattern in an almost world-wide sense are inevitable; moreover, such alterations may be made simply not because of recommendations of *Dietary Goals*, nor those of other authoritative bodies.

Increases in world food production are not keeping pace with increases in world population. In Africa, between 1968 and 1983 the population to be fed will increase by 76 per cent, whereas food production is likely to increase by only 45 per cent (Food and Agriculture Organization, 1975). Hence, in time, certainly in developed countries, and probably in some developing countries, restrictions in the production of animal products will be *mandatory*, to permit greater production and consumption of higher yielding plant products, virtually entirely for reasons of economy of land usage and the increased number of mouths that may be fed. That the agricultural changes envisaged will occur and will effect the food policies of Western populations is authoritatively appreciated. In a Leading article (1977b) in the *British Medical Journal* on 'Sensible eating' it was stated, 'few nutritionists now dispute that Western man eats too much meat, too much animal fat and dairy produce, too much refined carbohydrate, and too little dietary fibre. Epidemiological studies of heart disease suggest that some at least of the deaths in the middle-aged from myocardial infarction could be cut by a move towards a more prudent diet—which means more cereals and vegetables and less meat and fat. . . . *Our farm land is productive enough to support 250 million people on a vegetarian diet*' (the author's italics), i.e. five times the present population. Of course, to Western nations it will not be *compulsory* to make significant changes in diet for a very considerable time. Yet, as Hardin (1977) has frankly asked, can Americans be well nourished in a starving world?

Conclusion

From knowledge of the diet–disease situations of:

1. our Western ancestors;
2. migrating populations;
3. urban dwellers in developing countries;
4. particular populations (e.g. in wartime, also religious groups, vegans);
5. evidence from short-term studies on humans; and
6. animal experiment studies;

there is no doubt that it lies within man's ability and choice to lessen significantly morbidities and mortalities from several important diseases. But it is
equally clear, from our knowledge of the trends of changes in diet and lifestyle that have occurred, or are occurring, that in the masses there is neither
enough will nor conviction to make changes of sufficient magnitude to
engender a meaningful improvement in present ill health situations in
developed and, to a lesser extent, in developing populations.

References

Adams, H., Geefhuysen, J. and Hansen, J. D. L. (1978). A survey of admissions and deaths in a Black Paediatric Department. *South African
Medical Journal*, **53**, 703–705

Banks, H. L. and Magee, H. E. (1945). Effects of enemy occupation on the
state of health and nutrition in the Channel Islands. *Monthly Bulletin
of the Ministry of Health, London*, **4**, 184–188

Booyens, J. and de Waal, V. M. (1969). The food intake, activity pattern and
energy expenditure of male Indian students. *South African Medical
Journal*, **43**, 344–346

Bradshaw, E. and Harington, J. S. (1975). The changing pattern of cancer
mortality in South Africa, 1949–69. *South African Medical Journal*, **49**,
919–925

Bremner, C. G. and Ackerman, L. V. (1970). Polyps and carcinoma of the
large bowel in the South African Bantu. *Cancer*, **26**, 991–999

Burch, G. E. (1974). Trends in the incidence of disease in the United States.
American Heart Journal, **88**, 807–808

Burkitt, D. P. (1976). Varicose veins: Facts and fantasy. *Archives of Surgery*,
111, 1327–1332

Burkitt, D. P. and Trowell, H. C. (1975). *Refined Carbohydrate Foods and
Disease*. Academic Press, London

Campbell, G. D. (1963). Diabetes in Asians and Africans in and around
Durban. *South African Medical Journal*, **37**, 1195–1207

Chatterjea, J. B. (1969). Anaemia in pregnancy: preventive aspects. *Journal
of the Indian Medical Association*, **53**, 31–33

Clarke, M. F. (1966). The relation of weight to stature in young women:
studies at two medical colleges. *Indian Journal of Medical Research*, **54**,
389–401

Dietary Goals for the United States (1977). Prepared by the Staff of the Select
Committee on Nutrition and Human Needs, United States Senate.
United States Government Printing Office, Washington

du Plessis, J. P., Wittmann, W., Louw, M. E. J., Nel, A., van Twisk, P. and
Laubscher, N. F. (1971). The clinical and biochemical effects of riboflavin and nicotinamide supplementation upon Bantu schoolchildren
using maize meal as carrier medium. *South African Medical Journal*, **45**,
530–537

Edginton, M. E., Hodkinson, J. and Seftel, H. C. (1972). Disease patterns in a South African rural Bantu population. *South African Medical Journal*, **46,** 968–976

Fleisch, B. (1946). Nutrition in Switzerland during the war. *Schweizerische Medizinische Wochenschrift*, **76,** 889–893

Food and Agriculture Organization (1975). *The State of Food and Agriculture, 1974*, p. 121. Food and Agriculture Organization, Rome

Gillis, L. S., Lewis, J. and Slabbert, M. (1973). Alcoholism among the Cape Coloureds. *South African Medical Journal*, **47,** 1374–1382

Giraud, R. M. A., Luke, I. and Schmaman, A. (1969). Crohn's disease in the Transvaal Bantu. A report of 5 cases. *South African Medical Journal*, **43,** 610–613

Gupta, O. P., Joshi, M. H. and Dave, S. K. (1978). Prevalence of diabetes in India. *Advances in Metabolic Disorders*, **9,** 147–165

Hardin, G. (1977). Beyond 1976: Can Americans be well-nourished in a starving world? *Annals of the New York Academy of Sciences*, **300,** 87–91

Harper, A. R. (1978). Dietary goals—a skeptical view. *American Journal of Clinical Nutrition*, **31,** 310–321

Hegsted, D. M. (1978). Dietary goals—a progressive view. *American Journal of Clinical Nutrition*, **31,** 1504–1509

Herrick, J. B. (1912). Clinical features of sudden obstruction of the coronary arteries. *Journal of the American Medical Association*, **59,** 2015–2020

Hill, M. J., Morson, B. C. and Bussey, H. J. R. (1978). Aetiology of adenoma–carcinoma sequence in the large bowel. *Lancet*, **i,** 245–247

Hunt, S. P., O'Riordon, J. L. H., Windo, J. and Truswell, A. S. S. (1977). Vitamin D status in different subgroups of British Asians. *British Medical Journal*, **2,** 1351–1354

Jackson, W. P. U. (1978). Epidemiology of diabetes in South Africa. *Advances in Metabolic Disorders*, **9,** 111–146

Jivani, S. K. M. (1978). The practice of infant feeding among Asian immigrants. *Archives of Disease in Childhood*, **53,** 69–73

Keller, P., Schatz, L. and Jackson, W. P. U. (1972). Immunoreactive insulin in various South African population groups. *South African Medical Journal*, **46,** 152–157

Konar, M. (1974). Infant mortality in India. *Journal of the Indian Medical Association*, **62,** 100

Lal, H. B. and Caroli, R. K. (1967). Acute myocardial infarction in higher income group patients. *Indian Heart Journal*, **19,** 12–25

Lauer, R. M., Connor, W. E., Leaverton, P. E., Reiter, M. A. and Clarke, W. R. (1975). Coronary heart disease risk factors in schoolchildren: The Muscatine study. *Journal of Pediatrics*, **86,** 697–706

Leading article (1974). Can I avoid a heart attack? *Lancet*, **i,** 605–607

Leading article (1976). Prevention of coronary heart disease. *British Medical Journal*, **1,** 853–854

Leading article (1977a). Dietary goals. *Lancet*, **i,** 887–889

Leading article (1977b). Sensible eating. *British Medical Journal*, **2,** 80–81

Living Bible (1971). Exodus, Ch. 2, v. 4 and 5

Lubbe, A. M. (1971). Study of rural and urban Venda males: Dietary evaluation. *South African Medical Journal,* **45,** 1289–1297

Manning, E. B., Mann, J. I., Sophangisa, E. and Truswell, A. S. (1974). Dietary patterns in urbanized Blacks. *South African Medical Journal,* **48,** 485–497

Margo, G., Baroni, Y., Brindley, M., Green, R. and Metz, J. (1976a). Protein energy malnutrition in Coloured children in Western Township, Johannesburg. Part I. The ecological background. *South African Medical Journal,* **50,** 1205–1209

Margo, G., Baroni, Y., Brindley, M., Green, R. and Metz, J. (1976b). Protein energy malnutrition in Coloured children in Western Township, Johannesburg. Part II. Prevalence and severity. *South African Medical Journal,* **50,** 1241–1245

Margo, G., Baroni, Y., Green, R. and Metz, J. (1977). Anaemia in urban underprivileged children. Iron, folate and vitamin B_{12} nutrition. *American Journal of Clinical Nutrition,* **30,** 947–954

Margo, G., Baroni, Y., Wells, G., Green, R. and Metz, J. (1978). Protein energy malnutrition and nutritional anaemia in preschool children in rural KwaZulu. *South African Medical Journal,* **53,** 21–26

Mayet, F. G. H. (1976). The prevalence of anaemia and iron deficiency in the Indian community in Natal. *South African Medical Journal,* **50,** 1889–1892

Meade, T. W. (1975). Our lives and hard times. *Lancet,* **ii,** 1053–1057

Michael, C., Edelstein, I., Whisson, A., MacCullum, M., O'Reilly, I., Hardcastle, A., Toyer, M. G. and Jackson, W. P. U. (1971). Prevalence of diabetes, glycosuria and related variables among a Cape Coloured population. *South African Medical Journal,* **45,** 795–801

Mistry, S. D. (1965). Ethnic groups of Indians in South Africa. *South African Medical Journal,* **39,** 691–694

Morley, D. (1974). *Paediatric Priorities in the Developing World.* pp. 1 and 3. Butterworths, London

Mukerjee, A. B. (1975). Heart diseases in India. *Journal of the Indian Medical Association,* **65,** 156–158

Parkash, C., Puri, A. S., Mathur, O. C. and Sharma, R. (1968). Serum uric acid and serum cholesterol relationship in acute myocardial infarction. *Journal of the Indian Medical Association,* **50,** 561–562

Pedoe, H. T., Clayton, D., Morris, J. N., Brigden, W. and McDonald, L. (1975). Coronary heart-attacks in East London. *Lancet,* **ii,** 833–838

Reis, C. S. (1978). Demographic and epidemiological transition in Africa. *Tropical Doctor,* **8,** 229–233

Retief, D. H., Cleaton-Jones, P. E. and Walker, A. R. P. (1975). Dental caries and sugar intake in South African pupils of 16–17 years in four ethnic groups. *British Dental Journal,* **138,** 463–469

Richardson, B. D. (1970). Studies on South African Bantu and Caucasian pre-school children. Mortality rates in urban and rural areas. *Transactions of the Royal Society of Tropical Medicine and Hygiene,* **64,** 921–926

Richardson, B. D. (1977). Underweight, stunting and wasting in Black schoolchildren: malnutrition or adaptation? *Transactions of the Royal Society of Tropical Medicine and Hygiene,* **71,** 210–216

Richardson, B. D. and Pieters, L. (1977). Menarche and growth. *American Journal of Clinical Nutrition,* **30,** 2088–2091

Richardson, J. B. and Dixon, M. (1977). Varicose veins in tropical Africa. *Lancet,* **i,** 791–792

Robbs, J. V. and Moshal, M. G. (1979). Duodenal ulceration in Indians and Blacks in Durban. *South African Medical Journal,* **55,** 39–42

Robertson, M. A., Harington, J. S. and Bradshaw, E. (1971). Observations on cancer patterns among Africans in South Africa. *British Journal of Cancer,* **25,** 377–402

Rose, E. F. (1978). The role of demographic risk factors in carcinogenesis. In: *Prevention and Detection of Cancer,* **2,** 25–45. Editor H. W. Nieberg. Marcel Dekker, New York

Saunders, J. C. (1944). Wholemeal and laxatives. *Lancet,* **i,** 516

Scragg, J. N. and Rubidge, C. J. (1978). Patterns of disease in Black and Indian children in Natal. *South African Medical Journal,* **54,** 265–270

Seedat, Y. K., Seedat, M. A. and Nkomo, M. N. (1978a). The prevalence of hypertension in the urban Zulu. *South African Medical Journal,* **53,** 923–927

Seedat, Y. K., Seedat, M. A. and Reddy, K. (1978b). The prevalence of hypertension in the Indian population of Durban. *South African Medical Journal,* **54,** 10–15

Seftel, H. C. (1977). Diseases in urban and rural Black populations. *South African Medical Journal,* **51,** 121–123

Seftel, H. C. (1978). The rarity of coronary heart disease in South African Blacks. *South African Medical Journal,* **54,** 99–105

Seftel, H. C., Metz, J. and Lakier, J. B. (1972). Cardiomyopathies in Johannesburg Bantu. *South African Medical Journal,* **46,** 1707–1713, 1823–1828

Segal, I., Cooke, S. A. R., Hamilton, D. G. and Ou Tim, L. (1980a). The rarity of polyps in large bowel cancer in urban South African Blacks. *Gastroenterology,* (in press).

Segal, I. and Hunt, J. A. (1975). The irritable bowel syndrome in the urban South African Negro. *South African Medical Journal,* **49,** 1645–1650

Segal, I., Ou Tim, L., Hamilton, D. G. and Walker, A. R. P. (1980b) The rarity of ulcerative colitis in South African Blacks. *American Journal of Gastroenterology,* (in press)

Segal, I., Solomon, A. and Hunt, J. A. (1977). Emergence of diverticular disease in the urban South African Black. *Gastroenterology,* **72,** 215–219

Segal, I., Solomon, A., Ou Tim, L., Rabin, M. and Walker, A. R. P. (1980c) Hiatus hernia in Johannesburg Blacks. *South African Medical Journal,* **58,** 404–405

Spencer, I. W. F. and Coster, M. E. E. (1969). The epidemiology of gastro-enteritis in infancy: Parts 1 to 3. *South African Medical Journal,* **43,** 1391–1397, 1438–1442, 1466–1472

Truswell, A. S. and Mann, J. I. (1972). Epidemiology of serum lipids in Southern Africa. *Atherosclerosis*, **16**, 15–29

Wagstaff, L. A. (1976). Nutrition knowledge in urban Blacks. *South African Medical Journal*, **50**, 900–902

Waldmann, E. (1975). The ecology of the nutrition of the Bapedi, Sekhukhuniland. *Ecology of Food and Nutrition*, **4**, 139–151

Walker, A. R. P. (1961). Fibrinolytic activity of whole blood from South African Bantu and White subjects. *American Journal of Clinical Nutrition*, **9**, 461–472

Walker, A. R. P. (1966). Nutritional, biochemical, and other studies on South African populations. *South African Medical Journal*, **40**, 814–852

Walker, A. R. P. (1974). Survival rate at middle-age in developing and western populations. *Postgraduate Medical Journal*, **50**, 29–32

Walker, A. R. P. (1975). The epidemiological emergence of ischaemic arterial diseases. Editorial. *American Heart Journal*, **89**, 133–136

Walker, A. R. P. (1976). Gastrointestinal diseases and fiber intake with special reference to South African populations. In: *Fiber in Human Nutrition*, 241–261. Editors G. A. Spiller and R. J. Amen. Plenum, New York

Walker, A. R. P. (1978). Infant feeding practices in South Africa: An appraisal of their significance to health. *South African Medical Journal*, **54**, 820–822

Walker, A. R. P. and Arvidsson, U. B. (1953). Iron 'Overload' in the South African Bantu. *Transactions of the Royal Society of Tropical Medicine and Hygiene*, **47**, 536–548

Walker, A. R. P., Bernstein, R. E. and du Plessis, I. (1972a). Hyperinsulinaemia for glucose dose in South African Indian children. *South African Medical Journal*, **46**, 1916

Walker, A. R. P., Bhamjee, D., Walker, B. F. and Richardson, B. D. (1978a) Growth, school attendance, and serum albumin levels in South African Black children of 10–12 years. *Journal of Tropical Medicine and Hygiene*, **81**, 2–8

Walker, A. R. P., Richardson, B. D. and Walker, B. F. (1972b). The influence of numerous pregnancies and lactations on bone dimensions in South African Bantu and Caucasian mothers. *Clinical Science*, **42**, 189–196

Walker, A. R. P., Richardson, B. D., Walker, B. F. and Woolford, A. (1973a). Appendicitis, fibre intake, and bowel behaviour in ethnic groups in South Africa. *Postgraduate Medical Journal*, **49**, 243–249

Walker, A. R. P. and Segal, I. (1979). Epidemiology of non-infective intestinal diseases in various ethnic groups in South Africa. *Israel Journal of Medical Sciences*, **15**, 309–313

Walker, A. R. P. and Walker, B. F. (1977a). Weight, height and triceps skinfold in South African Black, Indian and White school pupils of 18 years. *Journal of Tropical Medicine and Hygiene*, **80**, 119–125

Walker, A. R. P. and Walker, B. F. (1977b). Effect of wholemeal and white bread on iron absorption. *British Medical Journal*, **2**, 771–772

Walker, A. R. P. and Walker, B. F. (1978a). High high-density lipoprotein cholesterol in African children and adults in a population free of coronary heart disease. *British Medical Journal,* **2,** 1336–1337

Walker, A. R. P. and Walker, B. F. (1978b). Blood pressure of South African Black schoolchildren aged 10–12 years. *Journal of Tropical Medicine and Hygiene,* **81,** 159–163

Walker, A. R. P., Walker, B. F., McKibbin, E., Martin, A. P. and Segal, I. (1980). Trends in death rates from coronary heart disease and cerebral vascular disease in ethnic populations in Johannesburg. *South African Medical Journal,* in press

Walker, A. R. P., Walker, B. F., Richardson, B. D. and Smit, P. J. (1972c). Running performance in South African Bantu children with schistosomiasis. *Tropical and Geographical Medicine,* *24,* 347–352

Walker, A. R. P., Walker, B. F., Wadvalla, M. and Daya, L. (1978b). Blood pressures of Indian and Coloured schoolchildren aged 10–12 years. *South African Medical Journal,* **54,** 315–318

Walker, B. F., Walker, A. R. P. and Wadvalla, M. (1973b). Cortical dimensions of second metacarpal in four ethnic groups of South African children. *Tropical and Geographical Medicine,* **25,** 65–70

19

Hawaii ethnic groups

Gary Glober and Grant Stemmermann

Ethnic groups

Hawaii, situated between Asia and North America, provides a unique, natural laboratory to test the concepts of westernization. Environmental 'experiments' on a grand scale have been going on for years, as different ethnic groups migrated to Hawaii to begin a new life. The majority of the Oriental immigrants came from rural areas to work in Hawaii's sugar and pineapple plantations and within a few decades moved from these agricultural areas to the cities.

In 1970, out of a total population in Hawaii of about 770 000, 36 per cent of the major ethnic groups were Caucasians, 29 per cent Japanese, 19 per cent Hawaiians and part-Hawaiians, 10 per cent Filipinos, 5 per cent Chinese and 1 per cent were Koreans. The majority of Hawaiians (95 per cent) were of mixed genetic backgrounds.

The Chinese were the first group of Oriental immigrants to come in significant numbers, the main migration of 46 000 lasting from 1852 to 1898. 180 000 Japanese came during the years 1886–1924. Although inter-racial marriages have become more common among the Japanese, they have remained less racially mixed than any of the other major ethnic groups in Hawaii. Approximately 100 000 Filipinos came to Hawaii during the period 1910–31. The Koreans first came to Hawaii in 1920.

In 1970, 50 per cent of the Caucasians were in professional, technical and managerial occupations compared with 48 per cent of the Chinese, 38 per cent Koreans, 30 per cent Japanese, 18 per cent Hawaiians and 10 per cent Filipinos. 14 per cent of the Caucasians, 15 per cent Koreans, 12 per cent Chinese and 12 per cent of the Japanese were labourers compared with 45 per cent of the Filipinos and 25 per cent of the Hawaiians. In 1977, the median family income for the Chinese was $21 183, Koreans $19 702, Japanese $19 431, Caucasians $19 005, Hawaiians $13 615 and Filipinos $12 683.

Diets

Researchers at the Cancer Center of Hawaii (L. Kolonel, J. Hankin and A. Nomura) are investigating ethnic diet patterns in men and women 45 years

319

and older. Their study population has been derived from a Hawaii Department of Health survey (1975–76) based on random household samples; the methods consist of seven-day dietary intake histories and have included 1500 interviews. Preliminary findings exhibit many similarities but also certain ethnic differences in diet (Tables 19.1–19.3). Fibre and carbohydrate totals are not available at present.

Table 19.1   Nutrient intakes of Hawaii ethnic groups, age-adjusted means

Nutrients		Caucasian (g/d)	Japanese (g/d)	Chinese (g/d)	Filipino (g/d)	Hawaiian (g/d)
Total protein	male	72	64	57	61	69
	female	56	50	49	48	53
Animal protein	male	52	41	37	40	48
	female	40	32	34	31	37
Saturated fats	male	31	22	23	22	27
	female	23	18	18	16	21
Unsaturated fats	male	46	36	36	31	42
	female	36	29	29	24	32
Meat with nitrites	male	25	26	19	20	27
	female	16	17	15	13	18

Source: Kolonel, L., Hankin, J. and Nomura, A. (unpublished observations of 1500 interviews of Hawaii Health Survey 1976–78)

Coronary heart disease

Have these economic and dietary characteristics affected the various ethnic groups? The most publicized effect of westernization has been the rapid increase of coronary heart disease. The age-adjusted mortality rate per 100 000 of coronary heart disease in Hawaii increased from 2·9 in 1910 to 105·0 in 1960 (Epidemiology Program, Cancer Center of Hawaii, unpublished observations).

Higher rates in Japanese immigrants

An international study of heart disease was initiated in 1965 to observe coronary heart disease risk factors in contrasting environments among people of the same genetic background. The three populations studied were men of Japanese ancestry, born between 1900 and 1919, resident either in Japan, Hawaii, or California (Kagan *et al.*, 1974). Using a 24-hour diet

Table 19.2 Cigarettes, alcohol and coffee taken by Hawaii ethnic groups, age-adjusted means

		Caucasian	Japanese	Chinese	Filipino	Hawaiian
Cigarettes						
Non-smokers (%)	male	39	47	63	52	43
	female	50	74	81	71	53
Lifetime use (pack years)[1]	male	27	22	18	18	23
	female	19	11	10	11	14
Alcohol						
Non-drinkers (%)	male	54	66	75	71	64
	female	72	93	95	96	83
Lifetime consumption (oz.)	male	4267	2321	912	2004	3130
	female	1692	225	214	241	1003
Beer						
1 can + per week (%)	male	34	30	20	26	33
	female	9	3	1	2	12
12 cans + per week (%)	male	15	12	3	10	22
	female	2	0	0	1	4
Hard liquor						
1 jigger + per week (%)	male	18	8	6	7	7
	female	15	3	2	1	5
12 jiggers + per week (%)	male	7	2	2	1	4
	female	4	1	0	0	2
Coffee						
cups per day	male	3	2	1	1	2
	female	2	1	1	1	1

Source: Kolonel, L., Nomura, A. and Hirohata, T. (unpublished observations of 10 000 interviews of Hawaii Health Survey 1975–76)
[1] Computed on 1 pack a day on average per year

Table 19.3   Foods eaten by Hawaii ethnic groups, times eaten per week, age-adjusted means

Food		Caucasian	Japanese	Chinese	Filipino	Hawaiian
Beef	male	4·2	3·8	4·5	3·6	4·2
	female	4·0	3·7	3·7	3·5	4·0
Pork	male	0·9	1·1	1·8	2·1	1·4
	female	0·7	0·9	1·7	2·1	1·4
Poultry	male	1·5	1·8	2·0	2·2	1·8
	female	1·5	1·7	1·7	2·2	1·7
Salted fish	male	0·1	0·2	0·1	1·1	0·3
	female	0·1	0·2	0·1	0·9	0·3
Other fish	male	1·2	1·6	1·2	2·5	1·9
	female	1·2	1·5	1·3	2·4	2·2
Pickled vegetables	male	0·8	2·9	0·9	1·4	1·7
	female	0·7	2·9	0·7	1·0	1·3
Raw vegetables	male	5·7	6·3	4·6	4·4	5·8
	female	6·1	6·6	5·3	4·4	6·0
Fresh fruit	male	5·2	5·0	5·6	4·6	4·7
	female	5·7	5·6	6·8	5·1	5·0

Source: Kolonel, L., Nomura, A. and Hirohata, T. (unpublished observations of 10 000 interviews of Hawaii Health Survey 1975–76)

recall method, significant dietary differences were found between the Japanese living in Hawaii and those still resident in Japan. In Hawaii, the Japanese men ate more calories, more saturated and unsaturated fats, more animal protein and less vegetable protein, more cholesterol, more simple, but less complex carbohydrates, and ingested less alcohol, than did the Japanese men in Japan (Kagan *et al.*, 1974).

The incidence of coronary heart disease in Hawaii-Japanese men was twice that of Japan and the rate for Japanese men in California was nearly 50 per cent higher than for Hawaii Japanese (Robertson *et al.*, 1977). The Hawaii Japanese weighed more than their Japanese counterparts and had higher serum cholesterol, triglyceride, uric acid and glucose levels. There were no differences in blood pressure. In Japan and Hawaii, men with coronary heart disease had significantly higher values for relative weight, serum cholesterol, serum triglyceride, serum uric acid, systolic blood pressure and diastolic blood pressure. However, using regression analyses, only systolic blood pressure, serum cholesterol, relative weight and smoking remained as independent variables. Cigarette smoking appeared to be the most significant risk factor in Hawaii but was unrelated to the incidence of coronary heart disease in Japan. The authors postulated that cigarette smoking in Hawaii was perhaps additive to, or possibly potentiated by, serum cholesterol levels, whereas cigarette smoking may not be as important in countries with relatively low levels of serum cholesterol (Robertson *et al.*, 1977).

The Honolulu Heart Study found, in a prospective study, that the Hawaii-Japanese men who eventually developed coronary heart disease had consumed fewer total daily calories than the control group (Yano *et al.*, 1978). Their intake of carbohydrates and starch also were lower. This coronary heart disease group ate as much sucrose as the control group, but less of the other sugars, than did the rest of the men. No positive association was demonstrated between the risk of coronary heart disease and dietary fats. The lower total calorie consumption of the coronary heart disease cases was largely due to decreased alcohol and carbohydrate intake; it could not be accounted for by either under-reporting food consumption among obese men, or diminished physical activity in the heart disease cases (Yano *et al.*, 1978).

In general, Japanese men in Hawaii followed a more Japanese lifestyle until World War II. Prior to 1940, 48 per cent of the Japanese men ate Japanese diets. By 1965, the proportion eating Japanese-style diets had dropped to 14 per cent (Yano *et al.*, 1978). The implication is that the dietary experience of early life may be critical in the subsequent risk of coronary heart disease, to that diet studies in middle-aged people will not uncover coronary risk factors.

There was a strong negative association between moderate alcohol consumption (up to 60 ml per day) and the risk for coronary heart disease (Yano *et al.*, 1977). Alcohol consumption was weakly related to levels of serum cholesterol and triglyceride but was found to correlate more strongly with high density (positively correlated) and low density (negatively correlated) lipoproteins.

Rates in other Hawaiian groups

Between 1955 and 1964, Hawaiians had a much higher coronary heart disease mortality rate than Japanese living in Hawaii (Bassett *et al.*, 1969). A study of Hawaiian and Japanese men hospitalized for myocardial infarction revealed, as did the Honolulu Heart Study, that the intake of total calories had been lower in heart cases than in controls of both ethnic groups (Bassett *et al.*, 1969). Although the Hawaiians had relatively lower calorie intakes they were more overweight than the Japanese. This paradox might be explained by the history of sporadic heavy feeding in Hawaiians (the so-called 'feast or famine' phenomenon) or by difference in physical activity. The Hawaiians had higher total fat and saturated fat intakes than the Japanese but there were no significant differences in fat intake between Hawaiian heart disease cases and controls. The Hawaiians smoked more, ingested more alcohol, but drank less coffee and tea, than did the Japanese. However, there were no differences in ethanol intake or cigarette smoking between cases and controls. The Japanese controls ate more sucrose and fructose as a percentage of their calorie intake but these sugars had no obvious effect on the risk of heart disease. There was a slightly higher crude fibre intake in Japanese (3·9 g) than Hawaiians (3·0 g) but no differences in fibre intake between cases and controls.

In Hawaii during 1950, the age-adjusted mortality rate per 100 000 for coronary heart disease in males was 280 among Caucasians, 78 among Japanese, 142 among Chinese, 80 among Filipinos, and 320 among Hawaiians and part-Hawaiians. By 1970, the mortality rate per 100 000 for coronary heart disease had risen to 236 among the Filipinos, whereas the rate climbed only to 160 in the Japanese, to 194 in Chinese, to 360 in Caucasians and to 380 in Hawaiians. During these twenty years the Filipinos experienced a rapid increase in social and economic status and many had moved from rural areas to the more densely populated regions of metropolitan Hawaii (Hackenberg et al., 1978). Filipino coronary heart disease rates increased 196 per cent during this period.

Cancer

Immigration

Each ethnic group in Hawaii experiences a different pattern of neoplastic disease. Some of the differences in cancer rate are substantial, yet lack an obvious explanation. Nevertheless, it is abundantly clear that cancer rates in certain ethnic groups change after immigration to Hawaii. Table 19.4 reports the average age-adjusted incidence of some of the major types of malignant tumours among five ethnic groups in Hawaii compared with rates in comparable ethnic groups in Japan, the United States and, as regards the Chinese, in Singapore. Table 19.4 is presented to highlight changes in cancer rate that occur after immigration.

There is a tendency for tumours which are common in the country of origin to decrease to the level of the host country. This downward trend is apparent for a stomach cancer among the Japanese, and for nasopharyngeal cancer among the Chinese; both decrease after immigration to Hawaii. Even after the initial decrease of cancer in the migrant population, the rates continue falling in succeeding generations. This suggests that environmental factors influence the level of risk.

There is also a tendency for tumours which are common in the host country to increase among the immigrants. Thus, cancer of the lung, colon–rectum, female breast and prostate become commoner among Japanese after immigration to Hawaii. The cancer rates, which increase or decrease after immigration, usually change more quickly in men than in women.

High rates and low rates

In Hawaii, both Caucasian and Hawaiians have the highest incidence of many common varieties of cancer. Male Hawaiian lung cancer rates are among the highest in the world; they are far higher than the rates among male Hawaii Japanese (Table 19.4), but the percentage of smokers and the lifetime use of

Table 19.4 Cancer rates[1] in Hawaiian ethnic groups; some are compared with their rates in other countries

Type of cancer		Japanese (Japan[2])	Japanese (Hawaii)	Caucasian (US[3])	Caucasian (Hawaii)	Chinese (Singapore)	Chinese (Hawaii)	Chinese (US[3])	Filipino (Hawaii)	Hawaiian (Hawaii)
Stomach	male	85	35	11	17	44	9	12	9	27
	female	40	22	6	7	18	10	10	6	25
Colorectal	male	12	39	44	37	22	49	43	31	24
	female	10	29	34	35	17	27	23	15	20
Lung	male	20	32	61	52	57	35	60	25	71
	female	7	8	19	19	18	17	22	19	21
Breast	female	13	44	80	80	19	54	44	22	66
Prostate	male	3	25	45	42	4	18	18	14	19
Nasopharynx	male	0	1	1	1	19	10	19	1	4
	female	0	0	0	1	7	5	6	1	2
Six totals		190	235	301	291	225	234	257	143	279

[1] Rate per 100 000 (age 15–75+): age-standardized to world population
[2] Miyagi, Japan
[3] San Francisco Bay area, United States
Source: Waterhouse et al. 1976

326   *Chapter 19   Gary Glober and Grant Stemmermann*

cigarettes have been reported to be similar in the two groups (Table 19.2). Other factors such as the daily consumption of alchol, might have influenced the duration and the degree of exposure to carcinogens. In Hawaii, the female breast cancer rates are highest in Caucasian women, followed by Hawaiian women; Filipino women have the lowest rates. Japanese women in Hawaii have much more breast cancer than Japanese women in Japan.

Exceptionally high rates for nasopharyngeal cancer are reported in Hawaii Chinese. This was expected because most of the Chinese of Hawaii are derived from Kwantung Province in South China, wherein this cancer is very common. The relatively high incidence of nasopharyngeal cancer among Hawaiians is also explained by the genetic link, for persons who have mixed Hawaiian and Chinese ancestries are designated as part-Hawaiian in census tables.

In Hawaii, Chinese men have the highest colorectal cancer rates, far higher than Caucasian men or women. Chinese women have a much lower rate than Chinese men. In the ethnic groups of Hawaii, male colorectal cancer rates are higher in three groups having the highest family income (page 319), first Chinese, second Japanese, third Caucasians. These cancer rates are lowest in two groups of men, Hawaiians and Filipinos, having the lowest family income.

In Hawaii low rates of many of the common cancers, especially lung and breast tumours, are found among Filipinos. They have the lowest family income (page 319) but have experienced a rapid increase of economic status and many have moved from rural to the more densely populated urban regions during the last 20–30 years (Hackenberg *et al.*, 1978).

Japanese cancer rates after immigration

Dietary changes after immigration

The most thoroughly studied shifts in the incidence of neoplastic disease have been those of the Hawaii Japanese. The most conspicuous environmental change experienced by these people has been in the types and the amounts of food consumed by them. As noted previously, the Hawaii Japanese diet contains larger amounts of fat and protein than does the indigenous Japanese diet and a larger proportion of each of these nutrients is of animal origin in Hawaii. The carbohydrate load is not only decreased in Hawaii, but a larger proportion of it is simple sugars rather than complex carbohydrates (starch foods); the latter contain minerals, micronutrients and fibre. A comparison of specific food items consumed by Caucasians and Japanese in Hawaii with those eaten by Japanese in a rural Japanese prefecture indicated that the Hawaii Japanese consume more rice and preserved meats than Caucasians but less milk. Both Hawaii populations consume more beef, fresh vegetables and coffee than do indigenous Japanese, and much less fish, rice and Japanese soup.

Stomach cancer

The incidence of stomach cancer has decreased considerably among second generation Hawaii Japanese, although high rates persist in the first generation. This is probably not the result of improved diagnostic or treatment methods, but can be explained on the basis of diminished consumption of traditional Japanese foods that are rich in salt and nitrates; accompanied by an increased use of fresh fruits and vegetables, both containing vitamin C (Stemmermann, 1977).

Differences in the male to female ratio of gastric cancer between Japanese and Caucasians, as well as the greater frequency of the diffuse type of gastric cancer among Japanese patients at all age levels, suggest that there is a strong host influence upon the morphology and behaviour of this cancer once induction has occurred. Hawaii Japanese demonstrate better survival with both the diffuse and intestinal types of gastric carcinoma than do the Hawaiians or Caucasians in Hawaii, probably because they have fewer tumours at stage IV at the time of diagnosis (Stemmermann and Brown, 1974).

Colorectal cancer

Carcinoma of the large bowel is one of the most common cancers in Hawaii Japanese, with male and female rates similar to those of Caucasians and roughly three times those reported from tumour registries in Japan (Table 19.4). The wide geographic variation in this form of cancer, and the rapidity of its increase among Hawaii Japanese, is the basis of the assumption that this tumour is dependent upon environmental factors.

The increase in colon cancer accompanies a rise in the frequency of other conditions in Hawaii Japanese associated with a Western lifestyle (e.g. obestiy, myocardial infarction, atherosclerosis, diverticulosis of the colon, and hyperplastic and adenomatous polyps of the large bowel). This has led to the generation of several inter-related hypotheses proposing that large bowel cancer is related to high fat diets, low stool weight, slow transit time and increased faecal bile salt excretion. These proposals were tested in Hawaii by the Japan Hawaii Cancer Study. The bowel transit times of Hawaii Japanese (31 hours) were as fast as those of indigenous Japanese (34 hours), in spite of much higher rates for colon cancer among the Hawaii Japanese (Glober *et al.*, 1977). Even though they had the same risk for large bowel malignancy, the Hawaii Japanese had faster transit times (31 hours) than the Hawaii Caucasians (56 hours). The stool weights in Japan were heavier (195 g) than those of Hawaii Caucasians (120 g) and Hawaii Japanese (121 g).

The Hawaii Japanese bile secretion was not substantially different from that of indigenous Japanese, nor have we been able to demonstrate a positive correlation between Western food items and the faecal content of secondary or modified bile acids (Mower *et al.*, 1978). Finally, Western-style meals, starch, legumes and beef were considered to be risk factors for colon cancer among the Hawaii Japanese as measured in a case control study (Haenszel *et al.*, 1973).

We have been able to demonstrate a significant increase in the frequency of direct acting mutagens in the faeces of Hawaii Japanese and have used a strain of *Escherichia coli* to demonstrate a *trans*-nitrosase exchange enzyme that appears to activate faecal nitroso compounds. This occurs in Hawaii Japanese faeces much more frequently than in faeces from indigenous rural Japanese (Stemmerman *et al.*, in press). These findings are consistent with the suggestion of Bruce *et al.* (1977) that one of the characteristics of high colon cancer risk populations is the presence of potentially carcinogenic nitroso compounds in the faeces.

Japanese and Caucasians had higher rates of survival from large bowel cancer than Filipinos and Hawaiians, while the Japanese had the highest survival rate overall (Hirohata *et al.*, 1977).

Hospital disease rates in Hawaii

Table 19.5 presents data concerning the prevalence of certain diseases in patients of six metropolitan hospitals in Hawaii for the period January 1974 to July 1978. The Castle, Kaiser, Kuakini, Queen's, St. Francis and Straub hospitals contributed statistics. These six hospitals have 67 per cent of all medical and surgical admissions in Hawaii.

Diverticulosis

Diverticulosis has been condidered to be a disease of westernization. Indeed, in a case control study of diverticular disease in an English hospital, patients with diverticulosis had a far higher incidence of varicose veins, hiatus hernias and gallstones than did the controls (Brodribb and Humphreys, 1976). Stemmermann and Yatani in Hawaii and Sato and his colleagues in Japan assessed the prevalence of diverticulosis, having employed the same observational methods. They found in autopsy material that 52 per cent of Hawaii Japanese had diverticulosis compared to the 1 per cent in Japanese in Japan (Stemmermann and Yatani, 1973; Sato *et al.*, 1976). An unusual feature of diverticulosis in Hawaii Japanese was the high frequency of right-sided diverticulosis, and at a younger age, than the left-sided form. Diverticulosis appeared to be associated with higher grades of atherosclerosis.

Comparing rates for diverticulosis from 1956 to 1962 (Chang, 1965) with those of 1974–78 presented in Table 19.5, there appears to be an increasing rise of this disease in the Japanese and a relative decrease for Caucasians. There has been no change during this period among the other ethnic groups.

Although the Hawaii Chinese men have higher death rates for coronary heart disease and colorectal cancer than the Hawaii Japanese men, the hospital in-patient rates for diverticulosis were lower in Chinese men. The Filipino men, who have had an amazingly rapid increase in coronary heart disease over the past twenty years, still have a low rate of diverticulosis reported among hospital patients.

Table 19.5 Disease rates[1] in hospital in-patients in Hawaii, sex and ethnic groups, January 1974–July 1978

Disease		Caucasian	Japanese	Chinese	Filipino	Hawaiian	Korean
Diverticulosis	male	810	529	468	321	297	217
	female	821	425	478	320	366	335
Hiatus hernia	male	523	73	137	115	81	39
	female	535	51	162	158	138	52
Oesophagitis	male	289	94	91	94	110	256
	female	264	67	169	187	82	395
Cholecystitis	male	531	541	915	538	297	959
	female	960	933	1637	1489	1382	2041
Appendicitis	male	209	267	202	350	331	751
	female	219	206	201	395	249	382
Varicose veins	male	57	8	11	25	96	0
	female	41	5	17	0	73	0
Haemorrhoids	male	79	92	178	136	118	101
	female	67	63	121	80	109	31

[1] Rate per 100 000 (age 15–75+): age-standardized to world population

Hiatus hernia

Hiatus hernia has been considered a disease of modern Western societies. The Hawaiians had a lower hospital rate for hiatus hernia than Caucasians (Table 19.5) in spite of diets similar in most respects (Tables 19.1–19.3). The oriental groups have the lowest rates for hiatus hernia; which suggests an inherited characteristic.

Varicose veins, haemorrhoids

Socioeconomic factors did not appear to play a role in the hospital rates of varicose veins or haemorrhoids in Hawaii (Table 19.5). Hawaiians are almost at the bottom of the economic scale (page 319) yet have the highest hospital rates for varicose veins and third highest for haemorrhoids. Although hospital statistics are based on conditions severe enough to require surgery, this bias probably has the same impact on all ethnic groups.

Gallstones

In terms of obesity and fat intake we anticipated that the highest rates of gallstones would be in the Hawaiians and Caucasians. However, the Koreans and Chinese led the list of hospital patients suffering from cholecystitis, and Caucasians and Hawaiians had relatively low hospital rates (Table 19.5).

Appendicitis

Walker and his colleagues (Walker *et al.*, 1973) in their review of the literature concluded that appendicitis had been rare in developing countries but incidence rose during improvement in socioeconomic circumstances. Appendicitis was rare in rural African Negroes who had high crude fibre intake (22 g/d) and short transit times. Transit times were comparable in urban groups of Negroes, Indians and Caucasians, but although crude fibre intakes differed slightly, urban Negroes 6·8 g/d, Indians 4·0 g/d and Caucasians 4·6 g/d, the latter had ten times more appendicectomies than the urban Negroes.

In Hawaii, the lowest hospital rates of appendicitis were among the Chinese and Caucasians (Table 19.5), although from a socioeconomic standpoint they would be considered as very 'westernized'. The Japanese males had higher rates than the Caucasian males even though the study of bowel transit times among Caucasians and Japanese revealed faster transit times in the Japanese (Glober *et al.*, 1977). The stool weights were the same. The Chinese and Caucasians have similar low hospital apprendicitis rates in spite of significant dietary differences (Tables 19.1–19.3). Finally, the highest hospital appendicitis rates were in the Filipinos and Koreans, even though they were at opposite ends of the socioeconomic scale (page 319).

Summary

In summary, the Hawaii Japanese exhibit significant westernization in disease patterns and diet as exemplified by their increased risk for coronary heart disease, cancers of the colon, breast and prostate; also diverticulosis and obesity when compared with the Japanese in Japan. Likewise, the Chinese in Hawaii, in contrast to the Singapore Chinese, have higher rates for these cancers. The Hawaii Japanese and Chinese were more 'Western' than the Filipino with regard to coronary heart disease, diverticulosis, cholecystitis, also colonic, breast and prostatic malignancy. However, the increasing rate of coronary heart disease in the Filipino males implies that this group will develop more of the other diseases as well.

Hospital rates for cholecystitis, hiatus hernia, appendicitis, varicose veins and haemorrhoids do not exhibit the expected effects of westernization. In general, diet studies in Hawaii did not point to any specific patterns that would explain the ethnic disease differences with the exceptions of alcohol and carbohydrates in coronary heart disease and nitrates and ascorbic acid in gastric cancer.

Acknowledgements

We are grateful to Sandra Baers, MPH, for technical assistance with regard to the disease rates and demographic statistics and to Patricia Yoshida, RN. We appreciate very much the cooperation of the medical record departments of Castle, Kaiser, Kuakini, Queen's, St. Francis and Straub hospitals and are grateful to L. Kolonel, MD (Cancer Center of Hawaii), A. Kagan, MD (Honolulu Heart Study) and A. Nomura, MD (Japan–Hawaii Cancer Study) for helpful editorial advice. Work was supported by the Honolulu Medical Group Research and Education Foundation and the National Cancer Institute: No1-CP-53511; No1-CP-61060 and 1-Ro1-CA20897.

References

Bassett, D. R., Abel, A., Moellering, R. C. Jr., Rosenblatt, G. and Stokes, III, J. (1969). Coronary heart disease in Hawaii: dietary intake, depot fat, 'stress', smoking and energy balance in Hawaiian and Japanese men. *American Journal of Clinical Nutrition, 2,* 1483–1503

Brodribb, A. J. M. and Humphreys, D. M. (1976). Diverticular disease, three studies. *British Medical Journal,* 1, 424–430

Bruce, W. R., Bargatse, A. J., Furrer, R. and Land, P. C. (1977). A mutagen in the feces of normal human. In: *Origins of Human Cancer,* 161–164. Editors H. H. Hiatt, J. D. Watson and J. A. Winsten. Coldspring Harbor Conference on Cellular Proliferation, Volume 4. Coldspring Harbor Laboratories Publications

Chang, W. Y. M. (1965). Colonic diverticulitis in Hawaii. *Hawaii Medical Journal,* 24, 442–445

Glober, G. A., Nomura, A., Kamiyama, S., Shimada, A. and Abba, B. C. (1977). Bowel transit time and stool weight in populations with different colon cancer risks. *Lancet,* **ii,** 110–111

Hackenberg, R. A., Gerber, L. and Hackenberg, B. H. (1978). *Cardiovascular disease mortality among Filipinos in Hawaii : rates, trends and associated factors. Research and Statistic Report,* Hawaii State Department of Health, September

Haenszel, W., Berg, J. W., Segi, M., Kurihara, M. and Locke, F. B. (1973). Large bowel cancer in Hawaiian Japanese. *Journal of the National Cancer Institute,* **51,** 1775–1779

Hirohata, T., Nomura, A., Rallahan, W., Burch, T., Harris, D. and Batten, G. (1977). Survival patterns from large bowel cancer in Hawaii. *Hawaii Medical Journal,* **36,** 343–347

Kagan, A., Harris, B. R., Winkelstein, W. Jr., Johnson, K. G., Kato, H., Syme, S. L., Rhoads, G. G., Gay, M. L., Nichaman, N. Z., Hamilton, H. B. and Tillotson, J. L. (1974). Epidemiologic studies of coronary heart disease and stroke in Japanese men living in Japan, Hawaii and California: demographic, physical, dietary and biochemical characteristics. *Journal of Chronic Diseases,* **27,** 345–364

Mower, H. F., Ray, R. M., Stemmermann, G. N., Nomura, A. and Glober, G. A. (1978). Analysis of fecal bile acids and diet among the Japanese in Hawaii. *Journal of Nutrition,* **108,** 1289–1296

Robertson, T. L., Kato, H., Gordon, T., Kagan, A., Rhoads, G. G., Land, C. E., Worth, R. M., Belsky, J. L., Dock, D. S., Miyanishi, M. and Kawamoto, S. (1977). Epidemiologic studies of coronary heart disease and stroke in Japanese men living in Japan, Hawaii and California. *American Journal of Cardiology,* **39,** 239–249

Sato, E., Ouchi, A., Sasano, N. and Ishidate, T. (1976). Polyps and diverticulosis of large bowel autopsy population of Akita prefecture compared with Miyagi. *Cancer,* **37,** 1316–1321

Stemmermann, G. N. (1977). Gastric cancer in the Hawaii Japanese. *Gann,* **68,** 525–535

Stemmermann, G. N. and Brown, C. (1974) A survival study of intestinal and diffuse types of gastric carcinoma. *Cancer,* **33,** 1190–1195

Stemmermann, G. N., Mandel, M. and Mower, H. (in press). Colon cancer: its precursors and companions in Hawaii Japanese. *Second Symposium on Epidemiology and Cancer Registries in the Pacific Basin.* Editor B. Henderson. *NCI Monograph,* in press

Stemmermann, G. N. and Yatani, R. (1973). Diverticulosis and polyps of the large intestine: a necropsy study of Hawaii Japanese. *Cancer,* **31,** 1260–1270

Walker, A. R. P., Richardson, B. D., Walker, B. F. and Woolford, A. (1973). Appendicitis, fibre intake and bowel behaviour in ethnic groups in South Africa. *Postgraduate Medical Journal,* **49,** 243–249

Waterhouse, J., Correa, P., Muir, C. and Powell, J. (1976). *Cancer Incidence in Five Continents,* III. International Agency for Research on Cancer, Lyon

Yano, K., Rhoads, G. G. and Kagan, A. (1977) Coffee, alcohol and the risk of coronary heart disease among Japanese men living in Hawaii. *New England Journal of Medicine,* **297,** 405–409

Yano, K., Rhoads, G. G., Kagan, A. and Tillotson, J. (1978). Dietary intake and the risk of coronary heart disease in Japanese men living in Hawaii. *American Journal of Clinical Nutrition,* **31,** 1270–1279

Part VI

Far East

20

Japan

Shun-ichi Yamamoto

Historical background

1900–1950

During much of the first half of the twentieth century Japan was directly or indirectly involved in a series of major or minor wars. These included the Russo-Japanese War 1904–5, the First World War 1914–18, the Sino-Japanese War and the Second World War 1939–45. This was a period of social and economic unrest, and consequently the new epidemiological approach, that had been adopted during the second half of the nineteenth century, made little progress. Attempts were made, however, during this period to collect some data on disease prevalence and distribution. The compilation of demographic and biostatistical data by the government started in 1899 and has continued ever since—except for the last two years (1944–45) of the Second World War. These allow some conclusions to be drawn as regards changes in disease patterns during this period, but the major changes of diet and lifestyle did not occur until after the war.

During the Second World War food shortages became severe in many areas of Japan from 1942 onwards. Even after the cessation of hostilities in 1945 the average energy consumption per adult was below 8·5 MJ (2000 kcal) until about 1950. The wartime food shortages accelerated an increase of tuberculosis: death rates fell when food supplies increased and new drugs became available. As discussed later diabetes mellitus decreased in prevalence during the years of the food shortages. The crude mortality rate from stroke also decreased during the period of food shortages; the yearly crude mortality rate per 100 000 fell from an average of 178 in the four years 1939–42 to 128 in the four years 1947–50, no data being available for the intermediate years of 1944, 1945 and 1946 (Watanabe, 1954).

After 1950

During the allied occupation after the war the Japanese were quick to learn, and enthusiastic to apply the scientific knowledge possessed by Western

337

nations. Probably no other nation has ever applied advanced scientific technology to such an extent and in so short a time. Developments in medical technology paralleled those in other fields. All this resulted in profound changes in the whole lifestyle, particularly in urban communities.

Dietary changes were particularly pronounced. During the years 1945–50 when the food shortages were still severe, large quantities of wheat flour, corn-flour, maize and powdered milk were imported. Preference was given to the Japanese children in the distribution of these imported foods, and as a consequence the young generation grew up with a preference for many Western foods and bread even replaced to a large extent rice. Special efforts were made to increase the energy intakes until in 1967 the average Japanese man ate daily 10·5 MJ (2500 kcal), the average Japanese woman 9·4 MJ (2250 kcal) (Oiso, 1971).

Fortunately it was recognized that these large dietary changes, which occurred over a short period of time, mainly in the years 1950–65, provided an opportunity to study changes in the pattern of disease that are associated with Western diets. For the first time in Japanese history obese children were seen in the large cities, although less cereals and potatoes were consumed, but milk, fat and oil, also sugar consumption, had all risen. In adults athero-sclerosis, ischaemic heart disease and maturity-onset diabetes mellitus became more common (Oiso, 1971). The changes in average adult nutritional intakes in Japan from 1950 to 1975 are recorded in Table 20.1 (Kagawa, 1978).

Table 20.1   Changes in adult nutrient intakes in Japan 1950–75 (Kagawa, 1978)

	Averages per capita per day			
	1950	1960	1972	1975
Energy (MJ)	8·7	8·7	9·5	9·1
(kcal)	2100	2100	2280	2190
Protein, total (g)	68	70	83	80
Protein, animal (g)	17	25	40	39
Lipids (g)	18	25	50	52
Carbohydrate (g)	420	400	360	340
Cereal energy (%)	78	75	52	50

Ischaemic heart disease

It is desirable to sound two notes of caution before there is any discussion concerning whether the incidence of coronary heart disease (CHD) has risen in Japan during recent years and whether there was a possible associa-tion with westernization of diets and of lifestyle. First, it should be clearly recognized that even in the late 1970s age-specific CHD death rates in Japan, both men and women, were still very low, they were only one-tenth of the USA death rates (Shirasaki, 1978). Second, recent dietary changes in Japan are not easily summarized in a single term of 'westernization'.

The initial westernization of Japanese diets began to occur at the time of the Meiji Restoration in 1878; then it occurred in a dramatic, almost revolutionary manner. Western foods began to be eaten at least by upper-class urban residents; people started eating beef, pork, bread, milk and sugar. The consumption of sugar rose after the colonization of Taiwan in 1895; therein sugar plantations were developed by semi-government enterprises, so that sugar crept slowly into the national diet even in rural areas of Japan. The second dietary change occurred, as already discussed, after the Second World War from 1950 onwards (Table 20.1). This involved a massive change of the diet involving a large proportion of the whole population; they became more affluent and diet and lifestyle became westernized in many respects. The average adult diet began to contain far more fat and sugar, but less starch and cereals (Table 20.1).

In the middle 1950s Ancel Keys, in association with Japanese physicians, stated '. . . of all large countries with detailed vital statistics, Japan reports the lowest mortality rate from coronary heart disease' (Keys *et al.*, 1958). Keys and his distinguished Japanese colleagues were among the first to record that Japanese who had emigrated to Hawaii developed more CHD than Japanese in Japan, but there was the same degree of prevalence of hypertension in the two countries. Recent studies from Hawaii (page 320) have confirmed and extended these observations.

In Japan during 1933 cardiovascular disease deaths comprised 13·2 per cent of all death certificates, and among them were stroke 9·3 per cent, endocarditis and valvular diseases 2·0 per cent, but angina and coronary heart disease were only 0·4 per cent. During the 1950s Japanese cardiologists and physicians began to report that they were diagnosing more cases of myocardial infarction so that in 1962 a Committee on the Etiology of Myocardial Infarction was set up with Professor Ueda of Tokyo University as Chairman, and its twelve members were drawn from universities throughout Japan. A series of reports, starting in 1957, were published. That of 1975 summarized evidence that '. . . the incidence of myocardial infarction has increased recently'. The evidence was derived largely from the recently created cardiovascular departments of the modern teaching hospitals. Evidence was produced to the Committee that from 1936 to 1950 the percentage of patients suffering from mycardial infarction in 13 major hospitals had averaged 0·2 per cent; that after 1950 the percentage figure had increased steadily until about 1965 and subsequently had averaged about 3·0 per cent during the next decade (Committee Report, 1975).

The various reports of the Myocardial Infarction Committee have been criticized on several grounds, namely that a rise in the incidence of CHD among hospital patients during the 1950s might be due to increased use of the electrocardiogram, and increased knowledge of the disease by Japanese medical practitioners and the general public; the latter had increased accessibility to the hospital owing to the general implementation of the health insurance system. Milder cases of CHD began to be recognized because more patients were being referred to recently enlarged cardiac departments of the teaching hospitals.

Yano and Ueda (1963) reviewed the position in Japan and were able to cite during the years 1957–60 some six communications which reported an appreciable increase in the incidence of coronary heart disease in Japan. There had been, however, no large-scale study of the prevalence of coronary heart disease in a big sample of the population. During 1958–60 Yano and Ueda (1963) conducted a large-scale prevalence survey of coronary heart disease detected at the initial examination of a prospective longitudinal study under the auspices of the Atomic Bomb Commission, Hiroshima. All sybjects had been exposed to varying degrees of exposure to irradiation at the 1945 atom bomb explosion. No evidence had been obtained at that time, or since, that nuclear irradiation influences coronary heart disease. Japanese and United States physicians examined 2848 men and 2171 women, aged 30 years or more. The Framingham study in the United States had specified the diagnostic criteria and classification of coronary heart disease; these were adopted in the Hiroshima survey, so that the disease was recorded as either definite myocardial infarction, angina pectoris or possible infarction.

The coronary heart disease prevalence at Hiroshima of definite myocardial infarction, angina pectoris and possible infarction had been 1·4 per cent for men and 0·8 per cent for women. These total rates, and those of the various age groups, in men and women, were only about one-quarter of the corresponding Framingham rates. The difference had been most marked in the younger age groups. At Hiroshima statistically significant correlations were reported between high CHD prevalence rates and high systolic blood pressure, also diabetes mellitus in men and obesity in women. Serum cholesterol levels were considerably lower at Hiroshima than at Framingham, but there was no significant correlation between these levels in Japanese men or women and the prevalence of coronary heart disease. These studies were the first stage of the large studies of migrant Japanese in Hawaii and California, which will be discussed later.

Autopsy data have also suggested that coronary heart disease has increased in recent years in Japan. For instance, during the period 1958–62 myocardial infarction was reported in 1012 autopsies out of a total number of 60 928 derived from many different centres. It was considered that myocardial infarction deaths had increased two-fold during the five years covered by this review (Hashimoto *et al.*, 1965). It is, however, impossible to accept a two-fold increase of CHD deaths in a stable community within as short a period as five years. More information is required concerning the age and sex structure of the whole community.

To summarize: CHD was certainly an uncommon disease in Japanese men and women prior to about 1950; it is probable that CHD incidence has risen in recent years especially in urban areas, but CHD as a cause of death is still far less common in all parts of Japan than in North America or Europe. After 1950 diets in all parts of Japan and for most of the people started to become much more westernized, but it should be borne in mind that the quantities of Western-type foods are still far less than those eaten in the United States and northern European countries. In the period 1950–67 the intake of fat per capita in Japan increased from 18 g/d to 43 g/d, and the proportion of saturated fats to polyunsaturated fats increased; the consumption of animal products, especially milk and eggs, increased considerably, likewise sugar. The intakes of rice, cereals and potatoes have all decreased. Energy intakes have altered little since 1950 in Japan, but the composition of the diet has altered considerably (Oiso, 1971; Kagawa, 1978).

CHD among Japanese in Hawaii and in California

The study of the prevalence of disease in migrant populations may afford information concerning environmental factors. If the populations studied are large this minimizes the influence of genetic factors. A prospective study of CHD and stroke was initiated in 1965 on a cohort of men of Japanese ancestry aged 45–69 years living in Hiroshima and Nagasaki, Japan; in Honolulu, Hawaii, and in the San Francisco Bay area, California. More than 10 000 men were examined and comparable techniques were employed in all areas. A series of publications have reported the methods of examination, the physical and laboratory findings and the methods employed in the dietary survey.

The Japanese California men were slightly heavier than the Japanese Hawaiian men, who were on average 8 kg heavier than those living in Japan. Skinfold thickness varied in a similar manner. Blood pressure levels were almost similar in Japan and Hawaii, but were higher in all age groups in California. Serum cholesterol levels were lower in all age groups in Japan, and averaged 4·7 mmol/l (180 mg/dl); these levels were higher and almost similar in all age groups in Hawaii and Japan, and averaged 5·7 mmol/l (220 mg/dl). Serum glucose levels at one hour after oral glucose 50 g were lower in all age groups in Japan than in age groups in California; in Hawaii levels followed an intermediate position. In Japan blood uric acid levels were lower in all age groups than in Hawaii and California, which had similar levels (Kagan *et al.*, 1974).

Special but similar techniques in the dietary survey were employed in all three areas. Four different methods revealed striking differences in the dietary patterns as the Japanese men had become progressively westernized in their diet in Hawaii, and even more so in California. In spite of the differences in body weight, which increased markedly in Hawaii and California, the energy intakes of the three groups had been very similar. It was therefore suggested that Japanese men in Japan had a higher energy expenditure than those in Hawaii and those in California. As westernization of the Japanese diet in Japan has accompanied the appearance of obesity in Japanese children, a new feature in the large cities (Oiso, 1971), it is possible that more consideration should be paid to the fattening properties of Western foods, rich in fat and sugar; these confer palatability, and are energy dense. The principal difference in the diets of the three Japanese cohorts lay in the starch foods (complex carbohydrates). In terms of total energy percentages the diet in

Japan was high starch 52 per cent, moderate sugar 11 per cent, but low in total fat 15 per cent; saturated fats were specially low and polyunsaturated fat constituted a fair proportion of the total fat. The Japanese Hawaii diet showed moderate westernization: it had low starch 33 per cent, more sugar 16 per cent, more fat 33 per cent, largely due to a four-fold increase in saturated animal fats. The Japanese California diet showed increased westernization, starch decreased to 30 per cent, sugar rising to 17 per cent, also fat rising to 38 per cent and saturated fats again increased. Cholesterol intakes were very similar in all three groups, from an average daily intake of 460 mg in Japan, to 540 mg in California. The dietary surveys acknowledged that it was impossible to quantify salt intake in free-living populations, but assessed sodium chloride daily intake to average in men aged 40–49 years 12–13 g in Japan, and 8–9 g in Hawaii and California. The pattern of smoking was studied in all three groups. A much larger proportion of men in Japan were mild smokers (10–20 cigarettes daily), but Hawaii had the largest number of heavy smokers (more than 40 cigarettes daily). A large number of publications set forth this survey of the effect of westernization of diets and lifestyle in Japanese migrants (Tillotson *et al.*, 1973; Kagan *et al.*, 1974). This large study of migrants demonstrated that westernization increased recognized CHD risk factors and that CHD prevalence increased.

Cerebrovascular disease and stroke

Cerebrovascular disease and stroke, especially that due to cerebral haemorrhage, has been considered to be the major cause of death in Japanese adults. Actually the death rates, recorded on the death certificates, started to decline since 1940, even before the years of meagre food supplies during and after the Second World War (Watanabe, 1954). The slow decline continued into the 1970s in spite of an increased number of elderly Japanese. The incidence of stroke increases in all ageing populations. For instance in Britain the incidence of stroke per 1000 persons is 5 among those aged 45–64 years and rises to 23 among those aged 65–74 years (Marcus, 1977).

In Japan 25 per cent of all deaths have been ascribed on the death certificates to cerebrovascular disease, and this percentage was recorded as late as 1966. The position is being re-evaluated at several Japanese medical schools wherein the number of neurologists and neurosurgeons have grown in recent years, having previously been but few. Rapid loss of consciousness in an elderly person had been too frequently equated with cerebral haemorrhage; the patient had seldom been referred to a hospital, and necropsies on elderly persons had been uncommon. In 1966 among 28 431 total necropsies in Japan CNS vascular lesions were only 4·5 per cent and IHD deaths were 1·7 per cent. A careful study of 2526 necropsies from 1950 to 1965 at the Atomic Bomb Casualty Commission reported CNS vascular lesions 6·1 per cent, hypertensive heart disease 7·8 per cent, CHD 1·6 per cent (Netsky and Miyaji, 1976).

A prospective clinical and necropsy study from 1961 until 1966 in the village of Hisayama has reported a fatal cerebral vascular disease rate of 8·0 per 1000 population per year and cerebral thrombosis was ten times commoner than cerebral haemorrhage (Katsuki and Hirota, 1966). These investigators concluded that cerebrovascular disease rates in Japan were similar to those published in the United States.

Diabetes mellitus

Death rates

There is no little information concerning the death rates of diabetes mellitus in Japan before the Second World War. Maturity-onset diabetes kills mainly through its cardiovascular complications and the presence of the former disease may not be recorded on the death certificate, or included in mortality data. The latter are therefore an unreliable source of evidence concerning the prevalence of the disease in any country. Probably changes in mortality data within a *single* country may be more informative.

Kurihara *et al.* (1971) have analysed age-adjusted diabetes death rates per 100 000 population from 46 countries. In 1950–51 Japan had the lowest figure, 3·2 for men and 2·9 for women; in 1964–65 these figures had risen to 5·6 for men and 5·2 for women. This would suggest that the prevalence of diabetes has increased in Japanese men and women during the period 1950–1965. Nevertheless the 1964–65 death rates were still lower than those of Europe, North America and Australia: this may be due to the fact, discussed later, that the fatal cardiovascular complications of diabetes mellitus appear to be less frequent and severe in Japanese adults.

Wartime food shortages

The Second World War was accompanied by severe food shortages; these started in 1942 and became severe; they persisted after the end of hostilities in 1945 and lasted until about 1950 (page 337). During these years there was some evidence that the prevalence of diabetes mellitus decreased. For instance, both the number of diabetic patients attending the medical clinic of Tohoku University Hospital, also the proportion of diabetic out-patients to total out-patients, during the years 1945–48 inclusive, decreased to a quarter of the pre-war figures (Goto *et al.*, 1958). Other data came from Kyoto University Hospital: during all years 1945–48 inclusive, diabetes mellitus was not recorded at any autopsy; but from 1965 to 1969 inclusive, about 12 autopsies a year reported the presence of diabetes mellitus (Okamoto *et al.*, 1971). Many countries have reported decreased diabetes death rates during the periods of food restriction that accompany war; these have been ascribed to decreased intakes of energy, fat and sugar, also increased intakes of dietary fibre, a postulated protective factor.

Prevalence surveys

Nothing was known concerning the prevalence of abnormal carbohydrate metabolism in Japan until a research group from 17 universities and medical centres in Japan conducted a diabetes detection survey during 1957–60. The diagnostic procedures and the definitions of normal and abnormal carbohydrate metabolism, in terms of the normal and abnormal glucose tolerance test (GTT), were clearly defined and were employed at all centres. Screening consisted in detecting urinary sugar and in estimating the blood sugar after a large breakfast. The results were subsequently summarized by Kuzuya and Kosaka (1971) and are given here, for the original publication of the research group, cited by these two investigators, is not easily consulted. A diabetes-type GTT was reported in 5·7 per cent of men aged 50–59 years, and in 3·5 per cent of women of similar age; also in 8·4 per cent of men aged 60–69 years and in 4·8 per cent of women of similar age. Both of these figures are lower than the estimate of the 15 per cent abnormal diabetic-type GTT in persons aged over 50 years reported in a Birmingham diabetes survey in England (Malins, 1968). Since the incidence of diabetes possibly increased progressively with age, and there are different ways of performing and interpreting a GTT, it is impossible to compare too closely one set of figures with another. No clear line divides mild diabetes from normality. The Japanese figures suggest that the prevalence of diabetes mellitus in Japan during 1957–60 was probably lower than, but was approaching that of countries in Europe and North America.

Increased prevalence

There is, however, some evidence that the prevalence of diabetes mellitus in Japan has increased in recent decades. First, the 17 universities group large-scale diabetes detection survey of 1957–60, already discussed, continued until 1962 and the same procedures and definitions were employed. This research group reported that during the six years of the survey, 1957–62, abnormal diabetic-type GTTs had increased 60 per cent in persons aged 40–49 years and 50 per cent in those aged 50–59 years (Kuzuya and Kosaka, 1971). Dietary intakes in Japan had increased and food patterns had become more westernized about 12 years previously, that is about 1950 (Kagawa, 1978).

Second, rising prevalence was also reported in Japanese-sponsored medical surveys at Hiroshima. It should be recognized that these surveys were conducted on those who had been exposed to nuclear irradiation in 1945. There is, however, no evidence in man or in animals that this irradiation predisposes to diabetes (Rudnick and Anderson, 1962). Japanese authorities have sponsored annual medical surveys of the 80 000 Hiroshima inhabitants who had been exposed to the 1945 atomic bomb. They employed Tes-Tape for the screening urinary test and an oral GTT on all glycosurics. During the seven years 1963–69 inclusive, the prevalence of glycosuria had doubled both in men and in women in the three age groups, 17–39 years, 40–59 years, and those over 60 years of age. This increase had been reflected in an increased number of diabetes-type GTTs. Details of the various categories of abnormal carbohydrate tolerance were given by Kawate (1971). He considered also that the 17 universities group diabetes detection survey and the Hiroshima annual medical survey demonstrated that diabetes mellitus prevalence was increasing in many areas of Japan. Kuzuya and Kosaka (1971) agreed that diabetes prevalence increased after the Second World War, especially after 1955; it had been very marked in persons over 60 years of age.

Dietary factors

Kagawa (1978) analysed the effect of the partial westernization of the Japanese diet and its influence on the increased prevalence of diabetes in Japan. He noted that diabetic patients, per 100 000 population of the 55–64 years old group, had increased from 163 in 1965 to 293 in 1974. However, this might be due to the fact that patients were looking increasingly to hospital treatment. Kagawa (1978), however, considered that dietary changes had been a major factor, but that westernization of the diet had so far been only slight. In 1975 the Japanese per capita intakes of both sugar and fats were still only half the US levels; the biggest difference between these two diets lay in the cereals. Japanese cereal intakes were twice those of the US, and in Japan wheat, although increasing, provided only a quarter, but rice provided still three-quarters of the energy. The first characteristic of the Japanese diet was the fact that amylopectins had predominated over starch as the principal carbohydrate. With westernization the Japanese had to adapt to a different form of carbohydrate, and it might be desirable to investigate the digestion and absorption of these two substances. The second characteristic of the Japanese diet, according to Kagawa (1978), was the amount and the difference in the dietary fibre. Japanese derive little dietary fibre from cereals, but fair amounts from Japanese vegetables, mannans of Konnyaku and the polyuronides of seaweed; all of these are eaten in the traditional diet.

Unusual features

There is agreement that diabetes mellitus in Japan shows certain unusual features. Males still predominate over females; acetonuria is not common and deaths from cardio–renal–vascular lesions are far less common than in North America and Europe. Retinopathy and hypertension are among the commonest complications. Even in 1969 less than 5 per cent of diabetics died of myocardial infarction (Kuzuya and Kosaka, 1971). Dietary factors were considered to play a major role in the complications, high salt intakes related to frequency of hypertension, low fat intakes to the infrequency of cardio-vascular lesions.

Childhood diabetes

Childhood diabetes mellitus is certainly rare in Japan. Miki and Maruyama (1971) obtained data from nearly 300 paediatric departments and estimated the prevalence to be about one patient per 25 000 children. This is one-tenth of the prevalence in the United States.

Diverticular disease of the colon

Although the frequency of diverticular disease has been increasing in recent years, particularly in urban communities, the condition is much less common in Japan than in Western countries. In a series of barium enema examinations Sugawara and Igarashi (1958) reported that diverticular were demonstrated in 14 per cent of white patients in Japan but in only 3·5 per cent of Japanese.

It is well known that diverticula of the caecum and ascending colon are more frequently observed than in other nations (Stemmermann and Yatani, 1973). Many believe these to differ from diverticula of the distal colon (Hill *et al.*, 1978) and to be due to different causes. Kodeki and Miyagi (1966) circulated many clinics in Japan in an attempt to estimate the relative frequency of diverticula in different segments of the colon. The caecum and ascending colon were found to be the most commonly affected site (47 per cent), followed by the sigmoid colon (24 per cent). Miyanaga (1974) reported 74 per cent of diverticula in the caecum and ascending colon; Kabe *et al.* (1976) reported that in 48 of 73 patients with diverticula the right colon was involved.

The relative rarity of Western-type diverticula, that is diverticula of the distal left colon, is emphasized by the fact that in a series of over 4000 radiological lower gastrointestinal tract examinations diverticula were found in 8·4 per cent of men and 4·1 per cent of women (Yazawa *et al.*, 1975). Judging from other studies, in which approximately half of the diverticula were reported in the caecum and ascending colon, the percentage of barium enema examinations, showing lesions beyond the hepatic flexure, must have been about 4 per cent in men and 2 per cent in women; these figures were reported in particularly careful studies using the clyster method (Yazawa *et al.*, 1975). These authors reported an earlier series (1967–74) of over 25 000 radiological examinations of the gastrointestinal tract in which colonic diverticula were detected in only 6 patients (0·02 per cent).

Kubo *et al.* (1969) cite three large series of radiological studies of the large bowel before 1966 totalling 51 462 patients in which diverticula were found in only 7 (0·01 per cent). These authors observed 55 cases of diverticular disease in 2592 patients (2·1 per cent) between 1965 and 1968. The percentage detected in barium enema studies during these four years was 1·3, 1·2, 1·9 and 3·3, suggesting perhaps a rise in frequency. The sex ratio in this study was male:female, 3:1, a figure comparable to that of other studies. This is consistent with the observation that diseases which are the result of a change in dietary customs usually increase in prevalence in men before women, as men are usually the first to change their dietary customs.

Shikata *et al.* (1970) conducted a survey of operations on the colon and rectum in Japan and obtained figures from 150 hospitals totalling almost half a million operations. Just under 6000 (1·2 per cent of the total) were performed for lesions in the colon and rectum, and only 2 per cent of these operations, that is 119 patients (0·02 per cent of the total operations) were performed for diverticular disease.

It can be concluded that diverticula of the colon are uncommon in Japan and that those of Western type affecting the distal colon are rare.

Diverticular disease appears to increase in prevalence when Japanese immigrate into Hawaii. Stemmermann and Yatani (1973) reported 10 per cent in men and 5 per cent in women aged 50–59 years, and 26 per cent in men and 7 per cent in women aged 60–69 years. These figures are lower than those for other Americans.

Gallstones

Several changes with regard to the occurrence and clinical characteristics of gallstones have taken place in Japan during the present century. The most significant change is the replacement of pigment stones by those composed largely of cholesterol, the type of stone responsible for the vast majority of cases of cholelithiasis in Western countries.

Change from pigment to cholesterol stones

Higashi (1965) showed from a series of over 20 000 autopsies that whereas prior to 1955 pigment stones had occurred three times as frequently as cholesterol stones, the ratio had been reversed within the last ten years; cholesterol stones had become three times as frequent as pigment stones.

Nishimura (1971), reporting on data from the Department of Surgery, Kyushu University, stated that before 1947 pigment stones were nearly three times as frequent as cholesterol stones. From 1947 to 1955 they were just over twice as common; however, between 1955 and 1960 the situation became reversed, cholesterol stones became the commoner stone. During the period 1961–70 cholesterol stones were three times as frequent as pigment stones.

Kameda (1974) showed from figures collected from many areas in Japan that in rural communities pigment stones were still much more common than cholesterol stones, while the reverse situation occurred in urban communities (Table 20.2). Alterations in lifestyle introduced with the acceleration in economic development after the Second World War seemed to have been responsible. This could account for the observation of Kiya (1966) that pigment stones were commoner in older and cholesterol stones in younger people.

Shimura (1974) reported from the University of Tokyo that between the periods 1947–50, and 1967–70, there was a gradual steady increase in the proportion of gallstones composed of cholesterol. Before 1950 pigment stones predominated by 3 to 1. By the period 1955–58 the frequency of both types was approximately the same. By the period 1967–70 cholesterol stones were more than twice as common as those composed of pigment.

Change in sex ratio

This progressive change in the clinical composition of gallstones was

348   *Chapter 20   Shun-ichi Yamamoto*

Table 20.2   Percentage of bilirubin to cholesterol in gallstones isolated from the residents in five Prefectures of Japan (Kameda, 1974)

Prefecture	Individuals (No.)	Bilirubin	Cholesterol	Ratio b/c[1]
Tokyo	499	23	70	0·3
Tochigi	84	39	55	0·7
Nagasaki	53	66	23	2·9
Akita	193	68	16	4·3
Aomori	56	75	7	10·7

Percentage of chemical component spans Bilirubin and Cholesterol.

[1] Bilirubin/cholesterol ratio

associated with an alteration in sex ratio of the patients. When pigment stones predominated they were commoner in men than in women. When the change to cholesterol stones occurred women became affected more than men.

Kameda (1974) emphasized that the sex ratio change had been most pronounced in urban areas; there the change in composition of the gallstones had been most noticeable, specially in the upper socioeconomic groups among whom the increased prevalence of cholelithiasis had been most evident.

Increased incidence

During the 12 years 1927–34 in the Surgical Department of Kyushu University only 275 of 10 012 admissions were for gallstones (2·7 per cent). The male to female ratio of 1·4:1 reflected the fact that at that time even in urban communities pigment stones predominated. Maki (1962) reported that, whereas only 1 per cent of the surgical admissions during the period 1941–51 had been for gallstones, this had increased to 6·2 per cent of the surgical admissions by 1961. This author also noted that the frequency of gallstones observed at autopsy had risen from 2·7 per cent during 1948–54 to 4·7 per cent during the years 1955–61.

Tanaka (1941) reported an average incidence of gallstones of 4·7 per cent in four autopsy series totalling 11 722 subjects. Kameda (1974) also reported a series of over 9000 autopsies performed from 1949 to 1971; these showed that the gallstone rate rose from 3·5 per cent in the period 1949–54 to 7·1 per cent in the period 1945–71.

To summarize: pigment stones formerly were commoner than cholesterol stones in Japan and the former were commoner in men. Cholesterol gallstones now are commoner than pigment stones, and the incidence has increased in recent years; the former are commoner in women. The increased prevalence of cholesterol gallstones in recent years has been associated with westernization of the diet (page 338).

References

Committee Report (1975). The incidence of myocardial infarction in hospitalized patients and the risk factors of myocardial infarction. *Japanese Heart Journal,* 16, 465–479

Goto, Y., Nakayama, Y. and Yagi, I. (1958). Influence of World War II food shortage on the incidence of diabetes mellitus in Japan. *Diabetes,* 7, 133–135

Hashimoto, M., Hashimoto, N., Ishihara, K., Matsui, H. and Hokaku, M. (1965). Statistical observation on the autopsy cases of myocardial infarction. *Naika (Internal Medicine),* 16, 1147–1156

Higashi, S. (1965). Some statistical comments on cholelithiasis. *Nippon Shŏkakibyō Gakkai Zasshi (Japanese Journal of Gastrointestinal Disease),* 62, 655–678

Hill, M. J., Morson, B. C. and Bussey, H. J. R. (1978). Aetiology of adenoma–carcinoma sequence in large bowel. *Lancet,* i, 245–247

Kabe, Y., Kido, H., Sugawara, K., Okamura, H., Suzuki, T. and Morita, K. (1976). The evaluation of diverticular disease of the colon. *Nippon Shŏkakigeka Gakkai Zasshi (Japanese Journal of Gastrointestinal Surgery),* 9, 437–442

Kagan, A., Harris, B. R., Winkelstein, W., Johnson, K. G., Kato, H., Syme, S. L., Rhoads, G. G., Gay, M. L., Nichaman, M. Z., Hamilton, H. B. and Tillotson, J. (1974). Epidemiologic studies of coronary heart disease and stroke in Japanese men living in Japan, Hawaii and California: demographic, physical, dietary and biochemical characteristics. *Journal of Chronic Disease,* 27, 345–364

Kagawa, Y. (1978). Impact of Westernization on the nutrition of Japanese: changes in physique, cancer, longevity and centenarians. *Preventive Medicine,* 7, 205–217

Kameda, H. (1974). Characteristic feature of gallstone in Japan. *Naika (International Medicine),* 33, 392–397

Katsuki, S. and Hirota, Y. (1966). Cited by Netsky, M. G. and Miyaji, T. (1976)

Kawate, R. (1971). Seven-year follow-up observations on glycosuria and diabetes mellitus in inhabitants in Hiroshima. In: *Diabetes Mellitus in Asia, 1970.* Editors S. Tsuji and M. Wada. Excerpta Medica, Amsterdam

Keys, A., Kimura, N., Kusukawa, A., Bronte-Stewart, B., Larsen, N. and Keys, M. H. (1958). Lessons from serum cholesterol studies in Japan, Hawaii and Los Angeles. *Annals of Internal Medicine,* 48, 83–94

Kiya, T. (1966). Statistical observation on cholelithiasis and cholangitis. *Nippon Geka Gakkai Zasshi (Japanese Journal of Surgery),* 67, 1049–1065

Kodeki, K. and Miyagi, S. (1966). Diverticulosis of colon. *Nippon Iji-Shinshi (Japanese Medical Journal),* No. 2207, 7–10

Kubo, A., Fuchagami, A. and Fujii, A. (1969). Diverticula of the large intestine. *Naika (Internal Medicine),* 24, 949–955

Kurihara, M., Matsuyama, T. and Segi, M. (1971). Diabetes mellitus mortality in Japan compared with other countries. In: *Diabetes Mellitus in Asia, 1970.* Editors S. Tsuji and M. Wada. Excerpta Medica, Amsterdam

Kuzuya, N. and Kosaka, K. (1971). Diabetes mellitus in Japan. In: *Diabetes Mellitus in Asia, 1970.* Editors S. Tsuji and M. Wada. Excerpta Medica, Amsterdam

Maki, T. (1962). The recent situation around gallstone in Japan. *Nippon Iji-Shinshi (Japanese Medical Journal)*, No. 2000, 17–22

Malins, J. (1968). *Clinical Diabetes Mellitus.* Eyre and Spottiswoode, London

Marcus, A. (1977). *Strokes.* Update Publications, London

Miki, E. and Maruyama, H. (1971). Childhood diabetes mellitus in Japan. In: *Diabetes Mellitus in Asia, 1970.* Editors S. Tsuji and M. Wada. Excerpta Medica, Amsterdam

Miyanaga, T. (1974). Diverticuli of the colon. *Geka Shinryō (Surgical Clinics)*, 16, 263–268

Netsky, M. G. and Miyaji, T. (1976). Prevalence of cerebral haemorrhage and thrombosis in Japan: study of the major causes of death. *Journal of Chronic Diseases*, 29, 711–721

Nishimura, M. (1971). Gallstone in Japanese. *Nippon Shŏkakibyō Gakkai Zasshi (Japanese Journal of Gastrointestinal Disease)*, 68, 290–295

Oiso, T. (1971). Recent annual changes in nutrition in Japan. In: *Diabetes Mellitus in Asia, 1970.* Editors S. Tsuji and M. Wada. Excerpta Medica, Amsterdam

Okamoto, K., Hazama, F. and Yamasaki, Y. (1971). Pathology of diabetes mellitus in Japan. In: *Diabetes Mellitus in Asia, 1970.* Editors S. Tsuji and M. Wada. Excerpta Medica, Amsterdam

Rudnick, P. A. and Anderson, P. S. (1962). Diabetes mellitus in Hiroshima, Japan. *Diabetes*, 11, 533–543

Shikata, J., Arai, M. and Matsumura, T. (1970). Benign diseases of colon and rectum, from nation-wide statistics in Japan. *Geka (Surgery)*, 32, 493–507

Shimura, H. (1974), The chronological change in gallstone. *Rinshō-to-Kenkyū (Clinics and Studies)*, 51, 2756–2762

Shirasaki, K. (1978). Death from heart diseases in several countries. *Hoken-no-Kagaku (Health Science)*, 20, 245–251

Stemmermann, G. N. and Yatani, R. (1973). Diverticulosis and polyps of the large intestine. A necropsy study of Hawaii Japanese. *Cancer*, 31, 1260–1270

Sugawara, T. and Igarashi, M. (1958). Diverticulosis and diverticuli of the colon. *Nippon Shŏkakibyō Gakkai Zasshi (Japanese Journal of Gastrointestinal Disease)*, 55, 773

Tanaka, S. (1941). Statistical observation on cholelithiasis treated at Department of Surgery, Kyushu University. *Nippon Geka Gakkai Zasshi (Japanese Journal of Surgery)*, 42, 343–364

Tillotson, J. L., Kato, H., Nichaman, M. Z., Miller, D. C., Gay, M. L., Johnson, K. G. and Rhoads, G. G. (1973). Epidemiology of coronary heart disease and stroke in Japanese men living in Japan, Hawaii, and

California: methodology for comparison of diet. *American Journal of Clinical Nutrition,* **26,** 177–184

Watanabe, J. (1954). Trend of death from stroke in Japan. *Kōsei-no-Shihyō (Health Indices),* **1,** (2), 6–12

Yano, R. and Ueda, S. (1963). Coronary heart disease in Hiroshima, Japan. *Yale Journal of Biology and Medicine,* **35,** 504–522

Yazawa, T., Ozaka, T., Watanabe, O. and Hara, T. (1975). Gastrointestinal diverticulosis in Japan. *I-to-Chō (Stomach and Intestine),* **10,** 721–727

21

Taiwan and China

David Landsborough

The author was a physician in a general hospital in Fukien province on the mainland of China from 1940 to 1951. He was physician and neurologist in a general hospital in Taiwan from 1952 until he retired in 1980. The National Taiwan University Hospital (NTUH), Taipei, is the largest general hospital in Taiwan, with 962 beds and an annual admissions rate of 16 000. Two-thirds of the in-patients come from Taipei city and surrounding areas and one-third from the rest of the island. The long establishment and stability of the hospital and its in-patient statistics have provided a guide to the incidence of disease. The Peiping (Peking) Union Medical College (PUMC) Hospital was the leading teaching and research medical institution in the mainland of China up to the year 1950. The Department of Internal Medicine had at its disposal 78 beds in the general wards and 15–20 beds in the private pavilion (Snapper, 1965).

TAIWAN

The land and the people

Taiwan is a fertile volcanic island separated from the mainland of China by 150 kilometres of the Pacific Ocean; the Tropic of Cancer passes through its centre. The population racially reflects the population of the mainland, with a heavy representation from south-east China. In 1972 the total population was 15 million, of which 82 per cent were Fukienese and Hakka in origin, 16 per cent came from the rest of China, and 2 per cent were aboriginals of Malaysian race. These proportions have changed little from 1949 until the present. The total population rose from 6 million in 1946 to nearly 17 million in 1977.

Social trends

During the last three decades social and economic changes have been very marked and have modernized the life of the people. At the end of the Second

352

World War 70 per cent of the people of Taiwan were agricultural and 30 per cent urban. Due to the determined policy of industrialization, in 1964 half the people were agricultural and half urban; in 1977 only a third remained agricultural and two-thirds were urban. Compulsory free education was extended from 6 years to 9 years in 1968; over 98 per cent of school-age children attend school. In 1946 there was one university, in 1977 there were nine universities. Nowadays there are well developed railways, motorways, roads, bus services, international and internal air communications. For instance in 1956 there were about 17 000 registered motor vehicles; by 1977 the number had risen to nearly 3 million.

There is a rapid increase in the number of young married women remaining in employment. The well-baby clinic of NTUH found that in 1965, 30 per cent of babies in the first month of life were exclusively breast-fed, but in 1978 only 7·5 per cent were breast-fed. At 4–6 months, of age the abandonment of breast-feeding was even more marked (Chen, C. L., 1978, personal communication). In spite of the increasing interest in recreational sport and exercise the enormous increase in motor transport has reduced the amount of daily exercise of a large proportion of the population. The tempo of life has quickened; commercial effort is headlong. Stress is the price that is being paid for this westernization of life.

Dietary trends

The staple constituent of the diet is polished white rice. Formerly in the poorer areas along the sea coast the staple diet was sweet potato, with small amounts of white rice added. Formerly in the mountains sweet potato, millet and taro were the staple foods. During the last 15 years, with the general economic development of the whole island, white polished rice has largely replaced other foods. There is almost universal disinclination to eat brown (unpolished) rice, because white rice is more palatable, it bears kudos, cooking is easier and quicker, also it can be stored for a much longer period. It has been thought that the loss of the fibre through polishing is made up by the fibre of other foods (legumes and roots), also of fruit and vegetables which are taken freely in the diet. So far there has been no analysis of diets in Taiwan with respect to dietary fibre, a recent concept. Chinese do not relish sweet food: the average sugar consumption in Taiwan at present is 48 g/d, this supplies 7 per cent of the daily total energy. Starchy foods supply 55–60 per cent of the total energy (Huang, P. C., 1978, personal communication).

The Joint Commission on Rural Reconstruction (JCRR) prepares a yearly Taiwan Food Balance Sheet. Chiu (1976) quotes from these figures (Table 21.1). It will be seen that the daily available food energy per head has increased from 5·3 MJ (1280 kcal) in 1945 to 10·5 MJ (2670 kcal) in 1975. Daily total protein has increased from 24 g to 74 g; animal protein has increased from 3 g to 24 g. In spite of the enormous improvement in the availability of nutrients during the last 30 years, even in 1975 the supply of vitamin A (5000 IU), riboflavin (1·6 mg), calcium (420 mg) and iron (13 mg) still appear to be low, even insufficient.

354   *Chapter 21   David Landsborough*

Table 21.1   Taiwan average per caput daily available nutrients 1945–75 (Chiu, 1976)

Year	Energy (MJ)	Protein (g)	Fat (g)	Carbohydrate (g)	Calcium (mg)	Iron (mg)
1945	5·3	24	11	190	130	5
1955	9·3	53	37	320	260	9
1965	10·0	61	47	340	280	10
1975	10·5	74	68	350	420	13

Conversion: SI to traditional units, 4·2 MJ ≈ 1000 kcals

Lee *et al.* (1976) found that between 1950 and 1974 total fat intake had increased from 12 per cent of total energy to 25 per cent; polyunsaturated and saturated fatty acids had increased from 2·3 and 3·4 per cent respectively to 5·4 and 7·5 per cent. The P/S ratio increased very slightly from 0·68 to 0·72. Daily total cholesterol intake increased from 76 mg in 1950 to 201 mg in 1974; daily consumption in urban Taipei was 373 mg and in San-chih county was 117 mg. Cholesterol consumption is still low compared with Japan (400 mg/d) and the USA (600 mg/d).

Salt intake (per head) varies with the occupation and economic situation. Huang *et al.* (1973, 1976) recorded 9·5 g/d in urban dwellers and 13·2 g/d in country people. Crowley *et al.* (1956) found Chinese soldiers in Taiwan were consuming over 20 g/d. In the fishing people of south-west Taiwan, fish and other foods were preferably eaten salted, both because of taste preference and as a means of preservation. Their salt intake was even higher than that of the soldiers (Tseng, 1967).

Improvement in nutrition has affected the average height and weight of children. Chen (1975) reported average increases from 1952 to 1972 in the 12-year-old age group as follows: in height, males increased from 136 cm to 143 cm, females from 135 cm to 146 cm. In weight males increased from 30 kg to 34 kg, females from 32 kg to 36 kg.

Disease trends

The emphasis in this chapter is in regard to whether, and in what way, diseases which are considered to be characteristic of Western countries are increasing in prevalence following westernization of the diet and manner of life of the Chinese. 'Westernization' may be defined as industrialization, with social trends towards the pattern of life (living standards, recreation and conveniences) in Europe and North America. Marked social changes have taken place in Taiwan during the last three decades, yet this period may not be long enough for disease prevalence trends to change. Unfortunately in Taiwan earlier statistics which would be comparable in value with present statistics are rarely available. A rough guide concerning disease trends may be provided also from yearly in-patient statistics from large general hospitals serving the whole population, also the impressions of observant doctors in full-time clinical practice who have remained in the same country for a long period of time.

Ischaemic heart disease (IHD)

In an epidemiological survey of 1051 subjects over the age of 40 in San-chih county, a rural area outside Taipei, the prevalence of IHD was found to be 0·9 per cent in males and 0·2 per cent in females (National Health Administration, 1975). A survey of 641 city dwellers of Taipei revealed a prevalence of 3·0 in males and 2·4 per cent in females. These values are much lower than those found in the USA. The serum lipid levels of these two populations are recorded under Cerebrovascular disease (page 357). In a survey of 1296 Taiwan aboriginal people over the age of 40, Tsai *et al.* (1966) found a prevalence of 2·1 per cent in men and 1·0 per cent in women. The mean cholesterol concentration in the blood was 3·8 mmol/l (149 mg/dl) in men and 4·1 mmol/l (157·0 mg/dl) in women. There was practically no rise with increasing age. In 127 NTUH in-patients with angiographically proved coronary artery disease the serum cholesterol, triglyceride and lipoprotein levels were significantly higher than those of 442 apparently healthy normal subjects of similar age, randomly selected as controls. The severity of the coronary obstruction was closely related to the raised levels of serum cholesterol and triglyceride (Huang *et al.*, 1978).

Concerning whether the prevalence of IHD is increasing there are the following observations. In NTUH the annual number of IHD admissions from 1966 to 1977 showed a steady rise from 82 to 291, which is a 3·5-fold increase. The annual total hospital admissions over the same period of time increased from 11 769 to 16 331, which is only a one-third increase. In Taiwan from 1957 to 1970 the crude death rate from 'arteriosclerotic and degenerative heart disease' rose from 4·9 to 11·6 per 100 000 of population. From 1971 to 1976 the crude death rate from 'ischaemic heart disease' rose from 6·3 to 10·6 per 100 000 (Health Statistics, National Health Administration, HSNHA, 1976 and earlier years). Age-specific mortality rates for these diseases have been calculated (Lee, L. Y., 1979, personal communication) and reveal an increased prevalence of IHD. The opinions of cardiologists in Taiwan (Wu, T. L., 1979, personal communication) are that IHD has been increasing in Taiwan in recent years and now stands at about half the US incidence in age groups of over 40 years.

Cerebrovascular disease (CVD)

Whereas the incidence of IHD is much lower in Taiwan than in Western countries the incidence of stroke is higher. As shown in Fig. 21.1, the mortality rate from CVD in both sexes in the 55–64 age group from 1955 until 1974 has fallen in other countries, but has remained high in the population of Taiwan,

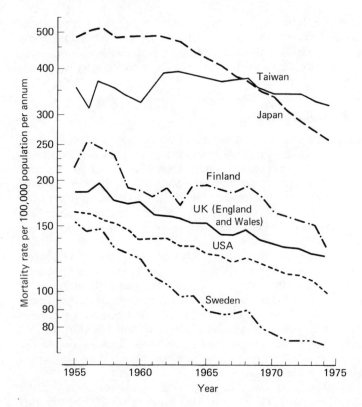

Fig. 21.1   Cerebrovascular disease mortality in Taiwan population of men and women aged 55–64 years from 1955 to 1974 (after Tseng, 1978a, b)

and now exceeds that of Japan, and probably that of any other country (Tseng, 1978a). A stroke register study in the Yen-ping area (population 50 160) of Taipei City, from January to December, 1975, following the methods suggested by the World Health Organization (1973), showed an incidence rate of 11·6 per thousand males in the 55–64 age group, and 25·8 for those over 65 years of age. The prevalence rates for males in the same two age groups were 21·1 per thousand and 74·0 respectively. These figures are higher than comparable figures from nine other countries and suggest the prevalence of stroke in Taiwan is extremely high (Tseng, 1978a). In 1963 Tseng (1978b) surveyed 17 953 subjects in rural south-western Taiwan and followed them up for the next 15 years. Those who were originally found to be hypertensive had received virtually no antihypertensive drug, 10·4 per cent of them had died from stroke; but among the non-hypertensives only 0·5 per cent had died from stroke, a 21-fold difference. It seems that hypertension is the major factor in causing stroke in Taiwan, whereas in IHD hyperlipidaemia is a major factor. The fact that blood cholesterol levels in Taiwan are generally low compared with those in the USA, while the prevalence of hypertension is the same, may explain the low prevalence of IHD compared with CVD in Taiwan.

Liu *et al.* (1973) performed 102 consecutive autopsies of stroke patients in Veterans General Hospital, Taipei, and compared them with an equal number of age-matched autopsies of non-stroke patients. The mean age of the former group was 54·7 years and of the latter 54·5. They found that in the stroke patients haemorrhage caused death in 71·4 per cent and infarction in 24·7 per cent. In the cerebral haemorrhage cases the cerebral arteries showed a more severe degree of atherosclerosis than did the coronary arteries. Those dying from cerebral infarction showed a greater degree of cerebral athero-sclerosis than those dying from haemorrhage. In the control group of 102 non-stroke autopsies 60·8 per cent were found not to have any athero-sclerosis of the coronary arteries, and 39·2 per cent were found to have a mild degree only.

Tseng *et al.* (1978) reported the serum cholesterol and triglyceride levels in subjects over 40 years of age in urban Taipei and rural San-chih county (1067 and 641 subjects respectively) and found the levels had not altered significantly in follow-up studies from 1973 to 1977. In subjects over the age of 40 the prevalence of hypercholesterolaemia, cholesterol over 6·47 mmol/l (250 mg/dl), was 5·5 per cent in Taipei, 4·3 per cent in San-chih. Hyper-triglyceridaemia, triglycerides over 2·26 mmol/l (200 mg/dl), was found in 13·5 per cent in Taipei and 7·7 per cent in San-chih.

The total mortality rate for CVD has risen from 48·8 per 100 000 in 1952 to 74·4 per 100 000 in 1975 (HSNHA, 1976). Among the ten leading causes of death in Taiwan CVD has climbed from fifth place in 1952 to first place in 1967, and has remained in that position.

Hypertension

Before the Second World War various reports on blood pressure in the Chinese on the mainland and in Taiwan had one point in common: Chinese were found to have much lower blood pressures than Westerners. After the last war Lin *et al.* (1958) made a survey in Taiwan of 9729 subjects over the age of 15 years in the city of Taipei. The mean values for systolic blood pres-sure in all age groups, and for diastolic pressure in age groups above 45 years, exceeded the values reported for Chinese before the war. The mean values for the blood pressure of 'Taiwanese' (descendants of the early Chinese settlers in Taiwan) were higher in all age groups than those of 'Mainlanders' (recent immigrants: the post-war influx of Chinese from the mainland). Hung (1961), studying this same group of 9729 subjects, suggested that 'diet, living pattern and stress brought about by social, economic and cultural transition' during and after the war in Taipei may have been a factor causing this difference. When the mean blood pressures of all these subjects were com-pared with Western mean blood pressures, the Western means were found to be higher in all the younger age groups, but over the age of 45 there was no significant difference between Western and Taiwan means. Tseng (1977) surveyed 6485 subjects over the age of 18 years in urban and agricultural areas of Taiwan. In the age groups below 45 years Tseng's figures were 3–5 mmHg higher than in the corresponding age groups in the series reported by Lin *et al.* (1958) and by Hung (1961). It appears that mean blood pressure levels for Chinese in Taiwan have gradually risen from the pre-war period until the present.

Criteria for the diagnosis of hypertension in a patient have not been uniform. The lack of comparable statistics for earlier periods and the present day hinder the assessment of any increased prevalence. In the following surveys the criteria were those recommended by WHO (1959), i.e. systolic pressure ⩾160 mmHg, or diastolic pressure ⩾95 mmHg. Tseng (1967) examined 14 304 subjects from a rural area of Taiwan and 5585 from a fishing (coastal) area; all were over 15 years of age. The total prevalence in the former was 11·4 per cent and in the latter 18·7 per cent. According to Tseng, when these figures are compared with data from a US national sample (National Center for Health Statistics, 1966) it appeared that the fishing population in Taiwan had a significantly higher prevalence of hypertension than the American sample; but there was no significant difference between the Taiwan agricultural population and the American sample. Chen *et al.* (1972) surveyed 5320 persons over the age of 15 in urban Taipei and found a prevalence of 10·7 per cent. Tseng (1977), in his survey of 6485 subjects in urban and rural areas, i.e. the Taiwan general population, found the total prevalence of hypertension was 14·1 per cent. Tsai *et al.* (1966) examined 1296 subjects of the Atayal aboriginal tribe in Taiwan over the age of 20 and found a total prevalence of 14·1 per cent. Whether the prevalence of hypertension has increased in Taiwan over the last three decades is not absolutely certain; but all the available evidence suggests that it has.

Other diseases

Peripheral vascular disease, intermittent claudication, etc.

Peripheral vascular disease, also intermittent claudication and non-embolic peripheral gangrene, i.e. arteriosclerotic gangrene, are very rare. When complicating diabetes, i.e. diabetic gangrene, it was found in 1·2 and 1·6 per cent of two different series of hospital admissions subsequently reported. Buerger's disease exists in Taiwan but is uncommon. Raynaud's phenomenon is very uncommon and Raynaud's disease is almost non-existent.

Deep vein thrombosis and pulmonary embolism

These are uncommon. Luh *et al.* (1967) reported 30 cases of pulmonary embolism from NTUH during eight years (1959–67). They observed that pulmonary embolism was rarely encountered postoperatively. The incidence of deep vein thrombosis and pulmonary embolism in Taiwan is much lower than in Caucasian races, even taking into consideration that the disease is diagnosed less often than it might be; there has been no obvious increase in incidence during the last three decades (Yang, S. P., 1978, personal communication).

Haemorrhoids

Haemorrhoids are very common in all groups in the community. Clinicians consider that the incidence has not changed. The age-adjusted prevalence rate has been found to be 18·77 per cent for males and 19·74 per cent for females (Lin, T. M., 1979, personal communication).

Varicose veins

Varicose veins are seen in all groups. Age-adjusted prevalence rates are 3·26 per cent for males and 10·21 per cent for females (Lin, T. M., 1979, personal communication).

Diabetes mellitus (DM)

There have been very few papers which have reported the incidence or prevalence of DM in Taiwan. Tsai (1970) studied the epidemiology of this disease among urban and rural people in northern Taiwan. In a total of 5863 subjects the prevalence of DM was 0·16 per cent for subjects below the age of 40, and 5·05 per cent for those aged 40 and over, with a total prevalence of 0·89 per cent. The mortality for DM, calculated from the Health Statistical Abstract, Taiwan Provincial Government (1957–66), has shown a steady marked increase. In 1957 it was 1·62 per 100 000 population; in 1961 it was 1·97; in 1966 it was 3·14.

Tsai (1975) also studied DM prevalence trends in two series of patients admitted to NTUH. The first series of 1552 DM patients during the years 1960–68 inclusive constituted 1·46 per cent of the admissions; the second series of 2104 DM patients during the years 1970–74 inclusive constituted 3·28 per cent of the admissions to the same units of the hospital. The two series of patients were derived from comparable groups of hospital patients; for instance patients aged 40 or more years averaged 91 per cent in the first series and 93 per cent in the second series. Markedly overweight patients had increased from 17 per cent in the first series to 33 per cent in the second series. This doubling of the proportion of middle-aged persons who were markedly obese during the 15 years 1960–74 and the increased number of DM patients reflected the growing affluence and dietary changes in the community. Juvenile diabetes (clinical onset before 15 years of age) is still uncommon among hospital patients; it constituted 0·8 per cent in Tsai's first series and 0·7 per cent in his second series. The author's impression, derived from clinical practice in Taiwan for 27 years, is that there has been a gradual increase in the incidence of diabetes mellitus.

Cholelithiasis

Formerly in Taiwan gallstones were predominantly pigment stones, but there has been a rapid increase in the incidence of cholesterol and mixed pigment stones during the last two decades. Chen *et al.* (1978) analysed 1318 cases of cholelithiasis among 35 741 general surgical cases operated upon in NTUH from 1950 to 1976 inclusive and 85 cases of cholelithiasis among 5141 autopsies from 1943 to 1977 inclusive. Before 1965 operations for gall-stones constituted only 1·45 per cent of the total general surgical cases. From 1965 to 1976 inclusive the percentage rose steadily to 8·79 per cent while the total annual number of surgical cases remained fairly constant. Autopsy cases over the age of 20 showed a 42 per cent increase in incidence of gallstone from 1966 to 1977 inclusive, compared with the earlier period 1943–65 inclusive.

Mixed pigment stones are rich in cholesterol, like cholesterol stones. The percentage of patients found to have mixed pigment stones, compared with the total number of gallstone patients, rose from 8·7 per cent in 1950–55 inclusive to 42·0 during 1976. Female preponderance, and increasing incidence with age, were found in both the surgical and the autopsy series. Increasing incidence with age was particularly true for cholesterol and mixed pigment stones. These trends are reported from NTUH, in which hospital two-thirds of the patients come from the Taipei area where the standard of living is higher than in the rest of the island.

Peptic ulcer (PU)

Sung *et al.* (1966) studied 1774 cases of PU in NTUH, diagnosed by positive x-ray findings and/or operation and biopsy, and found 79·4 per cent of cases were of duodenal ulcer (DU), 16·8 per cent were of gastric ulcer (GU), and in 3·8 per cent there were both gastric and duodenal ulcers present (GDU). The ratio of DU to GU was 4·7 : 1. Haematemesis occurred in 13·1 per cent of DU and 16·2 per cent of GDU, melaena occurred in 22·0 per cent of DU and 19·1 per cent of GDU. Perforation occurred in 16·6 per cent of DU and 32·4 per cent of GDU. Pyloric stenosis from chronic fibrosis around an ulcer occurred in 3·1 per cent of DU and 8·8 per cent of GDU.

The prevalence of PU in the population was indicated by Sung *et al.* (1976) in a sample mass survey of urban and rural populations in southern Taiwan. All subjects were government employees (non-labouring class); 5357 from Taiwan City and 3400 from Taiwan County, comprising a total of 8757. Routine barium meal ingestion with x-ray films taken in six different positions were followed by further study in hospital in all suspected cases. They found the prevalence of PU to be 6·01 per cent of the total number of subjects in city dwellers and 7·23 per cent in country dwellers; the prevalence of DU was 5·2 per cent and 6·7 per cent respectively. There has been no evidence of any increase of this disease during the last three decades.

Appendicitis

Admissions for acute appendicitis, about 20 per cent of all surgical emergencies admitted to NTUH during the period 1966–77, have not changed. The yearly death rates for acute appendicitis between 1952 and 1977 have fallen from about 8·5 to 4·7 per 100 000 of the population (HSNHA, 1976 and earlier years). Though more common than on the mainland the incidence of this disease has probably not altered in Taiwan in recent years.

Ulcerative colitis

The disease is identical with that in the West, but is very uncommon. From 1967 to 1976 inclusive among 4990 endoscopically examined patients in the gastroenterology section of internal medicine in NTUH 52 new cases (1·04 per cent) of ulcerative colitis were found (Sung, J. L., 1978, personal communication). There is no evidence that the incidence is increasing.

Crohn's disease

This disease is rare. In NTUH three cases have been diagnosed during the last ten years, with six suspected cases. There is no evidence that the incidence is increasing.

Diverticulosis of the colon

The incidence is very low, and does not seem to be increasing. Wang and Chou (1978) found 24 cases of diverticulosis in 1280 consecutive barium enemata at the Tri-Service General Hospital, i.e. in 1·9 per cent of cases. Clinicians and radiologists agree that most diverticula are found in the caecum and ascending colon and very few in the descending colon and pelvic colon. The aetiology of the disease is therefore thought to be different in Taiwan compared with that in Western countries.

Hiatus hernia

Symptomless, mild hiatus hernia found at x-ray examination is not uncommon. In routine barium meal examinations performed during the course of complete physical examinations (Yu, J. Y., 1979, personal communication) it was found approximately once in 50 cases (2 per cent). On the other hand in a radiological survey of 1367 government employees (non-labouring) in Kaohsiung City (Sung *et al.*, 1974) hiatus hernia was found in only 0·2 per cent of cases. Hiatus hernia producing symptoms is very rare. The incidence does not appear to be increasing.

Irritable colon

All clinicians agree that this disease is very common in Taiwan. There is no evidence that the incidence has increased.

Carcinoma of the colon and rectum

The incidence of colorectal carcinoma (CRC) in Taiwan is not as high as in Western countries, but it is gradually increasing. Hsu (1978) studies 1304 cases of carcinoma of the stomach and 1044 cases of CRC admitted to NTUH from 1954 to 1976 inclusive. While the annual incidence for both types of neoplasm rose with the increasing total annual admissions to the hospital, the rise in the incidence of CRC was more rapid than that of carcinoma of the stomach. Age-adjusted death rates for carcinoma of the colon and for carcinoma of the stomach between 1945 and 1973 show a progressive rise in the death rate for the former compared with the latter which has remained steady (Lin *et al.*, 1977).

Dental caries (DC)

Sugar consumption in Taiwan is increasing, especially among young people and in the rural areas; in the form of toffee it has become more popular. Eating between meals is more common. Hong *et al.*, (1979) surveyed 23 972 people of both sexes, in approximately equal number, randomly sampled over the whole island based on WHO recommendations. Three ethnic groups were studied: 'Taiwanese' (i.e. descendants of the early Chinese settlers in Taiwan), 'Mainlanders' (i.e. Chinese who came to Taiwan in the post-war influx), and aboriginals. For permanent teeth, Taiwanese over the age of 35 had double the DC prevalence rate of mainlanders and aboriginals of the same age group. Under the age of 20 the prevalence was about the same in the three groups. This suggests that the mainlanders and aboriginals had sustained a simple, low sugar diet habit for many years compared with the Taiwanese. The increased sugar consumption and between-meals eating of the youth of all three groups during the last two decades had resulted, however, in equal prevalence of DC. For deciduous teeth the prevalence was uniformly high, about 7 carious teeth per child at the age of 7 years.

Multiple sclerosis (MS)

This is rare in the Chinese race. Hung *et al.* (1976), while reviewing the very few reports of this disease from the mainland of China, reported 25 cases of

MS found in Taiwan in 20 years of neurological practice. There were two autopsies. The prevalence in northern Taiwan was estimated to be 0·8 per 100 000 population. Unless the disease is underdiagnosed it appears that MS is uncommon in Taiwan.

Pernicious anaemia (PA)

PA is very rare in the Chinese race. In Taiwan Liu *et al.* (1961) reported 11 cases of PA during the previous 11 years. Wang *et al.* (1978) reported 39 patients with megaloblastic anaemia seen at the Haematology Laboratory, NTUH, from 1950 until 1977. Twenty-nine of these patients were classical cases of PA (the 11 cases reported earlier were included in this group of 29). These workers see approximately one new case of PA a year which is a higher incidence than was found on the mainland before the Second World War (see under China, page 366).

Paget's disease of bone

This is excessively rare in the Chinese race. Snapper (1965) saw only one case in Peiping (Peking) in 20 years. It has never been reported in Taiwan.

CHINA MAINLAND

The land and the people

China embraces an enormous area. The United Nations estimate of the population for 1974 was 827 million. Whereas Taiwan is a reflection of ethnic Chinese mainly from south-east China, the people on the mainland include a number of different ethnic groups. In 1953 the percentage distribution of the population was Han 94, Mongolian 0·3, Tibetan 0·5, Manchu 0·4, Tribal 3·6, others 1·2 (Whitaker, 1978). Lin (1939) observed: 'Apart from the cultural unity which binds the Chinese people as a nation the southern Chinese differ probably as much from the northerners in temperament, physique and habits as the Mediterraneans differ from Nordic peoples in Europe.' The northern Chinese are tall, stable, phlegmatic and wheat-eating, the southern are lighter in build, enterprising, volatile and rice-eating. However, Latourette (1945) wrote: 'In spite of all the surviving variations in race the great mass of the Chinese people is remarkably homogeneous in physical appearance and culture.'

Social trends

When the author was in Fukien (1940–51) the majority of the people were farming, fishing and employed in physical labour. In the cities the people were shopkeepers and traders. There was hardly any industrialization. The tempo of life was slow, although domestic and economic stress was as prevalent as in any Chinese society at any time.

The author has not been able to obtain information about social changes covering the last 30 years, though these must have been very great. It can be assumed there has been a redistribution of wealth and the supply of food has been evenly distributed. China is essentially an agricultural and pastoral country; 80 per cent of the population are agricultural. The mineral wealth of the country is very great. If by 'westernization' is meant industrialization, with a trend towards the pattern of life in Western countries, then there is some degree of westernization. But compared with the degree of westernization attained in Taiwan that on the mainland of China is far less.

In 1966 all major educational institutions closed down at the start of the Cultural Revolution; a beginning was made in 1970 to enrol new students on a limited basis (Whitaker, 1978). All Chinese medical journals ceased publication for several years (Cheng, 1973). It has therefore been difficult to obtain information about recent disease trends on the mainland of China.

Dietary trends

Snapper (1965) of PUMC quoted an analysis by Guy and Yeh of Peiping (Peking) diets in 1938. There was a whole-cereal/legume/vegetable diet for poorer people and a milled-cereal/meat/vegetable diet for the richer people. The former diet provided 8·8 MJ (2100 kcals) per day, with 88 g protein, 47 g vegetable fat, 331 g carbohydrate. This 'poor' Peiping diet was found to provide at most calcium 0·4 g/d. The diet contained little or no vitamin D; rural workers in north China relied on the summer sunshine on their skins to supply their vitamin D, but for city dwellers this was insufficient. Hence the high incidence of osteomalacia in women; in 10 years 120 cases were admitted into PUMC. Peiping diets were also insufficient in vitamins A and C; symptoms of avitaminosis A and C were frequently seen. The diet of the poor people contained a small portion of salted turnips as a relish; Snapper did not mention the addition of salt to other foods.

It has been difficult to obtain clear knowledge of the nutritional situation on the China mainland during the last three decades. On a recent visit Cheng (1973) observed that the people of China were eating more and better food and that food was plentiful and available at very low cost. Bernard (1958) after a visit to China wrote: 'The food situation, at least in the provinces, appeared good; the workers and young children who can be seen everywhere half-naked and so numerous, appear in excellent health and well-fed.' The Food and Agriculture Organization of the United Nations (1977) published data on food supplies for China for 1961–74. This reported that the daily energy per caput had risen from 8·1 MJ (1900 kcals) in 1961 to 10·0 MJ (2300 kcals) in 1974. Total protein has increased from 53g/d to 63g/d; the animal protein has hardly changed, the increase was vegetable protein. According to Snapper (1965) the mainly vegetarian Chinese diet contains only small amounts of cholesterol but considerable quantities of unsaturated fatty acids.

Disease trends

Ischaemic heart disease (IHD)

Before the Second World War the rarity of arteriosclerosis in north China was shown by the large number of middle-aged patients dying from various diseases who were found to have hardly any arteriosclerosis at autopsy. 'Even in diabetes mellitus extensive arteriosclerosis must be infrequent because diabetic gangrene is as rare as senile gangrene'; angina of effort and coronary thrombosis also were rarely encountered (Snapper, 1965). Tung *et al.* (1958) when reviewing 3400 Chinese patients in Shanghai with cardiovascular disease, suggested that the low prevalence of clinical atherosclerosis in China was related to low serum cholesterol levels, due largely to the small amount of saturated animal fat in the Chinese diet.

IHD, formerly a rarity, has become recently quite common in China (Cheng, 1973). During a ward round in the former PUMC Cheng saw five patients with IHD in a ward of 40 patients. A routine ECG survey of workers over the age of 50 years in a Shanghai factory revealed 8 per cent had definite IHD and another 8 per cent had suspected IHD. All available evidence suggests that IHD is increasing.

Hypertension

Snapper (1965) quotes Tung who, before the Second World War, analysed the blood pressures of 123 northern Chinese males, and found the average pressure to be 102/64 for the age group 15–19 years, and 113/73 for the age group 50–53 years. Snapper stated that the symptoms of hypertension were sometimes present at blood pressures much lower than in the West. He observed that hypertensive patients did not usually die from coronary thrombosis but from heart failure or cerebral haemorrhage. More recently Cheng (1973) observed that, although aggressive treatment with antihypertensive drugs had lowered the frequency of renal complications in hypertension, yet hypertension still took its toll through cerebral haemorrhage.

Diabetes mellitus

Between 1921 and 1935 347 cases were studied in PUMC. Snapper (1965) considered diabetes to be fairly common among Chinese.

Deep vein thrombosis and pulmonary embolism

Snapper (1965) observed that these diseases were hardly ever encountered. Surgeons and gynaecologists operated without fear of a complicating thrombophlebitis or a fatal pulmonary embolism.

Cholelithiasis

Snapper (1965) reported that gallstones were rare in north China. Females and males were affected equally, whereas in the Western nations the ratio was 5:1. The average serum cholesterol levels were significantly lower than among Western people; this was to be expected in a population living mainly on a vegetarian diet. In Peiping (Peking) gallstones were a rare find in the autopsy room. If they were found they were not the white, yellowish or brown cholesterol stones found in the West, but black, containing calcium bilirubinate. These stones were usually radio-opaque.

Pernicious anaemia (PA)

Macrocytic nutritional anaemia was fairly common in China, but PA was rare. Williams (1932) reported one case; and Snapper (1965) with wide clinical experience in PUMC found only six patients between 1921 and 1941 in which the diagnosis of PA was justified.

Paget's disease of bone

As already stated this disease is exceedingly rare in the Chinese. Snapper (1965) saw one case: it affected the femur alone. He stated that this disease was rare in all oriental countries.

Conclusion

During the author's stay on the mainland of China (1940–51) many diseases, common in the West, were noted to be uncommon or rare. These were hypertension, obesity, diabetes, ischaemic heart disease, deep vein thrombosis and pulmonary embolism, peripheral vascular disease, gallstones and cholecystitis, diverticulosis of the colon. During his stay in Taiwan (1952–79) he noted that some of these diseases were becoming more common: hypertension, obesity, diabetes, ischaemic heart disease, gallstones and cholecystitis, also appendicitis.

Diseases which have remained rare both in mainland China and in Taiwan are deep vein thrombosis and pulmonary embolism, peripheral vascular disease, diverticulosis of the colon, ulcerative colitis, Crohn's disease, hiatus hernia, Paget's disease of bone, pernicious anaemia, multiple sclerosis.

Diseases which have remained common on the mainland and in Taiwan are cerebral vascular disease (more common in Taiwan), duodenal ulcer, varicose veins, haemorrhoids, irritable colon, ankylosing spondylitis, thyrotoxicosis (not uncommon), rheumatoid arthritis (not uncommon).

Acknowledgements

The author is grateful to the following persons for their generous assistance with the writing of this chapter: Professors Sze-piau Yang, Wen-ping Tseng, Tsu-pei Hung, Po-chao Huang, Ta-cheng Tang, Juei-low Sung, Tong-ming Lin, Jui-san Chen, Shu-chien Hsu, Chen-hui Liu, Yu-ching Hong, Teh-lu

Wu, Shih-hsien Tsai, Chiung-lin Chen, Juey-yun Yu, Yi-shiong Hang of NTUH; Dr. Ching-hwa Chiu of JCRR; Miss Hung-mei Lin for many hours of typewriting.

References

Bernard, J. (1958). Blood diseases in China (News and views). *Blood (Journal of Haematology)*, **14**, 605–606

Chen, C. M., Tseng, W. P., Tseng, Y. Z., Huang, P. T., Lin, C. C., Wang, Y. T. and Yang, H. C. (1972). Prevalence of heart disease in Taipei urban population. *Fifth Asian Pacific Congress of Cardiology, Free communication,* 271. Singapore Cardiac Society, Singapore.

Chen, J. S., Ho, K. J. and Hsu, S. C. (1978). Lipid metabolism from the studies of gallstones and bile in Taiwan for the last 25 years. *Symposium on Lipid and Lipoprotein,* 4–5. Imperial Chemical Industries, Taipei, Taiwan

Chen, M. L. (1975). Recent increments in physical development and nutrition of adolescents in Taiwan. *Journal of the Formosan Medical Association,* **74**, 67–69 (in Chinese)

Cheng, T. O. (1973). A view of modern Chinese medicine. *Annals of Internal Medicine,* **78**, 285–290

Chiu, C. H. (1976). Food supply and nutrition requirement in Taiwan. *Journal of the Chinese Nutrition Society,* **1**, 93–101

Crowley, L. V., Godber, J. T., Consolazio, C. F., Goldstein, D. R., Smith, E. P., Lewis, O. H., Ryer, R. R. and Pollack, H. (1956). Studies on nutrition in the Far East. IV. Mess practices in the Chinese Nationalist Army and the field test of a proposed enriched ration. *Metabolism,* **5**, 245

Food and Agriculture Organization of the United Nations, Rome (1977). Food Balance Sheets, China

Health Statistical Abstract, Taiwan Province (1957–66). Department of Health, Taiwan Provincial Government

Health Statistics, National Health Administration (1976). Taiwan, Republic of China

Hong, Y. C., Chang, C. K., Duh, F. G. and Knutson, J. W. (1979). Report on Taiwan Dental Survey, personal communication

Hsu, S. C. (1978). Follow-up study of colorectal cancer patients surviving more than ten years after surgery at the National Taiwan University Hospital. *Abstract, VIIIth Biennial Congress of the International Society of University Colon and Rectal Surgeons,* 59. Kyoto, Japan

Huang, P. C., Chen, S. H. and Chang, Y. F. (1976). Food consumption survey in San-Chih County, Taipei Prefecture. *Journal of the Chinese Nutrition Society,* **1**, 68–76

Huang, P. C., Wei, H. N. and Hung, M. H. (1973). Food consumption survey in Yen-ping District, Taipei City. *Journal of the Formosan Medical Association,* **72**, 427–433

Huang, P. J., Chen, J. S., Hsu, C. J., Chen, C. M. and Wu, T. L. (1978). Lipid abnormalities in Chinese with angiographically proved coronary artery disease. *Symposium on Lipid and Lipoprotein*, 6–15. Imperial Chemical Industries, Taipei, Taiwan

Hung, T. P. (1961). A study on the prevalence of elevated blood-pressure among urban Chinese in Taiwan. *Japanese Circulation Journal*, **25**, 1084–1100

Hung, T. P., Landsborough, D. and Hsi, M. S. (1976). Multiple sclerosis among Chinese in Taiwan. *Journal of the Neurological Sciences*, **27**, 459–484

Latourette, K. S. (1945). *The Chinese, their history and culture*, third edition revised, 499. Macmillan, New York

Lee, N. Y., Huang, S. C. and Huang, P. C. (1976). Study on dietary intakes of total lipids, fatty acids, cholesterol and vitamin E in Taiwan. *Journal of the Chinese Nutrition Society*, **1**, 82–91

Lin, T. M., Chang, L. C. and Chen, K. P. (1977). A statistical analysis on mortality of malignant neoplasms in Taiwan. *Journal of the Formosan Medical Association*, **76**, 656–668

Lin, T. Y., Hung, T. P., Chen, C. M., Hsu, T. C. and Chen, K. P. (1958). A study of normal and elevated blood pressures in a Chinese urban population in Taiwan (Formosa). *Clinical Science*, **18**, 301–312

Lin, Y. T. (1939). *My Country and My People*, 16. Heinemann, London

Liu, C. H., Lee., T. K., Wang, C. H., Yang, T. H., Shih, T. C., Chen, H. K. and Tsai, W. J. (1961). Pernicious anemia and related megaloblastic anemias in Taiwan. *Journal of the Formosan Medical Association*, **60**, 739–769

Liu, H. C., Chu, B. Y., Chiang, B. N. and Wang, S. P. (1973). Stroke, a clinico-pathological study. *Chinese Medical Journal, Republic of China*, **20**, 170–177

Luh, K. T., Lin, Y. W. and Yang, S. P. (1967). Pulmonary embolism and pulmonary infarction. *Journal of the Formosan Medical Association*, **66**, 410–424

National Center for Health Statistics (1966). Hypertension and hypertensive heart disease in adults, United States, 1960–62. Vital and Health Statistics. *P.H.S. Pub. No. 1000, Series 11, No. 13*. US Public Health Service, Washington, DC

National Health Administration and National Taiwan University Hospital (1975). *Joint Study Report*

Snapper, I. (1965). *Chinese lessons to Western Medicine*, second edition. Grune and Stratton, New York and London

Sung, J. L., Wang, T. H., Chen, C. S., Lin, P. H. and Chen, C. H. (1976). Epidemiological study on peptic ulcer and gastric cancer in the Chinese. *Journal of the Formosan Medical Association*, **75**, 116–119

Sung, J. L., Wang, T. H., Lu, T. H., Wu, S. C., Hsu, T. W. and Lee, T. H. (1974). Epidemiological study on peptic ulcer and gastric cancer in the Chinese. *Rendiconti di Gastroenterologia*, **6**, 111–115

Sung, J. L., Yang, T. H., Yu, J. Y., Hsu, S. C., Wang, C. H. and Huang, Y. C.

(1966). 1774 cases of peptic ulcer. *Journal of the Formosan Medical Association,* **65**, 436–446

Tsai, H. C., Tseng, W. P., Yen, T. S., Cheng, J. T., Wang, L. T., Hsieh, Y. Y., Wu, T. L. and Chen, J. S. (1966). Coronary heart disease and hypertension in Taiwan aborigines. *American Journal of Epidemiology,* **86**, 253–263

Tsai, S. H. (1970). Epidemiology of diabetes mellitus in Taiwan. Proceedings of a symposium, Diabetes Mellitus in Asia, *Excerpta Medica International Congress Series No. 221*

Tsai, S. H. (1975). Clinical features of diabetes mellitus in Taiwan. Proceedings of the Second Symposium, Diabetes Mellitus in Asia, *Excerpta Medica International Congress Series No. 390*

Tseng, W. P. (1967). Blood pressure and hypertension in an agricultural and a fishing population in Taiwan. *American Journal of Epidemiology,* **86**, 513–525

Tseng, W. P. (1977). Epidemiological study of stroke in Taiwan. Paper presented at International Congress on Hypertension, Bombay, India

Tseng, W. P. (1978a). Epidemiological study of hypertension and stroke in Taiwan. Paper presented at International Symposium on Prophylactic Approach to Hypertensive Diseases, Matsue, Japan

Tseng, W. P. (1978b). Epidemiology of stroke in Taiwan. *Journal of the Formosan Medical Association,* **77**, 727–728 (in Chinese)

Tseng, W. P., Chen, J. S., Hsu, C. J. and Chen, C. M. (1978). Lipid study in Taipei urban and San-chih rural populations. *Symposium on Lipid and Lipoprotein,* 1–3. Imperial Chemical Industries, Taipei, Taiwan

Tung, C. L., Wu, K. H. and Wang, C. Y. (1958). The relative incidence of atherosclerotic heart disease in east China and its relationship to cholesterol. *Chinese Medical Journal,* **77**, 596–602

Wang, C. H. and Chou, C. C. (1978). Diverticular disease of the colon in Taiwan. *Abstract, VIIth Biennial Congress of International Society of University Colon and Rectal Surgeons,* Kyoto, Japan

Wang, C. H., Shen, M. C. and Liu, C. H. (1978). Megaloblastic anemia. *Transactions of the Hematological Society of the Republic of China,* 96–101

Whitacker's Almanac (1978). 110th Annual Volume, 835–839. London

Williams, T. H. (1932). Pernicious anemia in Szechwan. *Chinese Medical Journal,* **46**, 673–675

World Health Organization (1959). *Hypertension and Coronary Heart Disease: Classification and Criteria for Epidemiological Studies.* Technical Report Series, No. 168. WHO, Geneva

World Health Organization (1973). Community control of stroke and hypertension. Report of a WHO meeting. Part 1. Geneva

Part VII

Regression of certain Western diseases

22

Diabetes mellitus

James Anderson

Introduction

Diabetes mellitus is rapidly emerging as a major health problem in most Western countries. In the United States, for example, an estimated 5 per cent of the population have diabetes and it is considered to be the third-ranked cause of death from disease (Anonymous, 1975). While the prevalence of ischaemic heart disease is declining (Walker, 1977), diabetes is on the increase (Anonymous, 1975). Dietary factors may be contributing to this increase in the prevalence of diabetes. Between 1880 and 1976, the intake of cereal fibres has declined by 90 per cent in the United States (Scala, 1975). Two recent dietary trends in the United States are the growing popularity of fast-food restaurants and the increasing use of highly processed foods (Page and Friend, 1978); both trends reduce dietary fibre intake. These dietary changes are consistent with the dietary fibre hypothesis of the aetiology of diabetes formulated by Trowell (Trowell, 1975). Epidemiological studies (Tulloch, 1962; Tsuji and Wada, 1971; West and Kalbfleisch, 1971; Baba *et al.*, 1976) document that the prevalence of diabetes is much lower in primitive villagers than in urban residents of big industrialized areas. Usually the intake of unrefined carbohydrate and dietary fibre by primitive people is quite high, while urban residents consume diets which are low in fibre, lower in carbohydrate and much higher in fat. These studies suggest that fibre-depleted diets may contribute to the high prevalence of diabetes in certain societies.

The importance of the diet in the management of diabetes has been recognized for many centuries. Because diabetes is characterized by hyperglycaemia and glycosuria, a restriction of dietary carbohydrate seemed logical. In the three decades before the discovery of insulin, very high fat and very low carbohydrate diets were used to treat persons with diabetes (Wood and Bierman, 1972). After insulin became available, some physicians liberalized the intake of carbohydrate, but carbohydrate restriction remained the mainstay of the diet for the next half a century. Consequently most persons with diabetes in Western countries have been treated with high fat diets which were restricted in simple and complex carbohydrate and were very low in dietary fibre. Despite impressive evidence that high fat diets impaired

373

glucose metabolism (Himsworth, 1933–34) and reports (Rabinowitch, 1935; Singh, 1955) that high carbohydrate, low fat diets reduced insulin requirements, carbohydrate restriction has perseverated as the principal feature of diets for persons with diabetes.

In the last decade the role of carbohydrate restriction has been reassessed and in 1972, the American Diabetes Association recommended that the carbohydrate intake of persons with diabetes could be liberalized (Bierman *et al.*, 1971). In 1976, two groups (Jenkins *et al.*, 1976; Kiehm, *et al.*, 1976) reported that a generous intake of dietary fibre might be beneficial for persons with diabetes. Recent studies (Anderson, 1977a, b, 1979; Anderson and Ward, 1978) have reconfirmed that high carbohydrate, low fat diets are beneficial for persons with diabetes. This emerging evidence has led to the suggestion that a high carbohydrate diet containing generous quantities of dietary fibre may be a prudent diet for most persons with diabetes mellitus (West, 1975; Anderson and Ward, 1978).

Traditional diabetic diets

The diets widely used in most Western countries for treating diabetes are designed to maintain the status quo. Excluding weight-reducing diets used for obesity, traditional diabetic diets are directed at promoting a consistent intake of nutrients from day to day; the distribution of nutrients throughout each day should be consistent. Thus, with constant diets and predictable activity levels, most patients are maintained on fixed insulin doses. There is no evidence that weight-maintaining traditional diabetic diets lead to improved glucose metabolism or reduced insulin requirements in lean individuals. The impact of a traditional diet on five non-insulin treated patients with diabetes was carefully documented by Kuhl (Kuhl, 1956). These diets provided 39 per cent of energy as carbohydrate, 44 per cent fat and 17 per cent protein (Fig. 22.1). When these individuals were fed weight-maintaining diets for 18–30 days, there were no significant changes in blood glucose concentrations. Other investigators (Strouse and Soskin, 1932; Hallgren and Svanborg, 1962; Stone and Connor, 1963) have also documented that moderate changes in the quantities of carbohydrate or fat intake do not alter insulin requirements. We have documented that weight-maintaining conventional diabetic diets do not alter insulin doses in lean patients hospitalized for up to three months (Anderson, J. W., unpublished observations).

Unfortunately, traditional diabetic diets may have substantial disadvantages for persons with diabetes. The prevalence of ischaemic heart disease is significantly higher in diabetic than in non-diabetic individuals (Santen *et al.*, 1972). Atherosclerotic cardiovascular disease accounts for approximately three-quarters of all deaths in persons with the maturity-onset (insulin-independent) type of diabetes (Bradley, 1971). Most persons with diabetes have been encouraged to eat more saturated fat and cholesterol than their non-diabetic peers eat. This generous intake of saturated fat and cholesterol

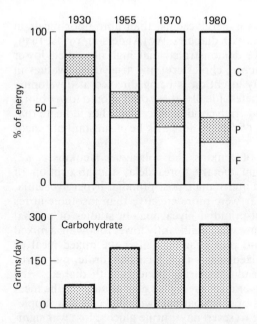

Fig. 22.1 Changing nutrient content of diabetic diets. The carbohydrate (C), protein (P) and fat (F) content are expressed as percentage of energy in top panel. The total available carbohydrate from a 2000 kilocalorie diet is presented in lower panel. The 1980 diet is the 'Prudent Diabetic Diet' discussed in text

may aggravate the risk for atherosclerotic cardiovascular diseases. Traditional diabetic diets are also low in dietary fibre. This may further contribute to the risk for vascular disease (Trowell, 1972; Morris *et al.*, 1977). Disturbances of cholesterol and triglyceride metabolism are common in persons with diabetes (Chase and Glasgow, 1976; Bennion and Grundy, 1977). Restrictions of cholesterol and saturated fat intakes are widely used to treat hypercholesterolaemia. Furthermore, the same restrictions have been recommended as a prudent diet for persons at risk for ischaemic heart disease (Anonymous, 1972). Regrettably, the traditional diabetic diets used widely for the last 50 years may have fostered unhealthy levels of serum cholesterol and increased the frequency of vascular disease.

Effects of fibre

High fibre diets have favourable effects on glucose and lipid metabolism. Walker and colleagues (Walker *et al.*, 1970) pointed out that high fibre diets were associated with lower fasting blood glucose values and less hyperglycaemia after oral glucose loads than values in individuals on low fibre diets. Jenkins and colleagues (Jenkins *et al.*, 1976, 1978a) documented that fibre rich meals were followed by less hyperglycaemia than fibre poor meals in normal individuals and in patients with diabetes. We (Anderson, 1977a, 1979; Anderson and Ward, 1978) have demonstrated that high fibre diets lower insulin requirements, blood glucose, cholesterol and triglyceride values in patients with diabetes. Currently attention is being directed at developing better diets for persons with diabetes. Ideally, these diets should lower blood levels of glucose, cholesterol and triglycerides. Recent studies indicate that the intake of generous quantities of dietary fibre may be of substantial benefit in achieving these aims.

The pioneering experiments of Jenkins and colleagues (Jenkins *et al.*, 1977a, 1978a) demonstrated that dietary fibres delay the absorption of glucose from the small intestine and reduce post-prandial hyperglycaemia. Water-soluble fibres such as guar were more effective than insoluble fibres such as bran in decreasing post-prandial glycaemia. In studies of normal individuals, the glycaemic response was significantly lower following a mixed meal plus guar or a glucose load plus guar than after the mixed meal or glucose alone. When similar mixed meals (106 g carbohydrate, 9·6 g protein, 17·8 g fat) were fed to insulin-requiring patients with diabetes, the glucose rise was significantly lower after meal plus guar than after the meal alone (Fig. 22.2). When the diets of seven patients with diabetes was supplemented with 25 g of guar for five to seven days, urine glucose loss was significantly lower (Fig. 22.3) than values on the control diets. Miranda and Horwitz (1978) also documented that high fibre diets were associated with significantly less hyperglycaemia than were low fibre diets. Their low fibre diets contained approximately 16 g of dietary fibre per day, while their high fibre diets provided approximately 48 g of dietary fibre per day (calculated from values provided by Anderson *et al.*, 1978). When eight insulin-treated patients with diabetes were given low fibre or high fibre diets for 10 days in a random sequence, post-prandial glucose values were significantly lower on the high fibre diets.

Thus, in short-term studies, when dietary fibre is ingested with carbohydrate the resulting glucose and insulin rises are significantly lower than when an equivalent carbohydrate load is ingested without fibre (Jenkins *et al.*, 1976, 1977a, 1978a; Haber *et al.*, 1977; Monnier *et al.*, 1978). The mechanisms responsible for these changes have not been delineated. Soluble fibres such as guar may form gels in the small intestine and delay the absorption of carbohydrate. The insoluble fibres do not appear to form gels and their influence on glucose absorption has not been determined (Anderson and Chen, 1979). Dietary fibres appear to enhance tissue sensitivity to insulin since lower glucose values are observed with lower plasma insulin levels. The mechanisms responsible for this apparent increase in sensitivity to insulin are not clear.

In long term studies (Jenkins *et al.*, 1978b, 1979) insulin doses were significantly lower on guar-supplemented diets than on control diets. These patients with diabetes were provided an average of 18 g of guar daily as guar crispbread. On control diets the insulin doses of six patients averaged 46 ± 6 units per day; after eight weeks on guar crispbread, insulin doses

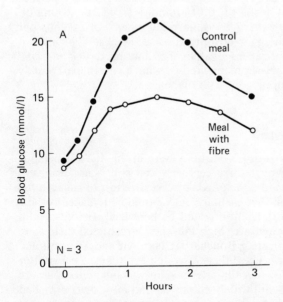

Fig. 22.2 Effects of fibre on post-prandial glucose values. These studies (Jenkins *et al.*, 1976) are described in text

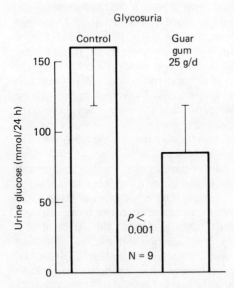

Fig. 22.3 Glycosuria of diabetic patients on control and guar-supplemented diets. Patients received control and guar-supplemented diets for five days in an alternating sequence (Jenkins *et al.*, 1977b)

averaged 36 ± 5 units per day ($P < 0.05$). During this eight-week period, urine glucose excretion fell from 61 to 17 mmol/l (1098 to 306 mg/dl, $P < 0.05$). Five patients with average insulin requirements of 41 units per day on control diets took the guar crispbread for 20 weeks. Their insulin doses decreased progressively to average values of 28 units per day ($P < 0.02$). These studies indicate that fibre-supplemented diets have a useful part to play in the dietary management of persons with diabetes.

High carbohydrate diets

The controversy over the quantity of carbohydrate in the diet for persons with diabetes has raged for over three centuries and still is not resolved. Recognizing that diabetes was characterized by excessive loss of sugar in the urine, some early workers felt that carbohydrate should be replaced; others reasoned that carbohydrate restriction would be beneficial. Before insulin became available, low carbohydrate, high fat, energy-restricted diets were championed by most authorities (e.g. Bouchardat, Naunyn, and Allen, quoted by Wood and Bierman, 1972). These diets provided less than 10 per cent of energy as carbohydrate. In the decade after insulin was introduced, severe carbohydrate restriction was still widely employed and most diets provided only 13–18 per cent of energy as carbohydrate (Fig. 22.1). This conventional wisdom that severe carbohydrate restriction was essential in treating diabetes, however, was attacked from several sides. Prominent clinicians (Sansum *et al.*, 1926; Gibson, 1929; Richardson, 1929; Geyelin, 1935; Rabinowitch, 1935) reported that their patients could tolerate diets containing 40–60 per cent of energy as carbohydrate. In a randomized study, Rabinowitch (1935) documented that high carbohydrate (59 per cent of energy) diets were accompanied by reductions in insulin doses in 50 patients over a five-year period, whereas conventional diets (23 per cent carbohydrate, 66 per cent fat) did not alter insulin doses in the other 50 patients. These high carbohydrate diets were accompanied by better diabetic control and lower serum cholesterol values than were the conventional diets. However, the high carbohydrate diets were consistently lower in calories and the role that weight loss may have played in the reductions in insulin doses in these patients cannot be evaluated.

In a remarkable study, Ellis (1934) administered glucose orally and insulin subcutaneously at hourly intervals to insulin-requiring patients and measured blood glucose values at 1- or 2-hour intervals. These patients tolerated up to 600 g of glucose daily without significant alterations in the blood glucose concentrations or insulin doses. Card (1938) evaluated the effect of low carbohydrate (19 per cent of energy from carbohydrate) and moderate carbohydrate (36 per cent) diets on nine insulin-treated patients. In the first period of approximately seven days' duration their carbohydrate intake averaged 100 g per day, whereas during the second period of approximately 21 days' duration their carbohydrate intake averaged 194 g per day. Insulin doses and blood glucose values were similar on the two diets. When the carbohydrate intake was increased, some patients transiently had more glycosuria (as noted previously by Woodyatt, 1924) but average urine glucose values on the moderate carbohydrate diets (3600 mmol or 20 g/d) were fairly similar to values on the low carbohydrate diets (2340 mmol or 13 g/d). These two studies coupled with other clinical observations (Sansum *et al.*, 1926; Gibson, 1929; Richardson, 1929; Geyelin, 1935; Rabinowitch, 1935) clearly indicated that most patients with diabetes can tolerate moderate to large amounts of carbohydrate without worsening of their diabetic control or increases in their insulin requirements.

As concern about the detrimental effects of carbohydrate intake have diminished, there has been a gradual increase in the amount of carbohydrate provided for patients with diabetes. By 1955, many diets in the United States provided about 40 per cent of energy as carbohydrate (Kuhl, 1956; Daughaday, 1958). By 1970 this had increased to approximately 45 per cent (Fig. 22.1). Several investigators (Bierman and Nelson, 1975; West, 1975, 1976; Anderson and Ward, 1978) have suggested that a prudent diet should be restricted in animal fat and cholesterol to provide about 55 per cent of energy from carbohydrate. This is consistent with the guidelines provided by the American Diabetes Association (Anonymous, 1977). This diet would also provide a moderate amount (approximately 40 g/d) of dietary fibre. Most clinicians in North America (Bierman and Nelson, 1975; West, 1975, 1976) and Great Britain (Truswell *et al.*, 1975) no longer restrict carbohydrate intake for persons with diabetes. However, in Great Britain, Australia, and South Africa some investigators (Turtle, 1970; Jackson and Kalk, 1972; Wall *et al.*, 1973; Doar *et al.*, 1975; Hadden *et al.*, 1975; Perkins *et al.*, 1977) still maintain that carbohydrate restriction (30–40 per cent of energy from carbohydrate) is the mainstay in the dietary management of diabetes.

The prudent diet recommended for Western people with diabetes (Fig. 22.1) still has less carbohydrate and dietary fibre than diets conventionally used in India, Japan and tropical countries (Tulloch, 1962; Tsuji and Wada, 1971; Baba *et al.*, 1976). In Western countries the intake of animal fat and cholesterol is considerably higher than that usually eaten in India, Japan and tropical countries. Available evidence indicates that the prevalence of ischaemic heart disease is lower in patients with diabetes in Japan, India and the West Indies (Tulloch, 1962; Tsuji and Wada, 1971; Baba *et al.*, 1976; Bierman and Nelson, 1975; West, 1975). Diabetic gangrene, common in Western people, is unusual in diabetic groups in Japan and the West Indies (Tulloch, 1962; Tsuji and Wada, 1971; West, 1975; Baba *et al.*, 1976). The low fibre intake and high animal fat and cholesterol intake of persons with diabetes in Western countries may contribute to the higher prevalence of arteriosclerotic vascular disease in these individuals.

The short report of Singh (1955) provides the strongest evidence that a high carbohydrate (approximately 60 per cent of energy) diet may lower insulin requirements of patients with diabetes. These high carbohydrate diets also provide generous quantities of dietary fibre from whole wheat chapatties. He studied 63 lean and 17 obese patients for between six months and five years. With these high carbohydrate, high fibre diets insulin therapy could be discontinued in 74 patients and doses were substantially lowered in the remaining

6 patients. More recent studies have supported the concept that high carbohydrate diets may have a beneficial impact on the control of diabetes (Kempner
et al., 1958); Patel *et al.*, 1969; Brunzell *et al.*, 1971, 1974; Gulati *et al.*, 1974;
Viswanathan, 1978; Anderson and Ward, 1978, 1979).

High carbohydrate, high fibre diets

Diets providing large amounts of unrefined carbohydrate and dietary fibre
are beneficial in the management of many persons with diabetes (Singh,
1955; Gulati *et al.*, 1974; Viswanathan, 1978). We have systematically
studied the effects of weight-maintaining, high carbohydrate, high fibre
(HCF) diets in lean individuals with diabetes (Kiehm *et al.*, 1976; Anderson
and Ward, 1978, 1979). The composition of representative diets is given in
Table 22.1. We have usually fed control diets for 7–11 days and then fed HCF
diets for 12–28 days. Patients have then been instructed in maintenance diets
for home use. The carbohydrate, protein and fat contents of the control diets
are similar to conventional diabetic diets; however, the control diets have
less cholesterol and more dietary fibre than most conventional diets. The
HCF diets provide 70 per cent of energy from carbohydrate and have large
quantities of dietary fibres. The maintenance diets resemble the diets
recommended (West, 1975) as prudent diets for persons with diabetes. Our
experience with these HCF diets will be briefly summarized.

The response of a representative patient is presented in Fig. 22.4. On the
control diet, this man required 32 units of insulin daily to maintain fasting
plasma glucose values of approximately 9·2 mmol/l (165 mg/dl) and urine
glucose excretion of 33 mmol/d (6 g/d). On the HCF diet his plasma glucose
and urine glucose values declined and insulin could be reduced rapidly.
After 16 days on the HCF diet his insulin could be discontinued. After insulin
was discontinued, his fasting plasma glucose values remained under 10 mmol/l
(180 mg/dl) and his urine glucose excretion below 35 mmol/d (6·3 g/d). On
the maintenance diet at home he has had fasting glucose values ranging from
7·8 to 10 mmol/l (140–180 mg/dl) for nine months without insulin or
sulphonylurea therapy.

Whereas weight-maintaining conventional diets or other isocaloric diets
do not greatly alter glucose metabolism or insulin requirements (Kuhl, 1956;
Hallgren and Svanborg, 1962), these HCF diets are accompanied by prompt
reductions in insulin doses. Twelve lean men were treated with control diets
for 7–11 days; there were no significant changes in insulin doses (Fig. 22.5).
They then received weight-maintaining HCF diets and insulin doses could
be lowered quickly. However, fasting plasma glucose and urine glucose
values were significantly lower on HCF diets than values on control diets.
Our experience with 33 insulin-treated patients is summarized in Fig. 22.6.
Seventeen patients ((11 lean, 6 obese) were treated with 14–20 units of insulin
per day on control diets. On HCF diets insulin could be discontinued in 16
of 17 patients after an average of 14 days. Eleven lean men required 25–32
units of insulin per day on control diets. On weight-maintaining HCF diets,

Table 22.1   Composition of representative 1800 kilocalorie diets[1]

	Control diet		HCF diet		Maintenance diet	
	g/d	% kcal	g/d	% kcal	g/d	% kcal
Protein	92	20	98	21	90	20
Carbohydrate, total	193	43	314	70	261	58
Simple	79	—	91	—	65	—
Complex	114	—	223	—	196	—
Fat, total	74	37	18	9	44	22
SAT[2]	26	—	5	—	12	—
MUS[2]	39	—	5	—	18	—
PUS[2]	9	—	7	—	12	—
Cholesterol	0·48	—	0·065	—	0·10	—
Dietary fibre	26	—	65	—	51	—

[1] From Anderson and Ward (1978, 1979)
[2] SAT, saturated; MUS, monounsaturated; and PUS, polyunsaturated fatty acids

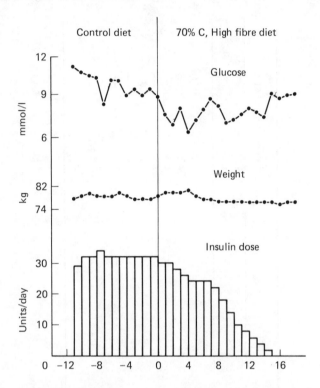

Fig. 22.4   Response of diabetic man to control and high carbohydrate, high fibre diets. Fasting plasma glucose values are presented in top line (Anderson and Ward, 1979)

insulin was reduced by an average of 1 unit per day and could be discontinued in five of these patients. For example, one man had been treated with 35–40 units of insulin per day for the previous six years. He required 32 units of insulin to maintain fasting plasma glucose values of approximately 8·3 mmol/l (150 mg/dl) and urine glucose values of 17–33 mmol/d (3–6 g/d). On the HCF diet, insulin was reduced by 2 units on alternate days and was discontinued after 33 days. Without insulin on the HCF diet his fasting plasma glucose values averaged 8·9 mmol/l (160 mg/dl) and his urine glucose excretion was less than 28 mmol/d (5 g/d). These studies suggest that HCF diets may have distinct therapeutic advantages for many patients with the maturity-onset (insulin-independent) type of diabetes.

Five lean adults with the juvenile-onset (insulin-dependent) type of diabetes have been treated with weight-maintaining HCF diets. These patients required an average of 44 units per day (range 40–55 units/d) on control diets. On HCF diets, plasma glucose and urine glucose values were slightly lower than values on the control diets and insulin doses were reduced to 34 units per day (range 20–46 units/d). The management of three patients was

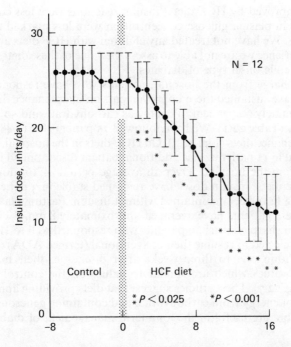

Fig. 22.5 Insulin requirements of lean diabetic men on control and HCF diets. These studies of Anderson *et al.* (1978) are described in text

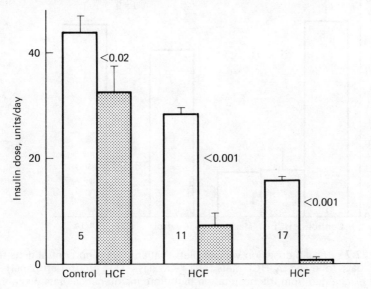

Fig. 22.6 Insulin doses of diabetic patients on control and HCF diets. These studies of Anderson *et al.* (1978) are described in text

distinctly improved by HCF diets: insulin reactions were less common and fluctuations in plasma glucose concentration were less marked than on the control diets. We have not treated any children with HCF diets and from our limited experience we are not able to assess the value of these diets for patients with the juvenile-onset type of diabetes.

After discharge from the hospital, patients who have responded well to HCF diets have sustained these improvements on maintenance diets providing approximately 60 per cent of energy as carbohydrate and 50 g of dietary fibre per day (Table 22.1). We have followed 15 patients for 6–48 months on these maintenance diets (Fig. 22.7). On HCF diets in the hospital, insulin was discontinued in 11 patients; one additional patient discontinued insulin after discharge from the hospital. Over an average period of 16 months on the maintenance diets, insulin doses have remained stable in 3 patients and the remaining 12 have been maintained without insulin. Fasting plasma glucose values in these patients have averaged approximately 8 mmol/l (144 mg/dl) (Fig 22.8). In sharp contrast, 9 patients who responded well to HCF diets in the hospital elected to resume their conventional (termed ADA) diets as out-patients. Within one to three weeks after discharge, their insulin doses returned to values which are similar to values on the control diet in the hospital (Fig. 22.7). These studies suggest that diets providing approximately 60 per cent of energy from carbohydrate and containing generous quantities of dietary fibre are useful in the long-term management of diabetes. These

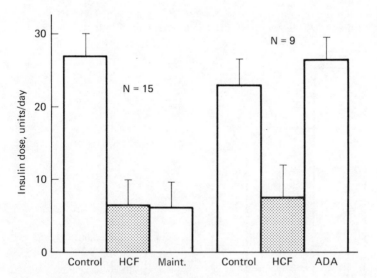

Fig. 22.7 Insulin doses on various diets. Patients were on control diets for 5–11 days followed by HCF diets for 14–33 days. One group (left panel) were discharged from the hospital on high fibre maintenance diets while the other group (right panel) resumed conventional (ADA) diets as out-patients. These studies of Anderson *et al.* are described in text

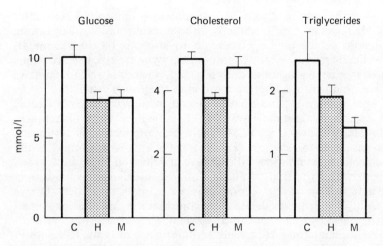

Fig. 22.8 Responses to control (C), HCF (H) and maintenance (M) diets of diabetic patients. Fasting plasma glucose and serum lipids were measured by Anderson *et al.* as described in text

diets have been well tolerated and not associated with appreciable gastro-intestinal side effects. We have made serial measurements of haemoglobin, serum calcium, phosphorus, alkaline phosphatase, iron, magnesium, caro-tene, folate, prothrombin and partial thromboplastin times on these patients and have not detected alterations on these maintenance diets.

At the present time we do not understand the mechanisms responsible for the improved glucose metabolism and reduced insulin doses on HCF as compared to control diets. Other studies (Anderson, 1979) suggest that changes in the carbohydrate and fat content of these diets might play a major role and that dietary fibre might have a minor role in the improved glucose metabolism. The intake of most of the carbohydrate in the unrefined form (i.e. in its natural fibre packages), probably does reduce post-prandial plasma glucose concentrations. These diets appear to increase tissue sensi-tivity to insulin since insulin doses were reduced in patients with the insulin-dependent type of diabetes. Our studies of insulin binding to circulating monocytes demonstrated that monocytes bound more insulin and have significantly greater numbers of insulin binding sites ($P < 0.001$) when patients were on HCF diets than observed on control diets (Anderson, 1979). Many patients respond rapidly to HCF diets (Fig. 22.5) and then have a slow adaptive response similar to that reported by Jenkins and colleagues (Jenkins *et al.*, 1978b, 1979). Two lean patients who were on 32 units of insulin on control diets illustrate this slow response. The first patient, as outlined above, required 33 days of treatment with the HCF diet before insulin could be discontinued. The second patient had received 30–40 units of insulin per day for 19 years and was reasonably well controlled on 32 units on the control diet. During a 21-day period on the HCF diet, his insulin gradually was reduced to 8 units per day. On the maintenance diet at home, he was able to reduce slowly the insulin dose and discontinue insulin ten weeks after discharge. He now has gone 18 months without insulin and has had fasting plasma glucose values ranging from 7·2 to 10 mmol/l (130–180 mg/dl) without insulin therapy. Obviously those patients who are able to discontinue insulin have residual endogenous insulin secretion which is able to maintain their glucose homoeostasis after discontinuing exogenous insulin.

Serum lipid responses have been evaluated in over 60 patients treated with HCF diets on our metabolic ward. Every patient has had a reduction in serum cholesterol values (Fig. 22.8). The average reduction in serum tri-glycerides has been 16 per cent ($P < 0.01$). Patients with normal serum triglyceride concentration show little change in values on HCF diets. How-ever, patients with hypertriglyceridaemia almost invariably have a distinct reduction in fasting serum triglyceride values while on the HCF diets. Twelve patients with hypertriglyceridaemia on control diets had fasting values ranging from 3·5 to 33·6 mmol/l (312–2970 mg/dl, average 1147); after 12 days on weight-maintaining HCF diets, serum triglyceride values were lower in every patient and average values were 63 per cent lower ($P < 0.01$). The dietary fibre content of these diets seems to be responsible for this triglyceride lowering effect since patients fed low fibre, high carbohydrate diets develop hypertriglyceridaemia with regularity (Anderson, 1977a). After discharge from the hospital, serum triglyceride values usually are even lower on the maintenance diets (Fig. 22.8). Thus, high fibre diets may have a substantial role in the management of hypertriglyceridaemia. Our experience indicates that HCF diets lower average cholesterol and triglyceride values in patients with diabetes and that these reductions are sustained on the home main-tenance diets. These improvements in lipid metabolism may lessen the risk for arteriosclerotic vascular disease in these patients with diabetes.

Conclusion

In most Western countries, traditional diabetic diets have been restricted in carbohydrate and dietary fibre. These diets have provided more animal fat and cholesterol than the usual diets of non-diabetic individuals in these countries. The large intake of animal fat and cholesterol may have contri-buted to the high prevalence of arteriosclerotic vascular disease among persons with diabetes in Western countries. Carbohydrate intake has been restricted for empirical reasons and there are no careful metabolic studies which demonstrate that low carbohydrate diets bestow any benefits on persons with diabetes.

High carbohydrate diets have been used in some Western countries and in India and Japan to treat patients with diabetes. The available data indicate that high carbohydrate diets lead to improved glucose metabolism and lower insulin requirements for most persons with diabetes. These high carbohydrate diets are accompanied by lower serum cholesterol and triglyceride values than observed when high fat diets are used to treat diabetes. Recent evidence suggests that dietary fibre intake is associated with improved glucose metabolism, lower insulin requirements, and lower serum lipid values than observed on low fibre diets.

High carbohydrate, high fibre diets are accompanied by dramatic reductions in insulin requirements and in serum lipids in selected patients with diabetes. These regressions in diabetes have been sustained for over three years in patients who have successfully followed these modified diets. These observations suggest that fat restricted diets providing generous quantities of complex carbohydrate and dietary fibre may have therapeutic usefulness for most adults with diabetes. High carbohydrate, high fibre diets may slow the progression of arteriosclerotic vascular disease in individuals with diabetes.

Acknowledgements

The assistance of Wen-Ju Lin Chen, PhD, and Beverly Sieling, RD, is appreciated. This work was supported in part by grants from the Veterans Administration and the National Institute of Arthritis, Metabolism, and Digestive Disease (Am 20889).

References

Anderson, J. W. (1977a). Effect of carbohydrate restriction and high carbohydrate diets on men with chemical diabetes. *American Journal of Clinical Nutrition,* **30,** 402–408

Anderson, J. W. (1977b). High polysaccharide diet studies in patients with diabetes and vascular disease. *Cereal Foods World,* **22,** 12–15

Anderson, J. W. (1979). High carbohydrate, high fiber diets for patients with diabetes. *Proceedings of Fourth International Symposium on Early Diabetes.* Plenum, New York

Anderson, J. W. and Chen, W. L. (1979). Plant fiber. Carbohydrate and lipid metabolism. *American Journal of Clinical Nutrition,* **32,** 346–363

Anderson, J. W., Lin, W-J. and Ward, K. (1978). Composition of foods commonly used in diets for persons with diabetes. *Diabetes Care,* **1,** 293–302

Anderson, J. W. and Ward, K. (1978). Long term effects of high carbohydrate, high fiber diets on glucose and lipid metabolism: A preliminary report on patients with diabetes. *Diabetes Care,* **1,** 77–82

Anderson, J. W. and Ward, K. (1979). High carbohydrate, high fiber diets for insulin-treated men with diabetes mellitus. *American Journal of Clinical Nutrition,* **32,** 2312–2319

Anonymous (1972). Food and Nutrition Board, National Academy of Science—National Research Council and Council on Food and Nutrition, American Medical Association, Diet and coronary heart disease—A joint statement. *Preventive Medicine,* **1,** 559–561

Anonymous (1975). National Commission of Diabetes. Report to the Congress of the United States. *Diabetes Forecast,* **28** (Supplement 1), 1–60

Anonymous (1977). *A Guide for Professionals: the Effective Application of 'Exchange Lists for Meal Planning'*. American Diabetes Association and American Dietetic Association, New York and Chicago

Baba, S., Goto, Y. and Fukui, I. (1976). *Diabetes Mellitus in Asia*. Excerpta Medica, Amsterdam

Bennion, L. J. and Grundy, S. M. (1977). Effects of diabetes mellitus on cholesterol metabolism in man. *New England Journal of Medicine,* **296,** 1365–1371

Bierman, E. L., Albrink, J. J., Arky, R. A., Conner, W. E., Dayton, S., Spritz, N. and Steinberg, D. (1971). Principles of nutrition and dietary recommentations for patients with diabetes mellitus. *Diabetes,* **20,** 633–634

Bierman, E. L. and Nelson, R. (1975). Carbohydrates, diabetes and blood lipids. *World Review of Nutritional Dietetics,* **22,** 280–287

Bradley, R. F. (1971). Cardiovascular disease. In: *Joslin's Diabetes Mellitus,* Eleventh edition. Editors A. Marble, P. White, R. F. Bradley and L. P. Krall. Lea and Febiger, Philadelphia

Brunzell, J. D., Lerner, R. L., Hazzard, W. R., Porte, D. Jr. and Bierman, E. L. (1971). Improved glucose tolerance with high carbohydrate feeding in mild diabetes. *New England Journal of Medicine,* **284,** 521–524

Brunzell, J. D., Lerner, R. L., Porte, D. Jr. and Bierman, E. L. (1974). Effect of a fat free, high carbohydrate diet on diabetic subjects with fasting hyperglycemia. *Diabetes,* **23,** 138–142

Card, W. I. (1938). The effect of different diets on the insulin sensitivity of diabetics. *Clinical Science,* **3,** 105–117

Chase, H. P. and Glasgow, A. M. (1976). Juvenile diabetes mellitus and serum lipids and lipoprotein levels. *American Journal of Diseases of Children,* **130,** 113–117

Daughaday, W. H. (1958). Dietary treatment of adults with diabetes mellitus. *Journal of the American Medical Association,* **167,** 859–862

Doar, J. W. H., Thompson, M. E., Wilde, C. E. and Sewell, P. F. J. (1975). Influence of treatment with diet alone on oral glucose-tolerance test and plasma sugar and insulin levels in patients with maturity-onset diabetes mellitus. *Lancet,* **i,** 1263–1266

Ellis, A. (1934). Increased carbohydrate tolerance in diabetics following the hourly administration of glucose and insulin over long periods. *Quarterly Journal of Medicine, New Series,* **3,** 137–153

Geyelin, H. R. (1935). The treatment of diabetes with insulin (after ten years). *Journal of the American Medical Association,* **104,** 1203–1208

Gibson, R. B. (1929). Latent tolerance in diabetes mellitus. A study of the effect of high sugar diets with insulin on controlled diabetics. *Journal of Laboratory and Clinical Medicine,* **14,** 597–604

Gulati, P. D., Rao, M. B. and Vaishnava, H. (1974). Diet for diabetics. *Lancet,* **ii,** 297–298

Haber, G. B., Heaton, K. W., Murphy, D. and Burroughs, L. F. (1977). Depletion and disruption of dietary fibre. Effects on satiety, plasma glucose and serum-insulin. *Lancet,* **ii,** 679–682

Hadden, D. R., Montgomery, D. A. D., Shelly, R. J., Trimble, E. R., Weaver, J. A., Wilson, E. A. and Buchanan, K. D. (1975). Maturity onset diabetes mellitus: Response to intensive dietary management. *British Medical Journal*, **3**, 276–278

Hallgren, I. E. and Svanborg, A. (1962). Short term study of effect of different isocaloric diets in diabetes. *Metabolism*, **11**, 912–919

Himsworth, H. P. (1933–34). The influence of diet on the sugar tolerance of healthy men and its reference to certain extrinsic factors. *Clinical Science*, **1**, 251–264

Jackson, W. P. U. and Kalk, J. (1972). Glucose intolerance retested. The importance of variability and a vindication of restriction of dietary carbohydrate. *South African Medical Journal*, **46**, 2065–2071

Jenkins, D. J. A., Leeds, A. R., Gassull, M. A., Wolever, T. M. S., Goff, D. V., Alberti, K. G. M. M. and Hockaday, T. D. R. (1976). Unabsorbable carbohydrates and diabetes: decreased post-prandial hyperglycaemia. *Lancet*, **ii**, 172–174

Jenkins, D. J. A., Leeds, A. R., Gassull, M. A., Cochet, B. and Alberti, K. G. M. M. (1977a). Decrease in postprandial insulin and glucose concentrations by guar and pectin. *Annals of Internal Medicine*, **86**, 20–23

Jenkins, D. J. A., Wolever, T. M. S., Hockaday, T. D. R., Leeds, A. R., Howarth, R., Bacon, S., Apling, E. C. and Dilawari, J. (1977b). Treatment of diabetes with guar gum. *Lancet*, **ii**, 779–780

Jenkins, D. J. A., Wolever, T. M. S., Leeds, A. R., Gassull, M. A., Haisman, P., Dilawari, J., Goff, D. V., Metz, G. L. and Alberti, K. G. M. M. (1978a). Dietary fibres, fibre analogues, and glucose tolerance: Importance of viscosity. *British Medical Journal*, **1**, 1392–1394

Jenkins, D. J. A., Wolever, T. M. S., Nineham, R., Bacon, S., Smith, R. and Hockaday, T. D. R. (1979). Dietary fibre and diabetic therapy: A progressive effect with time. *Proceedings of Fourth International Symposium on Early Diabetes*. Plenum, New York

Jenkins, D. J. A., Wolever, T. M. S., Nineham, R., Taylor, R., Metz, G. L., Bacon, S. and Hockaday, T. D. R. (1978b). Guar crispbread in the diabetic diet. *British Medical Journal*, **2**, 1744–1746

Kempner, W., Peschel, R. L. and Schlayer, C. (1958). Effect of rice diet on diabetes mellitus associated with vascular disease. *Postgraduate Medicine*, **24**, 359–371

Kiehm, T. G., Anderson, J. W. and Ward, K. (1976). Beneficial effects of a high carbohydrate, high fibre diet on hyperglycemic diabetic men. *American Journal of Clinical Nutrition*, **29**, 895–899

Kuhl, W. J. (1956). Metabolic studies with the arylsulfonylureas. *Metabolism*, **5**, 953–963

Miranda, P. M. and Horwitz, D. L. (1978). High-fiber diets in the treatment of diabetes mellitus. *Annals of Internal Medicine*, **88**, 482–486

Monnier, L., Pham, T. C., Aguirre, L., Orsetti, A. and Mirouze, J. (1978). Influence of indigestible fibers on glucose tolerance. *Diabetes Care*, **1**, 83–88

Morris, J. N., Marr, J. W. and Clayton, D. G. (1977). Diet and heart: A postscript. *British Medical Journal*, **2**, 1307–1314

Page, L. and Friend, B. (1978). The changing United States diet. *BioScience*, **28**, 192–197

Patel, J. C., Metha, A. B., Dhirawani, M., Juthani, V. J. and Aiyer, L. (1969). High carbohydrate diet in the treatment of diabetes mellitus. *Diabetologia*, **5**, 243–247

Perkins, J. R., West, T. E. T., Sonksen, P. H., Lowy, C. and Iles, C. (1977). The effect of energy and carbohydrate restriction in patients with chronic diabetes mellitus. *Diabetologia*, **13**, 607–614

Rabinowitch, I. M. (1935). Effects of the high carbohydrate–low calorie diet upon carbohydrate tolerance in diabetes mellitus. *Canadian Medical Association Journal*, **33**, 136–144

Richardson, R. (1929). High-carbohydrate diets in diabetes mellitus. *American Journal of Medical Science*, **177**, 426–430

Sansum, W. D., Blatherwick, N. R. and Bowden, R. (1926). The use of high carbohydrate diets in the treatment of diabetes mellitus. *Journal of the American Medical Association*, **86**, 178–181

Santen, R. J., Willis, P. W. and Fajans, S. S. (1972). Atherosclerosis in diabetes mellitus. *Archives of Internal Medicine*, **130**, 833–843

Scala, J. (1975). The physiological effects of dietary fiber. *American Chemical Society Symposium Series*. Lippincott, Philadelphia

Singh, I. (1955). Low-fat diet and therapeutic doses of insulin in diabetes mellitus. *Lancet*, **i**, 422–425

Stone, D. B. and Connor, W. E. (1963). The prolonged effects of a low cholesterol, high carbohydrate diet on the serum lipids in diabetic patients. *Diabetes*, **12**, 127–132

Strouse, S. and Soskin, S. (1932). Treatment of the same diabetic patient with widely varying diets. *Transactions of the Association of American Physicians*, **47**, 317–322

Trowell, H. (1972). Ischemic heart disease and dietary fiber. *American Journal of Clinical Nutrition*, **25**, 926–932

Trowell, H. C. (1975). Dietary-fiber hypothesis of the etiology of diabetes mellitus. *Diabetes*, **24**, 762–765

Truwell, A. S., Thomas, B. J. and Brown, A. M. (1975). Survey of dietary policy and management in British diabetic clinics. *British Medical Journal*, **4**, 7–11

Tsuji, S. and Wada, M. (1971). *Diabetes Mellitus in Asia, 1970*. Exerpta Medica, Amsterdam

Tulloch, J. A. (1962). *Diabetes Mellitus in the Tropics*. E. & S. Livingstone Ltd, Edinburgh

Turtle, J. R. (1970). Glucose and insulin secretory response patterns following diet and tolazamide therapy in diabetes. *British Medical Journal*, **3**, 606–610

Viswanathan, M. (1978). Dietary management of diabetes. *Journal of the Indian Medical Association*, **70**, 275–279

Walker, A. R. P., Walker, B. F. and Richardson, B. D. (1970). Glucose and fat tolerance in Bantu children. *Lancet*, **ii**, 51–52

Walker, W. (1977). Changing United States life-style and declining vascular mortality: cause or coincidence. *New England Journal of Medicine,* **297,** 163–164

Wall, J. R., Pyke, D. A. and Oakley, W. G. (1973). Effect of carbohydrate restriction in obese diabetics: Relationship of control to weight loss. *British Medical Journal,* **1,** 577–578

West, K. M. (1975). Prevention and therapy of diabetes mellitus. *Nutrition Reviews,* **33,** 193–198

West, K. M. (1976). Diet and diabetes. *Postgraduate Medicine,* **60,** 209–216

West, K. M. and Kalbfleisch, J. M. (1971). Influence of nutritional factors on prevalence of diabetes. *Diabetes,* **20,** 99–108

Wood, F. C. Jr. and Bierman, E. L. (1972). New concepts in diabetic dietetics. *Nutrition Today,* **7,** 4–12

Woodyatt, R. T. (1924). Some milder forms of diabetes with special reference to mild diabetes in elderly persons with arteriosclerosis. *Southern Medical Journal,* **17,** 145–153

23

Hypertension, hyperlipidaemia, angina and coronary heart disease

Hans Diehl and Don Mannerberg

'It is often necessary to make decisions on the basis of information sufficient for action, but insufficient to satisfy the intellect.'

I. Kant

Recent dietary changes

During the last 100 years far-reaching changes have occurred in the diet of the nations which became affluent. A substantial change has occurred in the composition of the average diet, such as that seen in the United States (Table 23.1).

Table 23.1   United States dietary trends 1860–1975

	Percentage of energy from major nutrients			
	1860	1910	1925	1975
Protein	12	12	12	12–15
Fat	25	32	35	40–45
Carbohydrates				
Complex (starch)	53	43	37	22
Simple (sugars)	10	13	16	24
Total	63	56	53	46

Source: Brewster and Jacobsen, 1978

Complex carbohydrates (starch) found in grain, vegetables, legumes and tubers, such as potatoes, have been reduced from being the mainstay of the diet to a minority role. Economic development, modern food processing, and national affluence are associated with diets that contain more total fat, saturated fat, processed vegetable fat, refined sugar, animal protein and cholesterol; this has occurred while consumption of cheap unrefined starch foods, rich in minerals, vitamins and fibre, has decreased considerably.

There are no hard data concerning the low CHD death rates during the last century in the United States 'but the attack rate appears to have increased substantially in the twentieth century' (Passamani *et al.*, 1978). This has coincided with the recent dietary change. Could it be possible that the rate of CHD might improve if the diet was changed back to that of 1860, for then the disease was apparently far less common in the United States?

CHD risk factors

Rich diets and affluence

Evidence from epidemiological, clinicopathological and animal studies have demonstrated that CHD is a multifactorial disease. It is not an inevitable consequence of ageing, but a matter of lifestyle with a confluence of affluence-related causes: rich diet, cigarette smoking, sedentary life patterns and a stress-filled way of life. Stamler (1978) has stated: 'It is further reasonable and sound to designate "rich diet" as a *primary, essential, necessary cause* of the current epidemic of premature atherosclerotic disease raging in the western industrialized countries. Cigarette smoking and hypertension are important secondary or complementary causes.'

Hyperlipidaemia

World Health Organization statistics have demonstrated the clear, quantitative association between certain blood lipid levels and the subsequent CHD incidence in the population. CHD risk rises progressively with serum cholesterol levels from the lowest to the highest values reported in the population (Passamani *et al.*, 1978). Serum cholesterol levels are the most prominent CHD risk factor (Stamler, 1978). Since two-thirds or more of the total serum cholesterol is carried by the low density lipoprotein (LDL) fraction, and since almost all triglycerides are carried in the very low density lipoprotein (VLDL) fraction, total serum cholesterol and triglyceride levels provide, from a practical point of view, a reasonable basis on which to formulate intervention therapy. Elevated serum triglyceride levels, especially those above 1·7 mmol/l (150 mg/dl), have been considered to be an independent CHD risk factor. Evidence for their *independent* role remains controversial; but much data suggest that the combination of elevated serum cholesterol and serum triglyceride levels increase CHD risk.

Recently many investigators have expressed misgivings concerning the high cut-off figures that divide normal lipid levels from hyperlipidaemia (Wright, 1976). Within the recommended range of 'normal' lipid levels there is a five-fold increased CHD risk. Necropsy studies of young American soldiers have demonstrated that almost no American man above 25–30 years is free of significant coronary atherosclerosis. Previously many accepted the National Institutes of Health cut-off levels of 'normal' blood lipid levels. Thus serum cholesterol levels in 'normal' men aged up to 59 years might range from 6·2 to 8·5 mmol/l (240–330 mg/dl) and serum triglycerides from 1·6 to 2·2 mmol/l (140–190 mg/dl).

Serum cholesterol levels of less than 3·9 mmol/l (150 mg/dl) and serum triglyceride levels of less than 0·9 mmol/l (80 mg/dl) are commonly seen in populations of developing countries in which CHD is rare and even in American strict vegetarians (Sacks *et al.*, 1975). It appears therefore desirable to regard these levels as therapeutic goals at least in persons having any manifestation of CHD (Pritikin, 1976; Wissler and Vesselinovitch, 1977; W. P. Castelli, personal communication, 1978; E. L. Wynder, personal communication, 1979).

Fat

In population studies serum cholesterol levels are closely related to the proportion of energy derived from fat, especially saturated fat (Stamler, 1978). Numerous metabolic studies in man have demonstrated that dietary cholesterol intake is related to serum cholesterol level. This question has been clarified by observations that the first 200–300 mg of dietary cholesterol have a much larger effect in raising serum cholesterol levels than higher intakes of dietary cholesterol 500 mg or more daily.

Polyunsaturated fats (PUF)

In the early 1950s it was discovered that serum lipid levels could be reduced if vegetable fats (PUF) were substituted for saturated animal fats. Accordingly large sophisticated dietary trials for the primary and secondary prevention of CHD were carried out in the United States and Europe: dietary cholesterol intake was reduced from 600 mg/d, to about 400 mg/d, and the total fat intake was usually reduced from 40 to 35 per cent energy, while much of the saturated animal fats were replaced with polyunsaturated vegetable oils. Serum cholesterol levels fell 7 to 16 per cent (Ahrens, 1976), but none of these extensive trials reported that mortality rates altered significantly (Borhani, 1977). Fears have been expressed that PUF may decrease usually serum cholesterol levels but raise tissue cholesterol levels (Wiggers *et al.*, 1977). PUF-rich diets favour gallstone formation in man (Bennion and Grundy, 1978) and possibly increase susceptibility to certain types of cancer (Carrol, 1975). An editorial article entitled 'The Potential Toxicity of Excessive PUF' criticized a dietary strategy based on 'personal impressions and fragmentary conclusions instead of *scientific* evidence' (Pinckney, 1973).

Lipid-lowering drugs

Four large prospective double-blind drug trials covering five-year periods have been reported. Serum cholesterol levels fell 5 to 10 per cent (Ahrens, 1976). Long-term survival after myocardial infarction did not improve; indeed excess mortality and unfavourable side effects resulted in more harm than good (Coronary Drug Project Research Group, 1975). British secondary CHD prevention studies reported some beneficial effect on angina mortality. The European Collaborative Primary Prevention Trial with clofibrate involving 16 000 men reported no decrease in CHD morbidity and mortality.

Instead there were excess deaths in the clofibrate-treated men due to diseases of the liver, gallbladder and intestines. 'The conclusions must be that clofibrate can no longer be recommended for general use' (Editorial, 1978). New directives from the National Institutes of Health stated that 'the widespread use of hypolipidemic drugs to treat or prevent CHD should be deferred until distinct benefits are demonstrated and significant toxicity can be excluded' (Rifkind and Levy, 1978).

Other risk factors

Prospective epidemiological investigations have confirmed the importance of *hypertension* as a risk factor in CHD and cerebrovascular disease. The prevalence of essential hypertension in the USA is estimated to range from 30 to 35 million, with more than 70 per cent of these affected individuals having mild hypertension in the diastolic range of 90–105 mmHg. Even this degree of elevation diminishes life expectancy.

Evidence that essential hypertension is caused by a high level of salt intake in salt-sensitive individuals has been summarized by many investigators (Freis, 1976; Meneely and Battarbee, 1976a, b). Moderate salt restriction to 3–6 g/d has resulted in significant blood pressure changes, often as effective as multiple drug therapy (Magnani *et al.*, 1976; Morgan *et al.*, 1978). Weight loss alone can cause highly significant reduction in blood pressure of overweight hypertensives. Regression equations predicting systolic and diastolic blood pressure falls of about 2·5/1·5 mmHg respectively per kg overweight lost have been calculated (Reisin *et al.*, 1978). Iacono *et al.* (1975) demonstrated that total fat intake reduction alone can affect blood pressure by influencing platelet and erythrocyte aggregation. Fat intake, reduced from 42 to 25 per cent in the diet for 40 days, produced a 10 per cent drop in systolic and diastolic blood pressure. Furthermore, isotonic graded exercise is known for its hypotensive effect by lowering peripheral vascular resistance.

In summary, a therapeutic lifestyle approach for essential hypertension should include moderate salt restriction, facilitation of ideal weight, which would be aided by exercise, and a redistribution of energy by reducing fat and animal products and increasing unrefined complex carbohydrates.

Physical inactivity, *obesity* and *smoking* are additional, well recognized CHD risk factors.

CHD protective factors

Unrefined complex carbohydrate (starch)

CHD prevention trials have mainly intervened in changing dietary P/S ratios and cholesterol intake. Total fat intake has not been aggressively lowered. If total fat was lowered, then what would take its place calorically? Some researchers have hesitated to advocate increased consumption of carbohydrates, especially in patients with hyperlipoproteinaemia type IV. This hesitation fails to recognize an important distinction in the carbohydrate foods (Ahrens, 1974). Refined simple carbohydrates induce high post-prandial serum triglycerides; on the other hand unrefined or lightly refined complex carbohydrate foods with high fibre content induce lower triglyceride levels; they increase carbohydrate tolerance in adults and in maturity-onset diabetics (Anderson and Chen, 1979) (page 380). Epidemiological data have reported that populations habitually consuming high intakes of unrefined high fibre foods, some eating even 85 per cent of daily energy, have low triglyceride levels, often less than 0·9 mmol/l (80 mg/dl).

Plant protein

Independent of the low fat, low cholesterol intake, vegetable protein *per se* may have a hypocholesterolaemic effect (Hamilton and Carroll, 1976). US vegetarians have lower plasma lipid levels than controls (Sacks *et al.*, 1975).

Physical exercise

Rehabilitation programmes for coronary patients usually discuss physical exercise in terms of restoring physical efficiency and increasing psychological morale (Hellerstein and Franklin, 1978). It is considered also that regular physical exercise has an important protective action in atherosclerosis (Simko, 1978).

Longevity Center, Santa Barbara[1]

Programme description and patients

The Longevity Center has advocated a comprehensive permanent lifestyle modification programme aimed at improving physiological function in those affected by degenerative cardiovascular diseases. The four-week residential intervention programme founded by Nathan Pritikin in 1976 in Santa Barbara, California, emphasizes a radical restructuring of the American way of life. It was designed simultaneously to reduce recognized CHD risk factors, increase CHD protective factors, alleviate symptoms and affect with time atherosclerotic processes. This new lifestyle involves a diet that resembles in its composition those of peasant communities in Africa and Asia among whom CHD is rare. It also includes increased regular physical exercise, mainly walking.

Every two weeks up to 50 patients, usually accompanied by the spouse, are admitted to the four-week residential programme. Patients are referred by physicians or elect to join. Prior to admission, all prospective patients are screened via submitted medical records. Conditions of acceptance are that the patient is ambulatory and self-sufficient and that the patient may be expected to benefit from the diet–exercise therapy. Over half the patients are 50–70 years of age, with a range of 20–91 years, and represent the middle and upper classes. As such, the patients are highly motivated, and amenable to

[1] Transferred in 1978 to Santa Monica.

the educational approach; most have been given no alternatives for the relief of their cardiovascular disease.

Diet

The diet contains much unrefined complex carbohydrate (starch) foods. Biochemical analyses of the diet have shown that 70 per cent of the daily energy is derived from starch as found predominantly in whole cereal grain products, tubers (potatoes), legumes (beans and peas) and vegetables. Refined cereal products are restricted, such as white flour, white rice and white pasta. Refined simple carbohydrates such as honey, molasses and sugar are not permitted. Simple sugars, as found in the plant foods, fruit and skim milk provide 5 per cent of daily energy. The diet is largely vegetarian with a small amount of white meat and fish (three ounces per week) taken as a condiment. Skim milk up to 250 ml/d (8 oz/d) is used, while egg yolks are avoided. Consequently, the cholesterol intake is negligible (less than 25 mg/d). Fat and oil intakes are very low, representing 10 per cent of daily energy with a P/S ratio of 1·84. The diet is moderate in protein (15 per cent of daily energy, or 85g/d), largely derived from plant sources such as grains, beans and peas, potatoes. The diet is high in dietary fibre (cellulose, hemicellulose and lignin) (50 g/d) and low in salt (3·65 g/d). No salt is added during cooking or at the table; salty foods are avoided. The potassium content of the diet is high (KCl 6·2 g/d) with a very low NaCl/KCl ratio of 0·6. The food is served in six small meals. The amount is influenced by weight status and clinical conditions. Low calorie foods such as raw vegetables and rice crackers may be eaten *ad libitum*. At first, many patients find the diet somewhat unpalatable, but by the end of the second week almost all accept the diet, for many are noticing improved health and lipid profiles and increased appetite. The average energy intake is 7 MJ/d (1700 kcal/d) and contains the adult US Recommended Dietary Allowance of all major nutrients, minerals, vitamins, also energy for age and degree of physical activity.

Medical care

An independent group of several full-time physicians attend to the needs of the patients at the Center. Objectives are to provide quality medical care, to monitor closely clinical changes and to rigorously document findings during the stay at the Center. Aside from the initial physical examination, which includes a comprehensive medical and lifestyle history, the patient is seen at least three times a week. Weight and blood pressures are taken daily prior to breakfast and exercising. The latter is recorded by a calibrated Sphygmetrics SR2 Automated Recorder, this is used to minimize intra- and inter-observer bias. Daily walking records are kept by the patient with close staff monitoring. Resting ECG and treadmill exercise tests utilizing 12 leads are performed on admission and discharge. Detailed blood chemistry profiles are obtained weekly during the residential stay, with analyses carried out by Bio-Science Laboratories at Van Nuys, California, a high grade independent laboratory.

Follow-up questionnaires and blood chemistry profiles are requested of all patients at six weeks after discharge and thereafter every six months for five years. Patients are referred back to their home physician.

Exercise, smoking, caffeine, alcohol and medication

Graded walking, and occasionally jogging, is prescribed according to the clinical examinations and treadmill stress test. Constant monitoring and testing allows the physician to modify exercise and to reduce medication if possible to complete elimination. Smoking cessation is strongly advocated; abstinence from alcohol and caffeine is encouraged.

Education

Detailed educational instruction is given to help patients, and family members, to understand the nature of their cardiovascular disease and the rationale of the Center's programme, and to increase motivation towards continuing adherence to the new recommended lifestyle under the supervision of their home physicians. The intensive 40-hour programme, employing various educational and behavioural techniques, including purchasing and preparation of food, has been designed to help patients to continue the modified lifestyle.

Methods and evaluation

A precoded data form was designed for use in tabulating the data needed from the patient files. A specifically written protocol was established to ensure replicability of the abstracted data. Great care was given in every step of data collection and processing to eliminate possible errors. Sample validity checks were carried out to ensure adherence to protocol in the abstraction process. After keypunching, the entire data set was machine verified, then a sample of the data was hand verified before storage in the computer file.

Evaluation of the short-term results of the treatment programme compared findings on admission and at discharge, utilizing paired t-tests. The biochemical baseline values were those obtained on the morning following admission. The discharge values were those obtained on the morning of departure.

Blood pressure baseline was the mean blood pressure taken on days 2, 3, 4 and 5 following admission. The discharge blood pressure was the mean of blood pressures recorded on the four days preceding the last day prior to discharge.

Status on admission

The Survey Research Service of Loma Linda University collaborated with the Longevity Center in an evaluation of the 26–30-day treatment of 893 consecutively admitted primary patients resident for at least 21 successive days from April 1976 to October 1977.

Table 23.2 records the status on admission, the main points of the history, any recommendations made by the referring physician within the previous two years, also the disease status when admitted, and the results of the treadmill exercise test. The percentages in Table 23.2 of disease status obviously exceed 100 per cent since most patients suffered from more than one disease.

Table 23.2   Status on admission of 893 patients

	Number	%
History		
Myocardial infarction	292	32
Cerebrovascular accident	36	4
Coronary bypass	77	9
Femoral bypass	27	3
Carotid endarterectomy	24	3
Coronary angiogram (no bypass)	193	22
Recent recommendations		
Coronary bypass	75	9
Coronary angiogram	56	7
Femoral bypass	9	1
Disease status		
Coronary heart disease	590	66
Angina pectoris	418	47
Hypertension	324	36
Claudication	198	22
Obesity	259	29
Diabetes mellitus	107	12
Gouty arthritis	57	6
Treadmill exercise test		
Positive	393	44
Negative	317	35
Equivocal	87	10
Excluded	96	11

The definition of hypertension was restricted to those diagnosed hypertensive in their medical history for at least one year *and* on antihypertensive drugs on admission; and to those diagnosed as hypertensive for at least one year *and* blood pressure on admission (average of days 1–3) of more than either 140 (systolic) or 90 (diastolic) mmHg in the absence of antihypertensive medication. The definition of obesity was applied to all those who had ⩾ 120 per cent of ideal body weight according to the Metropolitan Life Insurance table assuming medium frame. The definition of diabetes mellitus was restricted to those diagnosed thus in the medical history *and* on either oral hypoglycaemic drugs and/or insulin, and to those with fasting plasma glucose levels above 7·2 mmol/l (130 mg/dl) on at least two consecutive days while not receiving antidiabetic medication.

The 12 leads treadmill exercise test was performed according to the Bruce protocol. The test was performed on 797 patients on admission; it was considered positive in 393, negative in 317 and equivocal in 87 patients. Some 96 patients were excluded from the test; many of these patients had evidence of severe coronary heart disease, left ventricular failure or were taking digoxin. Others who were tested had documented histories of coronary heart disease and performed the initial test on admission with considerable caution.

Status on discharge

Blood lipids

Table 23.3 reports decrease of the group mean cholesterol level from 6·1 to 4·5 mmol/l (253–175 mg/dl), a mean decrease of 26 per cent, $P < 0.001$. These changes were accomplished without the use of hypolipidaemic drugs. The true changes would be larger, since 55 of the patients admitted were on clofibrate and cholestynamine which depressed their lipid values. All 55 patients were taken off these drugs during the first week of the treatment programme.

Table 23.3 Serum cholesterol levels of 878 patients at admission and discharge

| | Mean levels (mmol/l) | | | |
| | Admission | | Discharge | |
Number	Levels	Mean	Mean	Decrease (%)
28	<4·1	3·8	3·4	10
65	4·1–4·6	4·4	3·6	18
123	4·7–5·1	4·9	3·9	20
142	5·2–5·6	5·5	4·3	22
153	5·7–6·2	5·9	4·5	25
130	6·3–6·7	6·5	4·8	25
105	6·8–7·2	7·0	4·9	29
58	7·3–7·7	7·5	5·3	29
35	7·8–8·2	8·0	5·5	31
39	≥8·3	9·8	6·3	36
	Means	6·1	4·5	26

Conversion: SI to traditional units: cholesterol, 1 mmol/l ≈ 38·6 mg/dl

Table 23.4 Serum triglyceride levels of 873 patients at admission and discharge

| | Mean levels (mmol/l) | | | |
| | Admission | | Discharge | |
Number	Levels	Mean	Mean	Decrease (%)
194	<1·1	0·8	1·0	21 (Increase)
279	1·2–1·7	1·4	1·4	0
173	1·8–2·1	1·9	1·5	20
105	2·2–2·8	2·5	1·8	31
49	2·9–3·4	3·1	1·9	38
50	3·5–4·5	4·2	1·9	55
23	>4·6	8·3	2·6	68
	Means	2·0	1·5	25

Conversion: SI to traditional units: triglyceride; 1 mmol/l ≈ 88·5 mg/dl

Table 23.4 reports decrease of the group mean triglyceride level from 1·96 to 1·47 mmol/l (174–130 mg/dl), a mean decrease of 25 per cent, $P < 0.001$.

Diabetes mellitus and plasma glucose levels

Prior to admission 32 patients had been diagnosed as diabetic and were taking oral hypoglycaemic drugs. Fasting plasma glucose levels were monitored regularly and the dosage was decreased whenever improved carbohydrate tolerance occurred. On discharge only 6 of these patients were still taking hypoglycaemic drugs; 26 had normal plasma glucose levels and took no drugs. Prior to admission another 22 patients had been diagnosed as diabetic and been employing insulin injections. Eleven of these 22 patients were still taking insulin, usually in decreased dosage, when discharged; the other 11 patients had ceased insulin therapy completely and were discharged with normal plasma glucose levels. (Most of the diabetes patients were of the maturity-onset type even if they received insulin.)

Excluding the diabetic patients the mean fasting plasma glucose of the non-diabetic patients was 5·5 mmol/l (100 mg/dl) on admission and 5·2 mmol/l (94 mg/dl) on discharge.

Hypertension

Among the 324 hypertensive patients on admission (Table 23.2) 218 had been treated by antihypertensive drugs. Of these patients, 186, that is 85 per cent, left with normal blood pressure recorded as the mean figure for the four previous days, all of them had discontinued antihypertensive drugs. The admission mean blood pressure, systolic 134 and diastolic 77 mmHg, for these 186 male and female hypertensives reflected control through medication. As drug dosage was gradually lowered in response to decreasing blood pressure, slight transient increases for 1–3 days were noted. Eventually medication became unnecessary. On discharge the mean blood pressure, systolic 131 and diastolic 73 mmHg, reflected control through the regimen of diet and exercise. The remaining 32 hypertensives were discharged taking the appropriate dosage, usually decreased, of drugs to control the hypertension.

Weight

Most patients lost weight during the four-week diet and exercise programme, especially those who were obese (Table 23.5). Initially patients found the diet strange, a few patients even considered it unappetizing, for it is low in fat, sugar, salt and animal products. During the second week most patients noticed improved physical health and took more exercise. This stimulated appetite so that patients usually accepted the new diet as essential, and even enjoyable. However, they continued to lose weight slowly during their residential stay and usually for many months after discharge (page 407).

Exercise, angina and claudication

Prior to admission most patients had taken little physical exercise. At the Center, however, they were individually prescribed and encouraged to walk short distances several times daily, usually as a member of a group, and to increase the exercise time and distance gradually each day. The average group walking distance of 6·2 miles *per day* during the last two weeks of their stay represented a considerable improvement, especially for those suffering from CHD, angina and claudication.

Angina pectoris was present in 418 patients and intermittent claudication in 198 patients on admission. These patients were encouraged to continue walking in spite of moderate pain, but to stop if the pain became too severe

Table 23.5   Weight loss from admission until discharge of 893 patients

Number	Admission Weight status[1] (%)	Discharge Mean weight loss (kg)
259	⩾120 (obese)	6·0
212	110–119 (overweight)	4·5
226	100–109	3·0
113	90– 99	2·1
83	<90	1·4

[1] Ideal weight classification of Metropolitan Life Insurance

or they felt too exhausted. These patients usually found that they could increase physical activity while the physician also decreased the medication. As a result, 250 patients, 60 per cent of angina cases, were discharged having little or no pain on exertion, so that they required no medication. This improvement was also reflected in the treadmill exercise test and electrocardiogram data.

In a similar manner about half the claudication patients were discharged able to walk several miles daily with little or no pain while taking far less or no medication. In both claudication and angina patients improved tolerance of the treadmill test occurred. It was probably due to a combination of the training programme, weight loss, increased confidence on the part of the patient and increased cooperation with the staff, as well as the decrease of coronary heart disease risk factors by diet, exercise, and the cessation of smoking.

Smoking

On admission to the programme, 191 patients (17 per cent of the total) were smokers; of these 163 stopped smoking, usually on the first or second day of residence at the Center. Doubtless this aided recovery from cardiovascular degenerative disease, but as the large majority of claudication and angina patients were non-smokers on admission, the cessation of smoking in a small proportion of these patients did not explain the improved function and decreased pain in the whole group.

Treadmill stress test

The treadmill stress test at the end of the four-week programme usually revealed an improvement in functional capacity. RST segment depression occurred at the same heart rate on both the admission and the discharge tests. With rare exceptions, however, this RST segment depression occurred at a higher work load during the discharge test. Although the RST changes still occurred at the same heart rate, in many patients the angina had gone, or only occurred significantly at a higher heart rate. Apart from the training effect of exercise, variables between the first and second tests were:

1. decreased drug therapy (Inderal and nitrates);
2. weight reduction;
3. psychological improvement: for instance a depressed and frightened patient at the initial test had been transformed into a happier individual eager to compete in the second test.

These variables led to considerable difficulty in interpreting the significance of the improvement in the treadmill data. Statistical data therefore are not reported here lest these should be deemed to measure accurately the degree of improvement. One of us (D. M.) desires to state that he never noted reversal in the positive electrocardiograph changes of the 797 patients from the first to the second stress tests, as interpreted by him.

Discussion

Decision to publish preliminary report

The Survey Research Service of the Biostatistics and Epidemiology Department of Loma Linda University collaborated with the Longevity Center in the evaluation of the four-week treatment of 893 primary patients who attended at least 21 consecutive days from April 1976 to October 1977.

This is a preliminary report, requested by the two editors, both of whom visited the Center during the years 1977, 1978 and 1979. It is hoped that the publication of the short-term results (Trowell, 1977; Mannerberg, 1979) will encourage controlled trials of the diet and exercise programme in the treatment of essential hypertension, angina and claudication, and eventually even in CHD prevention trials. In the past large controlled trials involving the reduction of CHD risk factors have only been initiated if preliminary trials, often inadequately planned and lacking a control group, have produced suggestive evidence. It might be objected that no report should be issued until data have been accumulated over the next five to ten years of CHD morbidity and mortality in the Longevity Center patients. On balance, a preliminary report, however, appears justified.

Objections can be advanced in the interpretation of this preliminary data. The Center's patients were not selected to study a single defined disease category; they were self-selected patients with cardiovascular degenerative diseases, often associated with hypertension, diabetes and obesity. But such is life; coronary heart disease is usually associated with this group of diseases. Actually CHD was detected in only 66 per cent of all patients, and those who had severe myocardial failure were not admitted. Data from the Center even of specified disease groups cannot readily be matched by data of a comparable control group; indeed it is impossible to obtain persons for a control group.

It is considered justifiable to publish this preliminary report on the short-term results for two reasons. First, the diet was unusual; second, the results were surprising. The CHD literature is replete with short-term dramatic changes in a few patients, usually followed with equally dramatic relapse, but no report has been traced concerning even the short-term response of a large number of persons to a diet similar to that eaten by the Longevity Center patients. No other therapeutic diet has been as low in cholesterol, total fat, saturated fat, sugar and salt, or as high in unrefined complex carbohydrates (starch) or dietary fibre. Again, although there are no data on long-term CHD morbidity and mortality, there are data concerning the clinical regression of essential hypertension, angina pectoris and intermittent claudication in over half of the patients on discharge. By clinical regression one signifies that symptoms of these diseases have disappeared, simple clinical assessment records no evidence of abnormality, and the patient has ceased the pharmacological treatment of this disease.

Metabolic ward studies and follow-up of maturity-onset diabetes mellitus patients who ate a similar diet, reported much remission of this disease (page 380); this occurred in the diabetic patients at the Center. Clinical trials in England of a slightly modified diet in patients suffering from hypertension and/or angina reported that the majority of patients showed very considerable improvement (page 411). No claims are made that atherosclerosis is reversed or that coronary heart disease is prevented or reversed, although the disappearance of angina pain during prolonged walking, in over half the patients (page 402), is of considerable interest.

United States Dietary Goals

Taking evidence from many research scientists the United States Senate Select Committee on Nutrition and Human Needs (1977) recommended changes in the US diet to *prevent* degenerative cardiovascular disease. It recommended:

1. lower energy intake;
2. in terms of daily energy percentages, increased consumption of complex carbohydrate (starch) from 22 to 48 by increasing high fibre whole grain products, tubers, vegetables and fruit;
3. decreased consumption of refined sugars from 18 to 10;
4. decreased consumption of total fat from 42 to 30, saturated fat from 16 to 10;
5. decreased consumption of meat, whole milk and eggs;
6. no change in total protein intake;
7. reduced dietary cholesterol from 500–800 mg/d (in an adult) to about 300 mg/d;
8. reduced salt intake from 12–16 g/d (in an adult) to 5 g/d.

The Longevity Center diet to aid *regression* of degenerative cardiovascular disease exaggerates all of these recommendations and actually anticipated their publication, because the consensus of modern nutritional research provides the basis of the US Dietary Goals published by the Senate Select Committee.

CHD risk factors and protective factors

It is a sober reflection that, after at least three decades of intensive research in the primary and secondary prevention of CHD, 'unequivocal evidence is not yet at hand that cardiac infarction can be prevented, life prolonged, or death delayed by any means including multi-factor risk reduction, pharmacologic, or surgical' (Blackburn, 1978). This might suggest that coronary atherosclerosis is almost unique as a disease process, that it is inherently progressive, or at least stationary, rarely reversible, but at the same time both a common and a life-threatening complaint. The body has mechanisms that decrease and protect against all common slowly developing diseases, even against certain forms of cancer. In the 1930s Kenya Africans who ate a diet (page 10) very similar to that of the Longevity Center; even its low salt content, had atherosclerosis of the aorta, but little in the coronary arteries and no case of coronary thrombosis or middle-age stroke was reported in the first thousand autopsies (Vint, 1936–37).

The Longevity Center regimen encourages four measures that are probably CHD protective factors.

1. Physical exercise, even in the presence of pain and disability, is encouraged, unless it appears dangerous, since it is regarded not merely as a rehabilitation procedure but as a CHD protective factor (Simko, 1978).
2. Dietary fibre intake is very high; it is regarded as a possible protective factor. Morris *et al.* (1977) observed 377 healthy men in London from 1956 to 1976. The third of this group who ate the most cereal fibre developed only one-fifth of clinical CHD (5 cases) in comparison with the third who ate the least cereal fibre (25 cases), although serum cholesterol levels were similar in the two groups.
3. The diet is very low sodium (NaCl 3·6 g/d), high potassium (KCl 6·2 g/d). There is considerable evidence that low sodium, high potassium diets are protective against hypertension in man and certain experimental animals (Meneely and Battarbee, 1976a, b). No report has been traced of the trial of low sodium diets in CHD prevention trials.
4. Plant protein *per se* may be a protective factor (page 396).

Regression of atherosclerosis

Reviews of the regression of atherosclerosis in man have usually remained sceptical of the significance of the regression of experimental lesions in the arteries of animals fed unnatural diets, rich in cholesterol and saturated fats (Editorial, 1977). Serial coronary angiograms in man have occasionally reported regression, even disappearance, of coronary artery obstruction, but it remains a rare phenomenon. The first report of regression of atherosclerosis in man in patients medically treated for hyperlipidaemia was made in a serial study of femoral arteriography in 25 patients aged 22–65 years. Of these patients, all of whom had partially obstructed femoral arteries, 16 had no symptoms, 9 patients had a history of angina and/or myocardial infarction; only one patient reported claudication pain. Thirteen patients had hypercholesterolaemia (Fredrickson type 2), 12 patients had hypertriglyceridaemia (Fredrickson type 4). Patients were treated by dietary changes, including moderate reduction of fat, and hypotensive drugs. After an average period of 13 months, 9 patients showed significant regression, 3 had no change, and 13 showed significant progression of femoral obstructive atherosclerosis. All those who showed regression showed significant fall of serum cholesterol levels, serum triglyceride levels, also systolic and diastolic blood pressure readings. This was the first report of regression of atherosclerosis in man linked to the treatment of hyperlipidaemia by medical therapy (Barndt *et al.*, 1977).

Biological norms in ageing adults

There is growing evidence to suggest that many of the biological norms of ageing Western adults are not the norms of health, but that they are average figures in a population already developing the first signs of degenerative disease. This is reflected in rising body weight, higher blood pressure levels, higher serum cholesterol (Wright, 1976) and triglyceride levels, decreased carbohydrate tolerance.

It is for this reason that at discharge Longevity Center patients are referred to their own physicians and are advised to adhere to the 'regression diet' until serum cholesterol levels are below 3·9 mmol/l (150 mg/dl) and serum triglycerides below 0·9 mmol/l (80 mg/dl). Patients are then allowed to continue on a 'maintenance diet' which allows a small increase of some lean animal products.

Adherence to the Longevity Center diet

There remains the question of long-term adherence to the unusual diet. Six-monthly monitoring of serum lipids, blood glucose, body weight and blood pressure and the help of the patient's own physician, plus enquiries about the diet, assess compliance with the dietary regimen. Adherence is probably higher in painful life-threatening diseases such as angina, especially if pain disappeared when eating the diet at the Center. It would prolong this chapter unduly to list dietary compliance with the various diseases present. Diabetes is selected as a disease which is not usually painful and in which adherence might be low.

A 12-month follow-up of 81 discharged diabetics was conducted from Loma Linda University by means of a structured telephone interview and a 24-hour dietary recall as well as a dietary and lifestyle questionnaire. It elicited the following data. Out of 81 patients 74 had a total fat consumption of less than 25 g/d, 80 had cholesterol intake less than 200 mg/d, of these 51 less than 50 mg/d. The recidivism rate of ex-smokers within one year was 30 per cent; this compared favourably with other studies averaging 75–80 per cent (Schwartz, 1977). Of former patients, 61 per cent exercised more than 30 minutes daily. The group's mean body weight during 26 days at the Center decreased from 78 to 74 kg (173 to 163 lb); at one year mean body weight had decreased further to 71 kg (157 lb). It was moving downwards towards the mean ideal body weight for medium frame, that is 66 kg (147 lb). Although some patients may have tried to present themselves in a favourable light to the interviewer, the adherence trends are most encouraging.

Controlled CHD prevention trial recommended

The ultimate test of an aggressive attack to decrease all CHD risk factors and to increase all CHD protective factors can be demonstrated only by long-term morbidity and mortality data; these data are being compiled slowly for former patients of the Longevity Center. In our opinion the short-term results appear to justify a controlled trial in the secondary prevention of CHD.

Acknowledgements

Hans Diehl wishes to acknowledge the UCLA Center for Health Enhancement for supporting his post-doctoral fellowship in the UCLA Division of Epidemiology during which time the literature review and writing of this chapter was carried out. He also acknowledges the contributions made by Mr. Hy Bregar of the Blum-Kovler Foundation, which were earmarked for this project. Thanks go to Raymond Neutra, MD, DrPH, and Mervyn Hardinge, MD, PhD, DrPH, for their support and interest, and to the staff of the Longevity Center for their cooperation.

References

Ahrens, E. H. Jr. (1974). Sucrose, hypertension and heart disease, an historical perspective. *American Journal of Clinical Nutrition*, **27**, 403–422

Ahrens, E. H. Jr. (1976). The management of hyperlipidemia: whether, rather than how. *Annals of Internal Medicine*, **85**, 87–93

Anderson, J. W. and Chen, W. L. (1979). Plant fiber. Carbohydrate and lipid metabolism. *American Journal of Clinical Nutrition*, **32**, 346–363

Barndt, R., Blankenhorn, D. H. and Crawford, D. W. (1977). Regression and progression of early femoral atherosclerosis in treated hyperlipoproteinemic patients. *Annals of Internal Medicine*, **86**, 139–146

Bennion, L. J. and Grundy, S. M. (1978). Risk factors for the development of cholelithiasis in man (Second of Two Parts). *New England Journal of Medicine*, **299**, 1221–1227

Blackburn, H. (1978). The potential for preventing reinfarction. In: *Rehabilitation of the Coronary Patient*, 73. Editors N. K. Wenger and H. K. Hellerstein. Wiley, New York

Borhani, N. O. (1977). Primary prevention of coronary heart disease. *American Journal of Cardiology*, **40**, 251–259

Brewster, L. and Jacobsen, M. F. (1978). *The Changing American Diet*. Center for Science in the Public Interest, Washington, DC

Carroll, K. K. (1975). Experimental evidence of dietary factors and hormone-dependent cancers. *Cancer Research*, **35**, 3374–3383

Coronary Drug Project Research Group (1975). Clofibrate and niacin in coronary heart disease. *Journal of the American Medical Association*, **231**, 360–381

Editorial (1977). Regression of atheroma. *British Medical Journal*, **2**, 1–2

Editorial (1978). *British Medical Journal*, **2**, 1585–1586

Freis, E. D. (1976). Salt, volume and the prevention of hypertension. *Circulation*, **53**, 589–597

Hamilton, R. M. G. and Carroll, K. K. (1976). Effects of dietary protein from different sources upon plasma cholesterol levels in rabbits fed low fat, low cholesterol diet. *Atherosclerosis*, **24**, 47–62

Hellerstein, H. K. and Franklin, B. A. (1978). Exercise testing and prescription. In: *Rehabilitation of the Coronary Patient*. Editors N. K. Wenger and H. K. Hellerstein. Wiley, New York

Iacono, J. M., Marshall, M. W. and Dougherty, R. M. (1975). Reduction in blood pressure with polyunsaturated fat diets that reduce blood pressure in man. *Preventive Medicine,* 4, 426–443

Magnani, B., Ambrosioni, E., Agosta, R. and Racco, F. (1976). Comparison of the effects of pharmacological therapy and low sodium diet on mild hypertension. *Clinical Science and Molecular Medicine,* 51, 625–626

Mannerberg, D. (1979). Rehabilitation of cardiovascular diseases in a USA Centre. *Chest, Heart and Stroke Journal,* 3, 62–65

Meneely, G. R. and Battarbee, H. D. (1967a). High sodium—low potassium environment and hypertension. *American Journal of Cardiology,* 38, 768–785

Meneely, G. R. and Battarbee, H. D. (1976b). Sodium and potassium. In: *Nutrition Reviews' Present Knowledge in Nutrition,* 4th edition, 258. Nutrition Foundation, New York

Morgan, T., Gillies, A., Morgan, G., Adam, W., Wilson, M. and Carney, S. (1978). Hypertension treated by salt restriction. *Lancet,* i, 227–230

Morris, J. N., Marr, J. W. and Clayton, D. G. (1977). Diet and heart: a postscript. *British Medical Journal,* 2, 1307–1314

Passamani, E. R., Frommer, P. L. and Levy, R. I. (1978). Coronary heart disease: an overview. In: *Rehabilitation of the Coronary Patient.* Editors N. K. Wenger and H. K. Hellerstein. Wiley, New York

Pinckney, E. R. (1973). The potential toxicity of excessive polyunsaturates (editorial). *American Heart Journal,* 85, 723–726

Pritikin, N. (1976). Carbohydrates—maligned and misunderstood. *Journal of Applied Nutrition,* 28, 56–68

Reisen, E., Abel, R., Modan, M., Silverberg, D. S., Eliahou, H. E. and Modan, B. (1978). Effect of weight loss without salt restriction on the reduction of blood pressure in overweight hypertensive patients. *New England Journal of Medicine,* 298, 1–6

Rifkind, B. M. and Levy, R. I. (1978). Testing the lipid hypothesis. *Archives of Surgery,* 113, 80–83

Sacks, F. M., Castelli, W. P., Donner, A. and Kass, E. R. (1975). Plasma lipids and lipoproteins in vegetarians and controls. *New England Journal of Medicine,* 292, 1148–1151

Schwartz, J. L. (1977). In: *Research in Smoking Behavior,* Research Monograph 17, US Department of Health, Education and Welfare. Public Health Service, Washington, DC

Simko, V. (1978). Physical exercise and the prevention of atherosclerosis and gallstones. *Postgraduate Medical Journal,* 54, 270–277

Stamler, J. (1978). Lifestyles, major risk factors, proof and public policy. *Circulation,* 58, 3–19

Trowell, H. (1977). Cardiovascular disease and fibre. *Chest, Heart and Stroke Journal,* 2, 3–7

Turpeinen, O. (1979). Effect of cholesterol-lowering diet on mortality from coronary heart disease and other causes. *Circulation,* 59, 1–7

United States Senate Select Committee on Nutrition and Human Needs (1977). *Dietary Goals for the United States,* second edition. US Government Printing Office, Washington, DC

Vint, F. W. (1936–37). Postmortem findings in the natives of Kenya. *East African Medical Journal,* **13,** 332–340

Wiggers, K. D., Richard, M. J. and Stewart, J. W. (1977). Type and amount of dietary fat affect relative concentration of cholesterol in blood and other tissue of rats. *Atherosclerosis,* **27,** 27–34

Wissler, R. W. and Vesselinovitch, D. (1977). Regression of atherosclerosis in experimental animals and man. *Modern Concepts of Cardiovascular Disease,* **46,** 27–32

Wright, I. S. (1976). Correct levels of serum cholesterol. Average vs normal vs optimal (editorial). *Journal of the American Medical Association,* **236,** 261–262

24

Hypertension and angina

Paul Dodson and Daphne Humphreys

Dietary treatment of hypertension

The first diet employed by many investigators to treat essential hypertension was the rice–fruit diet of Kempner (1945). Blood pressure fell in about 70 per cent of patients, but even at the end of one month's treatment diastolic blood pressure often remained over 100 mmHg. Several reports confirmed these results in the United States and Britain. Analysis of the average adult diet for a day reported very low sodium, 5 mmol (NaCl 0·3 g) (Medical Research Council Report, 1950). In recent years adult requirements of sodium per day have been stated to be about 8 mmol (NaCl 0·5 g) (Meneely and Battarbee, 1976). At the end of one month's treatment Kempner's patients were in a state of sodium *depletion*, reflected in patients reporting that the diet was intolerable, insipid, in fact uneatable. It is impossible to provide this very low sodium diet if ordinary market foods are obtained.

These diets were therefore abandoned, especially when soon afterwards potent antihypertensive drugs were discovered. Misgivings must, however, be entertained concerning whether it is safe for a fair proportion of the population to take these potent drugs for many years. Possibly the dietary treatment of essential hypertension should be re-explored, if only to supplement drug therapy (Editorial, 1978). This journal also referred to the theory that essential hypertension might be a disease caused by excessive salt intake; this may affect salt-sensitive individuals while the majority apparently suffer no ill effect. Western diets provide daily for an adult sodium intake of 100–300 mmol (NaCl 6–18 g). Sodium is the only essential nutrient taken by man in 10–30 times the normal requirement; perhaps not everyone can adapt to this load of sodium.

During the past 30 years an increasing number of epidemiological studies of primitive populations have reported that blood pressure did not rise with age so that essential hypertension was very rare. Whenever it has proved possible to ascertain the salt content of their diets it has been reported that they added little or no salt to their food; their adult diets contained per day sodium 16–48 mmol (NaCl 1–5 g) (Gliebermann, 1973; Connor *et al.*, 1978; Trowell, 1978).

411

Blood pressure levels fell in hypertensive patients when daily sodium intake was reduced from 200 mmol (NaCl 12 g) to 75 mmol (NaCl 5 g) (Parijs *et al.*, 1971) and recent experiments emphasize that hypertensive patients vary considerably in their response to decreased intake of sodium. This led Kawasaki *et al.* (1978) to classify hypertensive patients into two groups, those who were salt-sensitive and those who were not salt-sensitive. They reported that blood pressure fell in *both* groups when daily sodium intake was reduced from that of an 'average' diet, 100 mmol (NaCl 6 g), to a low sodium 9 mmol (NaCl 0·6 g) diet. The salt-sensitive group blood pressure fell more than that of the non-salt-sensitive group. As these results were achieved in 7 days, it is possible that blood pressure might fall in some hypertensive patients even if sodium intake is reduced less drastically from 'average' levels to 50–70 mmol/d but for a longer period of time. This proposal provided the basis of the dietary treatment of hypertension that is about to be reported.

The diets of the primitive groups among whom blood pressure does not rise with age differ significantly from Western diets not only in being low sodium. Primitive diets are usually low fat, 10–25 per cent energy, high unrefined starch, 50–70 per cent energy, high dietary fibre, 30–50 g/d, and the potassium : sodium ratio is often over 1. Primitive populations, eating these diets and remaining physically active, seldom become obese (Van Itallie, 1978). Possibly a diet designed to treat hypertension should incorporate all, or many, of these features.

Morgan *et al.* (1978) have reported from an Australian out-patient hypertension clinic that a small but significant fall of blood pressure occurred in previously untreated patients suffering from mild hypertension, supine diastolic blood pressure 95–109 mmHg. Patients had been advised moderate salt restriction to sodium 70–100 mmol/d (NaCl 4·4–6·2 g/d) in their daily diet over a period of two years and had been compared with a control group who received no treatment or change of diet and with two other groups treated by different hypertensive drugs. At the beginning of the study all patients had a mean intake of sodium 191 ± 5 mmol/d (NaCl 12 g/d), range 50–400 mmol/d (NaCl 3–25 g/d). (Actually these figures of sodium intake were assessed from estimation of the urinary sodium for 24 hours.) Many of the patients advised a restricted sodium intake did not comply and their mean sodium intake fell only from 191 to 157 mmol/d (NaCl from 12 to 10 g/d). In spite of this meagre reduction of sodium intake the mean blood pressure of this group fell 7·3 mmHg during the two years of observation and 55 per cent of these patients slowly reached a diastolic blood pressure below 95 mmHg. The Australian physicians therefore recommended that any new patient presenting with diastolic blood pressure between 90 and 105 mmHg should be advised to reduce sodium intake to 70 mmol/d (NaCl 4·4 g/d).

Early in 1978 our attention was directed to a preliminary report from the Longevity Center, Santa Barbara (Trowell, 1977; Mannerberg, 1979). Hypertensive in-patients, many of whom had coronary heart disease, were treated by a low sodium diet, sodium 60 mmol/d (NaCl 3·7 g/d). Out of 218 *treated* hypertensive patients on admission 186, that is 85 per cent, were discharged 26 days later with mean diastolic blood pressure of 73 mmHg and had ceased all antihypertensive drugs. Angina also had disappeared in many patients.

The Longevity Center diet (page 397) resembled in its composition that of the Kenya Kikuyu in 1930 (Orr and Gilks, 1931). At that time Kenya Highland African blood pressure did not rise with age, essential hypertension was not reported, neither was coronary heart disease or angina (Vint, 1936–37; Trowell, 1978). East Africans subsequently adopted partially westernized diets, they started adding shop salt to their food, and hypertension is now common among them. Other features of the Longevity Center diet, and the 1930 Kenya Highland African diet, would probably prove unpalatable to English patients, for both contained little fat, sugar, cholesterol, and meat. A compromise diet was planned for hypertensive outpatients of the Royal Berkshire Hospital, Reading.

Patients, diet and methods

Patients

Thirty-two patients, already diagnosed and treated for essential hypertension by us (P. M. D. and D. M. H.), 24 men and 8 women, mean age 51 years, were selected for a trial of the dietary treatment of hypertension. They were recruited from the out-patients of the Royal Berkshire Hospital, Reading, because all of them still had supine diastolic blood pressure $\geqslant 90$ mmHg in spite of many months, even years, of treatment by drugs. Their supine diastolic blood pressure mean ($\pm$s.d.) was 98·3 ($\pm 8\cdot2$) mmHg. Every patient attending the clinic who had this level of supine diastolic blood pressure was regarded as a potential candidate. Those only were interviewed for recruitment who were considered to be those who would cooperate faithfully with a major change of diet. All gave informed consent after explanation of the diet.

In addition 11 angina patients were recruited for dietary treatment with the same diet. In addition they were encouraged to increase physical exercise by walking, as described shortly. Four of these 11 patients also had hypertension, so that 39 patients in all ate an experimental therapeutic diet.

Diet

With the aid of the hospital dietitian the diet was planned of which the mean features were that it would be low sodium, high potassium, low fat, high unrefined fibre-rich starch, low sugar. Although the menu sheets specified the recommended daily amounts of foods, all eaten at home, it is considered advisable to publish the probable range of food intake eaten by the average patient rather than a single mean figure. Overweight patients were encouraged to lose weight slowly, rarely more than 1 kg (2·2 lb) per month, by decreasing slightly the amount of food eaten. A few actually gained weight and details are given later.

The daily diet usually provided sodium 40–50 mmol (NaCl 2·5–3·5 g), potassium 80–90 mmol (KCl 6·0–6·7 g), K:Na ratio 1:0·5; daily energy 6·5–7·4 MJ (1600–1800 kcal), derived from protein 10–13 per cent, fat 15–20 per cent, starch 50–60 per cent, sugars 5–10 per cent, dietary fibre 30–35 g, cholesterol 500–600 mg. A detailed diet programme of meal menus, and recommended amounts of food at each meal, also a table of the sodium content per recommended portion of food, was issued by the doctor and explained to each patient. A list of forbidden heavily salted foods was issued and discussed.

Efforts were made to encourage a low sodium intake. It proved impossible to be certain that all urine passed during 24 hours would be collected by an out-patient, so attempts to secure analysis of urines, and thus an estimate of sodium intake, were abandoned. Patients were informed that the blood examination, obtained at every re-attendance, would provide a check of compliance with the prescribed diet. Patients were advised to add no salt during cooking or at table. A potassium-rich 'salt substitute' was recommended; this may have raised daily potassium intake to 100 mmol (potassium chloride 7·0 g). Heavily salted foods were forbidden, such as bacon, ham, sausages, tinned meat, fish and soup, also salted smoked fish, pickles, sauces, Bovril, Oxo, Marmite, salted peanuts and potato crisps. All tinned foods, except tinned fruits, were forbidden. Cheese, once weekly, was discouraged apart from low sodium cottage cheese. Wholemeal bread, plain biscuits, rye crispbread and skim milk, all containing moderate sodium, were permitted. Unsalted butter, although on the diet sheet, was discouraged, instead low fat margarine was recommended.

Fat was considerably reduced to about half of the customary amount, it provided 15–20 per cent of energy. The daily menu allowed low fat margarine 30 g (1 oz); also skim milk 350 ml (⅔ pint) for the breakfast cereal, tea and coffee. Low fat meats, such as chicken, also fish, were encouraged; all meat should be lean and visible fat should be cut away. Meat and fish should not be fried, but grilled, baked, stewed or boiled. Fatty meats were to be avoided, such as bacon, lamb, duck, goose, sausages and pâté. Full-fat cheese was allowed only occasionally, cake and pastry were not permitted. Ice cream, unless the low energy variety, was discouraged. Up to one egg was allowed daily.

Fibre-rich wholemeal bread and wholewheat breakfast cereals, to which hard wheat bran 25 g (1 oz) was added, potatoes and rye crispbread, were all encouraged; brown rice and pasta were also encouraged in the usual amount. Vegetables and fruit were eaten freely. Alcoholic drinks in moderation were allowed. Ordinary meals, and between-meals cups of coffee or tea with a plain biscuit, were taken as had been customary. On admission only two patients were smokers.

Methods

Patients were selected for the dietary trial from March 1978 until May 1979; three months later became the end of the period of observation, the results of which are presented in this communication. The group remains, however, still under observation and treatment. Patients attended usually every fortnight. They were weighed and blood pressures, systolic and diastolic at the 5th Korotkoff phase, were measured on a single mercury sphygmomanometer both in the supine and standing positions, usually by one doctor (P. M. D.), the other one (D. M. H.) assisting if the clinic was too busy. If blood pressure had fallen a reduction of antihypertensive drug dosage was considered.

Results

Hypertension

Improved control of blood pressure was achieved in 25 out of the 32 hypertensive patients during the period of observation, which lasted for a minimum period of three months up to a maximum of one year, with a mean of six months (Table 24.1). In 12 patients drug therapy was completely withdrawn because supine diastolic blood pressure, recorded on several occasions, was below 90 mmHg. All those who stopped antihypertensive drug therapy did so within three months. In 7 other patients drug therapy was considerably reduced, but not discontinued, as the supine diastolic blood pressure, although reduced, was seldom below 90 mmHg. In 6 other patients drug therapy had been substantially reduced but supine diastolic blood pressure remained about the same as at entry. In 7 other patients there was no significant change in drug therapy dosage or in supine diastolic blood pressure readings (Dodson, 1980).

The group of 32 hypertensive patients on entry to the dietary treatment took a total of 136 beta-blocker tablets daily, at the end of the period of observation the total number had fallen to 24 tablets daily.

Table 24.1 Diastolic blood pressure, supine and standing, during dietary treatment, mean levels mmHg

Time	At entry[1]	3 months	6 months	9 months	At end[2]
Supine	98·3	86·1	83·5	85·0	84·8
±s.d.	8·2	9·0	8·3	8·2	7·0
Standing	104·7	90·6	92·0	91·5	90·6
±s.d.	8·7	9·0	8·2	6·6	8·2
Number of patients	32	32	23	13	32

[1] Mean of all recordings during preceding 6–12 months, while under treatment with antihypertensive drugs
[2] Mean of all recordings at end of period of observation, many patients receiving reduced drug dosage or taking no drugs

Out of 32 hypertensive patients, 28 lost body weight, mean loss 5·9 kg (13 lb); in them supine diastolic blood pressure reduction averaged 12·6 (s.d. ± 8·2) mmHg. Four other patients gained weight, mean increase 2·5 kg (5·5 lb): their supine diastolic blood pressure reduction averaged 11·5 (s.d. ±7·9) mmHg.

Angina

Eleven patients, ten men and one woman, mean age 56 years, had been treated in the out-patient clinic for angina pectoris for at least six months, often for more than a year. They were recruited for the dietary trial in a manner similar to that used in the hypertension group. Four of the angina patients had been treated also for hypertension and their blood pressure results are included in those already presented. The angina group of patients was recommended to eat the same diet as that eaten by the hypertension group. In addition the angina patients were encouraged to increase physical exercise by walking several times daily within the limits of anginal pain. From day to day they also increased the length of the distance walked if improvement had occurred.

The first priority of treatment of the angina patients was the increase of exercise tolerance while reducing the number and severity of the angina attacks. When these objectives began to be realized the dosage of the angina drugs was slowly decreased. Within a month every patient had more than doubled his exercise tolerance.

Seven angina patients became completely free of all anginal pain even while walking 3 or more miles daily. In the other four patients the frequency and severity of the angina attacks decreased considerably and they were able to walk 0·5–2 miles daily. The glyceryl trinitrate tablets of the group decreased from 20 tablets daily on entry to 10 tablets daily at the end. Members of the group had almost ceased to take all other angina tablets. Five patients were able to discontinue thiazide diuretics prescribed previously for left ventricular failure following myocardial infarction; a sixth patient was able to halve the dosage. Beta-blocker drugs, taken for the associated hypertension, were reduced in this group from 32 tablets to 19 tablets daily. This reduction was not as large as that in the uncomplicated hypertension group, but therapy had been directed primarily to the relief of angina. In one patient suffering from severe angina and intermittent claudication, drug therapy remained unchanged but the patient's exercise tolerance increased over a period of three months from 300–800 yards; after even this exertion the angina pain was classified as mild.

Case History

Mr. F. J. aged 63 was admitted to hospital in 1970 with central retrosternal chest pain and a diagnosis of myocardial infarction was made. In October 1977, antihypertensive therapy with oxprenolol 80 mg thrice daily and

Navidrex-K one in the morning was commenced, but in January 1978 he developed increasing angina and was admitted to hospital and treated for a further myocardial infarction. Blood pressure on admission was 190/120 and subsequently at follow-up in May 1978 was 170/100 on clonidine 0·1 mg twice daily, oxyprenolol 80 mg thrice daily, bumetanide once daily and metolazone 5 mg in the morning. After January 1978 he was able to walk only 440 yards before developing severe angina and shortness of breath despite thiazide diuretics and beta-blockade. He entered the trial in June 1978, and after one month all drug therapy was withdrawn and he was able to walk 2 miles before the onset of anginal pain. After two months on the dietary regimen he was able to walk 4 miles free from angina despite variable blood pressure control. In March 1979 he is still free from angina, his blood pressure well controlled at 150/90 and he is now an active man.

Discussion

Dietary acceptance and adherence

Initially patients found the diet uninteresting and lacking in flavour. Patients attended at first at least every fortnight and they were encouraged to persevere with the diet. After about a month most patients became accustomed to the diet; they had improved physically, were taking more exercise, and appetite was keener. They recognized that the diet had improved their illness and that drug dosage was dropping and side effects were decreasing. Some patients not only became accustomed to the new diet, they even positively developed a dislike of salty foods.

It is difficult to see how a control series could have been recruited. We had previously treated unsuccessfully all patients for several months; then it became obvious that unexpected beneficial results were occurring in the large majority of diet-treated patients. It was not considered advisable, or indeed ethical, to randomize future potential candidates into a control group who would continue to be treated unsuccessfully, and a second group who would receive the beneficial dietary treatment.

Instead there were the previous records of unsuccessful treatment of our patients to be compared with the subsequent dietary treatment period. At the end of three months all patients were asked to resume their former diet, which some still considered to have been in certain respects more tasty. In this way patients would become their own controls. However, only 2 out of 39 hypertension and angina patients agreed to do so. The other 37 patients firmly declined because of marked improvement in their symptoms, general well-being, and they were glad to be taking fewer drugs. One of these two dissenting patients was an adult coeliac who, being on a gluten-free diet, eventually found the restrictions intolerable. While taking the new therapeutic diet her blood pressure had dropped from a previous average reading of 175/105 to 152/92 mmHg with total withdrawal of previous antihypertension therapy, clonidine 0·1 mg every morning and oxyprenolol 80 mg thrice daily. The second of these two dissenting patients had become free from angina after eating the therapeutic diet for three months, but then he resumed his previous diet during a period of family difficulties, and his angina returned after a period of two weeks. The two groups total of 39 patients is still being observed and treated to ascertain the degree of long-term adherence to the diet.

Regression of hypertension

The low sodium intake of 40–50 mmol/d (NaCl 2·5–3·5 g/d) is regarded as the essential recognized therapeutic factor in the antihypertension diet. On entry mean supine diastolic blood pressure was 98·3 (s.d. ± 8·2) mmHg. At the end of the period of observation, mean duration 6 months, this level had fallen to 84·8 (s.d. ± 7·0) mmHg, and 25 out of 32 patients (78 per cent) had achieved improved blood pressure control. Twelve patients (37 per cent) had achieved normal supine diastolic blood pressure and had ceased all anti-hypertension drugs; 13 patients (41 per cent) had considerably decreased drug dosage, half of these with a significant fall of blood pressure; 7 patients (22 per cent) showed no improvement.

It is impossible to compare these results with those achieved at the Longevity Center, Santa Barbara (page 400). There on admission some 218 hypertensive patients all treated previously by antihypertensive drugs had a mean diastolic blood pressure of 77 mmHg; 186 patients (85 per cent) were discharged after 26 days' dietary treatment with normal diastolic blood pressure mean of 73 mmHg, all of them having ceased antihypertensive drugs. Their diet had averaged sodium 60 mmol/d (NaCl 3·7 g/d). These patients had desired treatment for a wide variety of degenerative cardiovascular diseases, chiefly coronary heart disease: the Royal Berkshire Hospital patients were selected because their blood pressure had *not* been normalized by drugs. Experience in both institutions suggest that sodium intake in an adult of 40–60 mmol/d (NaCl 2·5–3·8 g/d) will probably normalize diastolic blood pressure in a large proportion of essential hypertension patients.

No report has been traced in the medical literature of a long-term trial of moderately low sodium diets, sodium 40–80 mmol/d (NaCl 2·5–5·0 g/d). The only trial that approximated to this low sodium intake was that of Parijs *et al.* (1971), who gave sodium 93 mmol/d (NaCl 5·6 g/d) to 22 essential hypertension out-patients for 28 days and found a moderate significant decrease of mean diastolic blood pressure of 4·4 mmHg. They remarked: 'It remains to be established if this trend will increase or decrease over longer periods of time.' This small decrease of diastolic blood pressure, compared with considerable decrease among Royal Berkshire Hospital and Longevity Center patients, suggests that other antihypertensive factors operated in the latter two dietary trials.

Meneely and Battarbee (1976) have summarized evidence that potassium may be a protective factor against experimental salt-induced hypertension in certain animals. There has been little investigation of this dietary factor in human hypertension. Western diets have a K:Na ratio of about 1:2. The diets of primitive populations among whom blood pressure does not rise with age have a K : Na ratio of 1 : 0·5, and the Royal Berkshire Hospital diet K : Na ratio was 1 : 0·5. Potassium intake by the Royal Berkshire Hospital patients of 80–90 mmol/d (KCl 6·0–6·7 g/d) was towards the upper level of intake present in many Western diets, but whether potassium acted as a protective factor in the Royal Berkshire Hospital diets remains an open question.

There is a relationship of obesity to hypertension. Most of our patients lost weight, but blood pressure fell as much among the minority who gained weight (page 416). A recent trial of weight-reducing diets for hypertension, by referral to a dietitian, reported far less reduction of blood pressure after attempting to follow a diet providing only 3·3 MJ (800 kcals) for a year (Ramsay *et al.*, 1978). In our opinion our patients seldom ate less than 6·0 MJ (1500 kcals)/d, but blood pressure fell far more than in those eating diets which provided only about half this energy.

Does low sodium intake alone explain the truly surprising results? It is hoped that future work, assaying first the blood pressure response to the *whole* diet, will determine the response of hypertension under more sophisticated conditions. If confirmed, it should be possible subsequently to determine the role of different factors in the diet, even the role of exercise.

Acknowledgements

The authors would like to thank Mrs. O. Patrick (Hospital Dietitian) for her help in preparation of the dietary formulation, and the Staff of Loddon Ward (Royal Berkshire Hospital) for their considerable assistance with this work.

References

Connor, W. E., Cerqueira, M. T., Connor, R. W., Wallace, R. B., Malinow, M. R. and Casdorph, H. R. (1978). The plasma lipids, lipoproteins and diet of Tarahumara Indians of Mexico. *American Journal of Clinical Nutrition,* **31,** 1131–1142

Dodson, P. M. (1980). Dietary fibre, sodium and potassium. *British Medical Journal,* **1,** 564. Correction, 720

Editorial (1978). Hypertension—salt-poisoning? *Lancet,* **i,** 1136–1137

Gliebermann, L. (1973). Blood pressure and dietary salt in human populations. *Ecology of Food and Nutrition,* **2,** 143–156

Kawasaki, T., Delea, C. S., Bartter, F. C. and Smith, H. (1978). The effect of high-sodium and low-sodium intakes on blood pressure and other related variables in human subjects with idiopathic hypertension. *American Journal of Medicine,* **64,** 193–198

Kempner, W. (1945). Compensation of renal metabolic dysfunction. Treatment of kidney disease and hypertensive vascular disease with rice diet. *North Carolina Medical Journal,* **6,** 61–87

Mannerberg, D. (1979). Rehabilitation of cardiovascular disease in a USA center. *Chest, Heart and Stroke Journal,* **3,** 62–65

Medical Research Council Report (1950). The rice diet in the treatment of hypertension. *Lancet,* **ii,** 509–513

Meneely, G. R. and Battarbee, H. D. (1976). Sodium and potassium. In: *Nutrition Reviews' Present Knowledge in Nutrition,* fourth edition. Nutrition Foundation, New York

Morgan, T., Adam, W., Gillies, A., Wilson, M., Morgan, G. and Carney, S. (1978). Hypertension treated by salt restriction. *Lancet,* **i,** 227–230

Orr, J. B. and Gilks, J. L. (1931). *The Physique and Health of Two African Tribes.* Special Report Series Medical Research Council, No. 155. Her Majesty's Stationery Office, London

Parijs, J., Joosens, J. V., der Linden, L. V., Verstreken, G. and Amery, A. K. P. C. (1971). Moderate salt restriction and diuretics in the treatment of hypertension. *American Heart Journal,* **85,** 22–34

Ramsay, L. E., Ramsay, M. H., Hettiarachchi, J., Davies, D. L. and Winchester, J. (1978). Weight reduction in the blood pressure clinic. *British Medical Journal,* **2,** 244–245

Trowell, H. C. (1977). Cardiovascular diseases and fibre. *Chest, Heart and Stroke Journal,* **2,** 3–7

Trowell, H. C. (1978). Hypertension and salt (letter). *Lancet,* **ii,** 204

Van Itallie, T. B. (1978). Dietary fiber and obesity. *American Journal of Clinical Nutrition,* **31,** S34–S52

Vint, F. W. (1936–37). Post-mortem findings in the natives of Kenya. *East African Medical Journal,* **13,** 332–340

25

Haemorrhoids, diverticular disease and deep vein thrombosis

Conrad Latto

Introduction

In 1971, following the reading of Surgeon-Captain Cleave's book *The Saccharine Disease* (Cleave *et al*., 1969), a clinical trial of the use of wheat bran was undertaken in a surgical ward at the Royal Berkshire Hospital, Reading. It was undertaken initially to determine whether its use diminished the incidence of postoperative constipation and deep vein thrombosis. The patients in an eighteen-bed, mainly urological, surgical ward were given bran, one heaped tablespoonful three times a day (wheat bran 50 g/d, dietary fibre 22 g/d), both preoperatively and postoperatively if the patients were able to take it.

This resulted in a rapid reduction of the incidence of postoperative constipation and as a result its use was soon adopted in most medical and surgical wards of the hospital. In addition, it became the standard treatment for uncomplicated diverticular disease and all the gastroenterologists soon advocated its use. It was not long before the message reached the general practitioners, some of whom became very enthusiastic, and the 'Bran Wave' rapidly burst over the community.

At a conservative estimate over 20 000 patients have been treated in hospital with bran, many taking it regularly even after discharge. A considerable number have adopted a diet rich in cereal fibre and often including wholemeal bread. In addition, a great number of non-patients, influenced by the widespread publicity, are now adding bran to their food and/or taking high fibre breakfast cereals.

Haemorrhoids

Experience in the Royal Berkshire Hospital in the management of haemorrhoids by bulking agents, in this case by bran, has been similar to that described by Webster *et al* (1978). First degree haemorrhoids have responded well and have seldom required injections. Although patients with second degree haemorrhoids have obtained considerable symptomatic relief, bran treatment has had little place in the management of those of third degree, apart from the relief of any associated constipation.

A review has been undertaken of the use of high fibre diets in the management of haemorrhoids by five other surgeons in the United Kingdom; this showed marked variation in the mode of management. The five standard methods of treating haemorrhoids—injections, banding, anal dilatation, cryosurgery and the St. Mark's ligation–excision operation—were all used. Personal communications from five surgeons, Frohn, M. J. (1976), Painter, N. S. (1975), Tovey, F. I. (1978), Burkitt, D. P. (1978) and Brodribb, A. J. M. (1978), state that all have modified their indications for surgery as a result of the introduction of bran. They all consider that the majority of first degree haemorrhoids can be satisfactorily dealt with by this alone, injections only very occasionally being required. Second degree haemorrhoids were dealt with by one or other of the standard surgical procedures listed above.

Following any of these procedures all the surgeons included bran in their postoperative management and are convinced that this improved the results of treatment. Although four of the five surgeons use the standard St. Mark's operation for third degree haemorrhoids, the number of these operations performed per annum has been considerably reduced.

A review of the effect of the massive introduction of bran and high fibre foods on the frequency of haemorrhoidectomy in the Reading community has also been undertaken. From 1970 to early 1978 the six general surgeons in the Royal Berkshire Hospital, Reading, used with few exceptions only two methods of treatment, injections or the St. Mark's operation. In 1978 banding and maximal anal dilatation were introduced widely. The waiting lists of all six surgeons have remained virtually without patients with haemorrhoids, suggesting that there is no hidden group of untreated patients. During the years 1970–77 the annual number of haemorrhoidectomy operations fell from 178 to 98, a reduction of 42 per cent. This reduction may well represent the effect of high fibre foods being used increasingly in the community. It might reflect a reduction in the incidence of the disease, or the conferring of sufficient symptomatic relief to render hospital treatment no longer necessary.

Diverticular disease

Since 1971 this disease has normally been treated with bran, other bulking agents being prescribed only occasionally. This has radically altered the management, surgical resection being rarely required except for complications which now seldom occur. In 1970 one resection for this disease was performed on average every two weeks, but now only one is performed each year.

Several hundred cases of diverticular disease are currently being treated with bran and high fibre diets. Since 1971 only one patient thus treated has been admitted to hospital with a surgical complication, rectal haemorrhage, presumed due to diverticular disease. Since the introduction of bran on a massive scale to the Reading and Berkshire community the number of admissions for perforated diverticulitis and peritonitis has fallen by half, from 16 to 8 per year. It would appear that a reduction in the incidence of surgical complications of diverticular disease is beginning to occur.

Several studies have been recorded from the Royal Berkshire Hospital. Brodribb and Humphreys (1976) reported symptomatic relief and a reduction in intracolonic pressures and normalization of transit times in 88 per cent of 40 patients after six months' treatment. Metabolic studies in these patients showed minimal significant changes apart from a slight fall in oral glucose tolerance curves.

Deep vein thrombosis and pulmonary embolism

During visits to many hospitals in Equatorial Africa and India during 1971–72 numerous clinicians were questioned regarding their experience of postoperative deep vein thrombosis (DVT) and pulmonary embolism (PE). All agreed that clinically manifest DVT was rare and that fatal PE was very rare even in elderly persons after major operations such as prostatectomy. Dhall *et al.* (1976) reported from Nairobi, Kenya, that 'the risk of thrombo-embolism in Africans is many times lower than in American negroes . . . (but) there has been a steady increase in the incidence of pulmonary embolism over the last decade'. The epidemiology of DVT and PE has been summarized by Burkitt (1972), who related a high incidence of both diseases to a low intake of dietary fibre which was postulated to be a cause of constipation, haemorrhoids, varicose veins and DVT.

It was therefore decided to record all cases of clinically manifest DVT and PE in a surgical ward of the Royal Berkshire Hospital, in which all patients were being asked to take, if possible, wheat bran 40–50 g/d after admission; a few had been taking it prior to admission. The investigation was planned in two stages. Initially the hospital records reported only clinically manifest DVT and PE, no special attempt being made to examine all patients for calf tenderness and oedema. The surgical ward had a large number of middle-aged and elderly men undergoing high risk surgical operations such as open prostatectomy. Over a six-year period only one case of clinically diagnosed DVT and no case of PE had been recorded in the hospital notes of this surgical ward.

It was subsequently recognized that many minor cases of DVT and small PE were not being recorded. To obtain a more accurate estimate of the effect of bran on the prevalence of DVT a prospective investigation employing ^{125}I-labelled fibrinogen was undertaken. Fifty patients, the majority of whom had had open prostatectomy operations, were tested for DVT by ^{125}I-labelled fibrinogen. Positive calf signs, indicating the presence of DVT, were detected in 22 per cent of patients, but in the majority of these positive signs were transient and disappeared within 48 hours. This would suggest that, although postoperative DVT occurred in nearly a quarter of the patients, the clots were probably small and were resolved rapidly by fibrinolysis (Latto, 1979). In this small series of 50 patients none developed any clinical signs of DVT, such as oedema, or any leg pain.

Following these preliminary studies it is hoped to undertake a more extensive controlled clinical trial in which more data on DVT will be collected and the blood will be examined for any factor such as hypercoagulability and fibrinolytic activity which might influence the incidence, severity, duration and complications of DVT. Brisk fibrinolysis has been reported in Africans and New Guineans and it has been suggested that this might be due to their high fibre diets (Trowell, 1975).

Speaking as a practical surgeon one can only ask for a thorough investigation of this apparently simple prophylactic measure. Other surgeons such as Frohn (1976) and Blacklock and Jameson (personal communication, 1978) report equally gratifying results in large series of surgical cases treated by them with bran.

Cleave, Campbell and Painter (1969) studied the epidemiology of haemorrhoids, deep vein thrombosis and pulmonary embolism; they suggested that these surgical disorders were due to constipation caused by a low intake of fibre. Painter contributed a chapter on diverticular disease to the book; subsequently he published his pioneer studies of the treatment of this disorder with high fibre wheat bran (Painter, 1975).

References

Brodribb, A. J. M. and Humphreys, D. M. (1976). Diverticular disease: three studies. *British Medical Journal*, **1,** 424–430

Burkitt, D. P. (1972). Varicose veins, deep vein thrombosis and haemorrhoids. *British Medical Journal*, **2,** 556–561

Cleave, T. L., Cambell, G. D. and Painter, N. S. (1969). *Diabetes, Coronary Thrombosis and the Saccharine Disease,* second edition. John Wright, Bristol

Dhall, D. P., Colin, J. F. and Rottcher, K. H. (1976). Pulmonary embolic disease. *East African Medical Journal*, **53,** 202–211

Frohn, M. J. (1976). Left leg varicose veins and deep vein thrombosis. *Lancet*, **ii,** 1019–1020

Latto, C. (1979). Post-operative deep vein thrombosis in Nigerians on high-fibre diets. *British Medical Journal*, **1,** 199

Painter, N. S. (1975). *Diverticular Disease of the Colon. A Deficiency Disease of Western Civilization.* Heinemann, London

Trowell, H. C. (1975). In: *Refined Carbohydrate Foods and Disease: Some Implications of Dietary Fibre.* Editors D. P. Burkitt and H. C. Trowell. Academic Press, London

Webster, D. J. T., Gouch, D. C. S. and Craven, J. L. (1978). The use of a bulk evacuant in patients with haemorrhoids. *British Journal of Surgery*, **65,** 291–292

Part VIII

Summary

26

Contributors' reports

Hugh Trowell and Denis Burkitt

Joint enquiry into Western diseases

All 34 contributors to this book were sent a 12-page memorandum prepared by the editors concerning a suggested list of Western diseases. In some 22 diseases, or disease groups—cancer being enumerated as a single group—existing evidence was usually consistent and occasionally weighty, as in coronary heart disease. These 22 diseases and disease groups are listed in the Preface. Contributors were asked to present data concerning the hypothesized list of diseases and opposing viewpoints were assured full publication, as occurred in some of the data from Hawaii (Chapter 19), also in multiple sclerosis (Chapter 5).

Epidemiologists can justifiably object that there exist valid age and sex group incidence data in only a minority of these diseases, that few of them have been clearly defined by international agreement, also that incidence has not been determined by agreed methods of investigation. These conditions have been fulfilled only for ischaemic heart disease and some varieties of cancer. There are much data concerning dental caries, also obesity and body weight, and increasingly for the different types of diabetes mellitus. Nevertheless it is probably true to state that whenever sophisticated surveys have been conducted to determine the incidence of any Western disease, the data have confirmed opinions held by experienced clinical workers. There is a modern tendency of excessive reluctance to accept evidence of anecdotal and incomplete nature. It is pertinent to remember that a substantial body of such evidence can be of great value. It was largely such evidence that elucidated the epidemiological and other features of kwashiorkor and Burkitt's lymphoma in which we were respectively involved.

Knowledge concerning the incidence of Western diseases is restricted at present to the commoner medical and surgical diseases of adults and specially of the elderly. Subsequent studies will certainly show that there are paediatric, orthopaedic, gynaecological and obstetrical, neurological, dermatological, ophthalmic and auditory diseases that may be regarded as Western diseases. A few of the possible candidates are mentioned briefly later in Chapter 27.

It is indeed ironical that there are still little data concerning the prevalence

427

of constipation in different communities. There is moreover no international agreement about definition, classification and methods of investigation of this disorder. Little is known about normal stool weight, consistency, composition, or intestinal transit times. There is convincing evidence that dietary fibre intakes, especially that derived from cereals, is the major factor in the production of a normal stool and of easy defaecation. If this is so, then ˙ constipation is the commonest Western disease.

It is not possible to present in a summary of this book all the facts contained in the preceding chapters concerning any reported change in the incidences of the commoner medical (Table 26.1) and surgical (Table 26.2) diseases that occur during westernization of the diet and lifestyle. The chapters concerned, enumerated in both tables, should be consulted to assess the nature of the observations, the experience of the contributor and the limitations and inaccuracies inherent in pioneer studies. Epidemiologists are indeed invited, and will we trust be stimulated, to visit and work in these countries and as a result contribute better disease incidence data.

Increased incidence of certain medical diseases during westernization

Table 26.1 summarizes the reported increased incidence of six common medical diseases, all of which are stated by many of the contributors to increase in incidence and prevalence during westernization: blood pressure rising with age and essential hypertension, obesity, diabetes mellitus (largely type II, non-insulin-dependent diabetes mellitus, usually obese) and coronary heart disease (CHD). These four diseases are discussed in Chapter 1. Gallstones (Chapter 3) and renal stones (Chapter 4) are also discussed. *None* of these six Western diseases have been reported in any hunter-gatherer or nomad group until after some degree of acculturation, except women of pastoral tribes who may take much milk, and become obese.

Blood pressure rising with age and essential hypertension

These have not been reported in hunter-gatherers or nomads unless they add salt to their food. Recently essential hypertension was reported to be common and severe among Gashgai nomads of Iran; they were only very lightly acculturated but added salt to their food (Page, 1979), as did some of the neolithic hunter-gathers (Brothwell and Brothwell, 1969). Blood pressure did not rise with age and essential hypertension appeared absent in Kenya Highland Africans in 1930 when shop salt was not a feature of their traditional diet, but essential hypertension emerged subsequently when shop salt became freely available and was widely used (Chapter 1). Essential hypertension was reported to be rare in rural peasant agriculturalists exposed for only a short time to westernization, as in the West Nile district of Uganda (Chapter 13), Papua New Guinea (Chapter 12) and certain Pacific islands (Chapter 15) and some Polynesians (Chapter 16).

Essential hypertension was common in the urban areas of Zimbabwe

(Chapter 14) and among South African Bantu (Chapter 18) when blood pressure observations commenced in the 1930s and 1940s. Salt had been added by Africans to food in these countries, first in South Africa, then in Zimbabwe, since at least the beginning of this century. It is therefore of considerable interest that no increase of hypertension was reported in Zimbabwe (Chapter 14) and only a doubtful increase in urbanized Africans in South Africa (Chapter 18); see Table 26.1.

Body weight, obesity and diabetes mellitus type II

Body weight increased and obesity became common in hunter-gatherers such as Eskimos (Chapter 8), North American Indians (Chapter 9), Australian Aborigines (Chapter 11), also in peasant agriculturalists of Uganda (Chapter 13), Pacific islands (Chapter 15), Polynesians and Maoris (Chapter 16) and South African Bantu, especially women (Chapter 18), likewise in the inhabitants of Taiwan (Chapter 21) during westernization. The incidence of diabetes mellitus paralleled this change; this disease has not been recorded in any hunter-gatherer until some time after first contact with more sophisticated groups (Truswell, 1980); it remained rare in many lightly acculturated peasant agricultural populations, but increased in incidence after westernization, even in Japan (Chapter 20) and Taiwan (Chapter 21) in recent years during post-war westernization.

Coronary heart disease (CHD) and angina

It is well recognized that CHD and angina are very rare in hunter-gatherers and in peasant agriculturalists, but appear eventually after many years of a high degree of acculturation. These are the last Western diseases to emerge; usually cases of angina are recorded even while myocardial infarction remains very rare. These diseases remained rare in Ugandans (Chapter 1 and 13), and among Zimbabwe Africans (Chapter 14), South African Bantu (Chapter 18), Papua New Guineans (Chapter 12), Pacific islanders (Chapter 15) and Polynesians (Chapter 16).

CHD incidence increased considerably in Australian Aborigines, North American Indians, New Zealand Maoris and South African Indians after a short period of westernization (Table 26.1).

'Overkill' after rapid and severe acculturation

If westernization occurs rapidly in time and is severe in degree, especially in previously lightly acculturated groups, then the incidence and severity of certain Western diseases rises rapidly until it may exceed the level found in Western white communities who made a comparable change over the course of a long period of time. This 'overkill' phenomenon is seen with regard to diabetes and gallstones in North American Indians (Chapter 9), diabetes in Nauruans (Chapter 15), also CHD in Maori women (Chapter 16). Gout, not summarized in Table 26.1, also has a high incidence in New Zealand Maoris

Table 26.1 Increased incidence of medical diseases during westernization

Increase +   doubtful increase ±   no change 0   no report (blank space)

Group (Chapter)	Hyper-tension	Obesity	Diabetes[1]	Gall stones[2]	Renal stones[3]	CHD[4]
Hunter-gatherers						
Eskimos (8)	+ +	+ +	+ +	+		+ +
Australian Aborigines (11)	+	+ +	+ +	+	+	+ +
North American Indians (9)						+ +
Agriculturalists in						
West Nile, Uganda (13)	+ +	+	+ +	+[5]	+[5]	+[5]
Zimbabwe (14)	0		+ +	+ +	+[5]	+ +
South Africa (Bantu) (18)	+ +	+ + +	+ +	+	+ +	+ + +
Papua New Guinea (12)	+ +	+ +	+[5]			+ + +
Pacific Islands (15)	+ +	+ +	+ +			+ + +
Sub Saharal Africa (1)	+ +		+ +			
Polynesia (16)	+ +		+			
Migrants						
Maoris (16)	+ +	+ +	+ +	+ + +		+ +
South African Indians (18)	+ +	+ +	+ +	+ +	+	+ +
Israelis (17)	±		±			+ + +
Far East						
Japan (20)	+		+ +	+ +		+ +
Taiwan (21)		+ +	+ +	+		+ +
Hawaiian groups (19)		+		0		+

[1] Type 2 non-insulin-dependent variety, formerly called maturity-onset type
[2] Cholesterol-rich variety, more data in Chapter 3
[3] More data in Chapter 4
[4] Coronary heart disease and angina
[5] Very rare in rural areas; no data concerning increased incidence

(Chapter 16) but not in North American Indians (Chapter 9). It is possible that the incidence of gout rises at an early stage of westernization but may fall later, as occurred probably in eighteenth century England.

Order of emergence of Western surgical diseases

For convenience of presentation, Western diseases have been put into Tables 26.1 (medical) and 26.2 (surgical), but surgeons also are concerned with gallstones and renal stones, and physicians interested in hiatus hernia. The division is somewhat artificial. The list of surgical diseases in Table 26.2 is presented in their characteristic order of emergence to become a common clinical disorder. This order of emergence applies particularly to sub-Saharal Africans; there are fewer data from other continents. These surgical diseases concern the gastrointestinal tract, especially the colon. Westernization of almost any diet involves two changes, first a reduced consumption of starch foods (complex carbohydrates), specially cereals; second the latter are increasingly refined to produce low fibre white wheat flour and polished white rice. The intake of dietary fibre, specially cereal fibre, falls considerably. This results in low stool weights, prolonged transit times, unnaturally firm faecal masses and resultant difficult defaecation. It is significant that the order in which these diseases normally appear with increasing age in Western communities is the same as that in which these disorders emerge as common clinical conditions in developing countries following westernization of the diets. This suggests that the incidence of these diseases may be in part the result of varying periods of exposure to a single environmental factor— decreased fibre intakes—or allied environmental factors (Chapter 2).

Order of emergence of Western medical diseases

The Western medical diseases reflect a more complex number of aetiological factors and it is not possible to trace a single order of emergence in developing communities comparable to that seen in the Western surgical diseases. Aetiological factors have been most clearly established with regard to coronary heart disease (CHD); even here there is a long list of accepted risk factors and there are also protective factors, but the latter have not been clearly identified. Until recently little was known about aetiological environmental factors in the other five medical diseases listed in Table 26.1.

Among the metabolic group of Western diseases obesity appears first; this occurs largely among upper class groups, but eventually often becomes more marked in the previously underprivileged lower classes. The rising incidence of obesity is paralleled closely by a rising incidence of diabetes mellitus type II. A hypothesis has been set forth in Chapter 1 which suggested that major aetiological factors in the production of obesity and diabetes mellitus type II, both in susceptible phenotypes, have been the increasing consumption of fat and low fibre cereal products and sucrose in modern Western-type diets.

These measures increase palatability and encourage high energy intakes and comfort-feeding and -drinking in susceptible persons.

There is some evidence, as from Japan (Chapter 20), paralleled by the experience of one of us in a paediatric ward for 20 years in Uganda (H. T.), that type I insulin-dependent ketosis-prone diabetes mellitus is very rare in *children* until much westernization of the diets has occurred for many years.

Among the cardiovascular diseases there is a definite sequence of emergence: essential hypertension emerges first, clinically this remains silent until cerebrovascular disease and stroke become common; subsequently cardiac and renal complications may prove the commonest manifestations. Eventually angina becomes clearly recognized and increases; finally myocardial infarction emerges (Walker, 1975), then increases until it becomes the main cause of death in the Western world, the incidence continuing to rise in young males for several decades, but total incidence tends to become stable but at a high level, until in the end, as in the United States, it falls gradually as risk factors are identified and decrease slightly and treatment improves.

The increasing incidence of these cardiovascular diseases reflects mounting exposure to multiple risk factors, high fat intakes, specially saturated fat, perhaps also more sucrose and cholesterol. Cigarette smoking is a new major factor. Salt intakes have been high for millennia, and in salt-sensitive persons cause high blood pressure, which now becomes often the major CHD risk factor in Western communities. The role of CHD protective environmental factors is uncertain, but exercise, polyunsaturated fats and cereal fibre decrease during westernization and all these have been suggested to offer some protection. The interplay of all these factors, acting on susceptible phenotypes from childhood onwards, coupled with the mysterious tendency towards thrombosis, venous or arterial, that is present in Western communities, produces the rising incidence of CHD (Chapter 1). To aid regression all these factors must be borne in mind (Chapters 23 and 24).

As there are different varieties of gallstones it is not possible to speak of the emergence of a single disease. Pigment stones, although not common, have been the dominant variety in the Far East, as in Japan, but cholesterol gallstones have increased with westernization of the diet (Chapter 20). Heaton (Chapter 3) has summarized the evidence that cholesterol-rich gallstones are a disease of modern Western civilization and that the disease is related to obesity, diabetes mellitus type II and hypertriglyceridaemia, with refined and fibre-depleted carbohydrates as the principal aetiological factors.

The increased incidence of calcium renal stone in Western communities is reviewed by Blacklock (Chapter 4); he summarized evidence that the 'stone wave' must be ascribed to the modern dietary changes.

Increased incidence of Western surgical diseases

Table 26.2 summarizes the reports of the preceding chapters concerning the increased incidence in various communities of six common surgical diseases in association with westernization of the diet and lifestyle. Impoverished

Table 26.2 Increased incidence of surgical diseases during westernization

Increase +   doubtful increase ±   no change 0   no report (blank space)

Group (Chapter)	Appendicitis	Haemorrhoids	Varicose veins	Colorectal cancer[1]	Hiatus hernia	Diverticular disease
Hunter-gatherers						
Eskimos (8)	+			+		+
Australian Aborigines (11)	+			+		+
North American Indians (9)	+					
Agriculturalists in						
West Nile, Uganda (13)	+	+	+	+		++
Zimbabwe (14)	+	+	++			++
South Africa (Bantu) (18)	+		++	+		
Papua New Guinea (12)	+		++			
Pacific Islands (15)	+	+		+[2]	+	+
Sub-Saharal Africa (1)	+	+	+			
Polynesia (16)	+				+	+
Migrants						
Maoris (16)	+	±		+[3]	+	++
South African Indians (18)						
Israelis (17)				+		
Far East						
Japan (20)	+	C[4]	C[4]	+	R[5]	+R[5]
Taiwan (21)						
Hawaiian groups (19)	0	0	0	+	0	+

1 See Chapter 7 for increased incidence of colorectal, breast, lung, prostate, ovary and pancreas cancers; some contributors also added these cancers to their list
2 Also increased incidence of polyps of large bowel
3 More data on other varieties of cancer in Chapter 17 (Israel)
4 Remained common, and 5 remained rare, after westernization

unacculturated ethnic groups are placed towards the top of the table; more affluent westernized ethnic groups are placed towards the bottom.

Hunter-gatherers and peasant agriculturalists constituted a large group of underprivileged communities, at least until recently, and the Maori and South African Indians moved from poverty to relative affluence over a short period of time. Putting all these 12 ethnic groups together one notes that there were 36 reports of increased incidence of the six surgical diseases (recorded as + in Table 26.2), one report of a doubtful increase (±). The reports of a stationary incidence (o) came only from Hawaiian ethnic groups and are discussed later.

All contributors had many years' experience in these communities and they considered that the increased incidence could not be explained in terms of the increased number of old persons, or the improved facilities of diagnosis and treatment attracting more patients; they all considered that there had been a true increased incidence of certain diseases. Certain contributors, very understandably, offered no information concerning the incidence or prevalence of haemorrhoids, also concerning hiatus hernia. It is hoped that future surveys with improved facilities will test the validity of all these data.

Certain diseases concern young persons; they are not the diseases of the elderly. Thus in these 16 ethnic groups appendicitis incidence was reported to have increased, usually considerably, in 10 groups, even in large towns where illness of employed persons makes a visit to a hospital clinic or a doctor's surgery obligatory. Varicose veins in 7 groups and diverticular disease in 9 groups were reported to have increased, colorectal cancer incidence was reported to have increased in 6 groups, haemorrhoids in 3 groups, likewise hiatus hernia in 3 groups.

Stationary incidence rates in more affluent ethnic groups

A profoundly different incidence of surgical diseases (Table 26.2) is reported in the more affluent acculturated ethnic migrant groups of Israel, also in the residents of Japan and the Chinese in Taiwan, likewise in the Hawaiian ethnic groups that came usually many years ago as migrants from Japan and other Asian countries.

The Israeli ethnic groups came mostly from the westernized countries of Europe, America, and the Middle East; amongst them the Western pattern of cancer has been seen; no comments were made concerning any change in incidence of other Western surgical diseases.

Taiwan has become increasingly westernized and affluent during the last 25–30 years; clinical observers have reported that appendicitis incidence has possibly increased, but there is no evidence that the incidences of varicose veins and haemorrhoids have changed. The Western diseases that emerge last, namely hiatus hernia and diverticular disease (Chapter 2), are still rare and there is no evidence of any change of incidence.

The various Hawaiian ethnic groups have been westernized for a longer period of time and have usually become more affluent than any other group reported in Table 26.2. Diverticular disease is reported to be commoner in

Japanese residents in Hawaii than in those resident in Japan; this disease is often right sided, thus differing from diverticular disease encountered in Europe and North America. There are no data concerning whether any of the other surgical diseases considered in Table 26.2 had a different incidence in Hawaiian ethnic groups than in the Asian countries from which they, or their forebears, came. Hospital in-patient figures for these six surgical diseases suggest that all of them are common and differ little in incidence among the six ethnic groups in Hawaii. These ethnic groups nowadays differ little in their family income and all of them are affluent in comparison with people living in European countries. These Hawaiian ethnic groups display the Western pattern of cancer.

It is considered that the data from the more affluent westernized ethnic groups in Israel, Taiwan, Japan and Hawaii, considered as a whole, do not undermine the hypothesis that certain surgical and medical diseases are characteristic of westernization. In the opinion of the editors the data from these affluent countries support the overall hypothesis.

Other Western diseases

Data concerning other Western diseases, the incidence of which rises with westernization, are found elsewhere in this book. The following varieties of cancer increase with westernization: colorectal, breast, lung, prostate and ovary (Chapter 7); other varieties are discussed in the data on Israeli migrants (Chapter 17). Increased incidence of cholesterol gallstones (Chapter 3), renal stone (Chapter 4), rheumatoid arthritis, other varieties of arthritis and gout (Chapter 6) are discussed elsewhere in the book.

The incidence of ulcerative colitis rises with westernization and supporting data come from Zimbabwe (Chapter 14), South African Indians and Bantu (Chapter 18) and Maoris (Chapter 16). Crohn's disease remains a rare disease in Taiwan (Chapter 21), also in other developing countries of Asia, Africa and South America (Trowell, 1975a). Deep vein thrombosis and pulmonary embolism incidence rises with westernization in sub-Saharal Africans (Chapter 2) and in Taiwan (Chapter 21). The prevalence of pelvic phleboliths correlates with the incidence of deep vein thrombosis (Chapters 2 and 8).

Multiple sclerosis (MS) is a rare disease in many developing countries. Shelley and Dean (Chapter 5) discuss its peculiar epidemiology and suggest that an unidentified viral infection occurring frequently in young children of developing countries due to low standards of hygiene, but at a later age in Western countries, might initiate the disease more frequently in the latter.

MS should not be considered a Western disease until there is clear identification of environmental factors (see also Chapter 27).

References

References of Chapters 26 and 27 are on pages 440–443.

27

Treatment and prevention: a note on autoimmune disease in sub-Saharal Africans

Hugh Trowell and Denis Burkitt

Treatment

High fibre diets (HF diets)

The preceding chapters report two lines of treatment. The addition of wheat bran to make a high fibre diet (HF diet) is an easy and effective measure to prevent and treat constipation and prevent any straining during defaecation. An alternative procedure involves eating wholemeal bread and high fibre cereals, also more vegetables and fruit. These measures have revolutionized the treatment of diverticular disease (Painter, 1975); they have offered considerable relief to a large proportion of patients having irritable bowel syndrome. First degree haemorrhoids may be successfully treated by HF diets, second degree haemorrhoids may require also surgical treatment; the reported reduced incidence of postoperative deep vein thrombosis and pulmonary embolism by HF diets (Chapter 26) awaits confirmation in further trials.

High carbohydrate, high fibre diets (HCF diets)

The second line of treatment is far more difficult; it involves a major change in the composition of the diet to resemble at least partially that of peasant agriculturalists. This therapeutic diet is a high carbohydrate (starch) high fibre diet (HCF diet). An HCF diet of high unrefined starch (complex carbohydrates) is of necessity also low fat and low sucrose. These HCF diets, unrefined starch 70 per cent energy, dietary fibre 50–70 g/d, have been used with considerable success to treat diabetes mellitus type II; many of these patients discontinue all oral therapy (Chapter 22). Type I diabetics treated thus have decreased insulin requirement but still remain insulin dependent. Both varieties of diabetics have lower blood triglyceride and cholesterol levels and it is hoped they will develop fewer cardiovascular complications.

HCF diets may also be combined with low salt intakes, sodium < 60 mmol/d (sodium chloride < 4 g/d) in the treatment of essential hypertension. Two medical centres report that many patients, who had been treated for essential

436

hypertension previously with hypotensive drugs, after eating this diet for a few weeks reached normal diastolic blood pressure and ceased drug therapy (Chapters 23 and 24).

If these low salt HCF diets are still further modified to contain little fat, < 10 per cent energy, no added sucrose, and very low cholesterol, < 20 mg/d, and are combined with more exercise as therapy for angina patients then performance improves and pain decreases. Many state that all pain has disappeared and fewer drugs are taken (Chapters 23 and 24); diet in the latter chapter contained more fat and much more cholesterol.

It must be clearly recognized that controlled trials, long-term assessment, and morbidity data, with regard to the dietary treatment of essential hypertension, angina, and even CHD, have not yet been undertaken. These diets resemble in their composition the 1930 Kenya Kikuyu diet eaten by Africans among whom hypertension, diabetes mellitus type I and type II, angina and all manifestations of CHD were extremely rare (Chapter 1).

Prevention

Western diseases and ageing

Western diseases are predominantly the degenerative diseases of ageing. Before prevention can be discussed one basic criticism of the general hypothesis concerning Western diseases must be met. Many who have never spent much time in developing countries have suggested that the apparent scarcity of Western diseases is explained because young persons do not come to hospital if they have, say, appendicitis, and the elderly languish and die of degenerative diseases at home, and in any case there are very few of them. Many surgeons in these countries can, however, produce lists of their surgical emergencies crowded with strangulated herniae and other acute abdominal conditions, but very few cases of appendicitis. Pathologists also publish papers on the diseases detected in the autopsies of elderly persons.

Forty per cent of South African Bantu aged 50 years survive until 70 years of age, but only 33 per cent of 50-year-old South African Caucasians survive to 70; the latter have better medical treatment, but the former have much less degenerative disease (Walker, 1974). In Uganda there are over half a million Ugandans aged 60 years or more; this represents 6 per cent of the total population. Among the 400 autopsies of Ugandans of this age conducted during 1968–72 at MakerereUniversity Medical School, Kampala, less than 5 per cent died of degenerative disease. Only 3 died of coronary heart disease (CHD), and 9 of hypertension. Most died of infective disease. 'CHD has emerged and can be identified over the age of 60' but not at an earlier age, according to this pathologist (Drury, 1973). A medical survey of a defined population of 12 000 rural Ugandans had their ages assessed by the 'milestones of local history': 729 persons were 50 years or more, 219 persons were over 70 years, but only 4 appeared to be suffering from senile dementia (Bennett, 1971). Little is known about the prevalence of senile dementia in peasant agriculturalists who had low salt intakes for most of their lives coupled with the typical diet of such a community; these communities have less atheroma and hypertension. Gordon (1936) stated that senile dementia was a 'notable absentee' in a Nairobi mental hospital.

By way of contrast many pathological changes develop slowly throughout life in modern Western man which are not directly due to ageing. These changes 'do not occur in primitive populations' stated Bierman (1976); he enumerated several of them thus. Body weight increases in men until 40–50 years, in women until 50–60 years, serum cholesterol and triglyceride levels also rise until a similar age, blood glucose after meals rises with age until many develop impaired glucose tolerance, insulin resistance rises with age so that the pancreas reacts by secreting more insulin after glucose challenge. This is the background of degenerative cardiovascular disease, of atherosclerosis, and of diabetes mellitus type II. Only the most susceptible phenotypes, however, will develop overt manifestations of disease.

This catalogue of diseases in modern Western man can be extended. Blood pressure rises with age in most populations but not in certain primeval groups who add little or no salt to their food; atheroma develops more extensively and more severely in modern Western man (Chapter 1). Haemorrhoids and varicose veins increase in frequency; colorectal cancer incidence rises, and hiatus hernia and diverticular disease eventually appear late in life and become common conditions in industrialized Western communities (Chapter 2).

Dietary goals to prevent certain degenerative diseases

Coronary heart disease has been attributed to certain factors in Western-type diets and lifestyle. These matters have been studied by at least 15 national committees of medical experts, nine of whom have recommended some dietary change for the general population.

A detailed study has been made by the United States Senate Select Committee on Nutrition and Human Needs (1977). Having collected evidence concerning CHD, obesity and other degenerative diseases from the medical experts of the National Institutes of Health and doctors elsewhere in the United States and from other countries, and have received criticisms of their first statement of *Dietary Goals for the United States* (1977), the second edition was published in December of that year. Their recommendations were:

1. reduce energy if overweight and increase exercise. In terms of energy percentages they recommended;
2. increase starch (complex carbohydrates) from 22 to 42, increase whole cereals, vegetables and fruit, these measures increase dietary fibre intake considerably;
3. reduce sucrose from 18 to 10;
4. reduce total fat from 42 to 30, decrease saturated fats but increase polyunsaturated fats;
5. reduce cholesterol to 300 mg/d;
6. reduce salt to 5 g/d from approximately 12–16 g/d.

These constituted the recommended Dietary Goals for the *whole* US population.

The therapeutic HCF diet, already mentioned (page 436), anticipated and even increased these numerous recommended changes in the US diet. These therapeutic HCF diets apparently aid the regression of diabetes mellitus type II (Chapter 22), hypertension, angina and hyperlipidaemia (Chapters 23 and 24): this adds considerable weight to the recommended US Dietary Goals. It is suggested that these HCF diets should be tried in the treatment of other Western diseases, especially at an early stage.

Other factors will increase the pressure towards dietary change, certainly in patients and eventually perhaps in the population as a whole. It is financially impossible to treat medically all the Western diseases and this treatment affords only limited relief and often occasions retirement from work. On the other hand major dietary change will be strongly resisted, specially by persons who consider themselves fit. Individuals will claim their rights to choose their own food; and in the years of peace and plenty this is permissible. A decreased consumption of any food will be strongly resisted by commercial interests. An enormous debate is just beginning. A fundamental problem lies in rendering palatable low fat, low sucrose, low salt foods, but no material problem should remain insoluble if mind and spirit combine to seek a solution.

Autoimmune diseases in sub-Saharal Africans

All diseases in which autoimmunity is recognized to be an important factor are reported rarely in sub-Saharal Africans. Some of these diseases are fairly common in Western communities, such as multiple sclerosis, but not a single case in 18 million South African Bantu (Chapter 5), and rheumatoid arthritis less common in rural than in urban South African Bantu (Chapter 6). Some autoimmune diseases are not common in Western communities; thus many of the autoimmune endocrine diseases are rare, and these might easily be missed and certainly under-reported in sub-Saharal hospitals. Other diseases such as ulcerative colitis might be missed if chronic dysentery is common, but few medical school pathologists, however, would miss this disease at an autopsy (Trowell, 1975a).

The rarity of many autoimmune and certain endocrine diseases was reviewed previously and some 40 articles from African medical journals were cited (Trowell, 1975b, 1960). Since that date articles have added considerable support, as the subsequent bibliography shows and as a more recent review suggested (Adadevoh, 1970). A list of nine of the commoner autoimmune diseases, some of which are endocrine disorders, was sent to all contributors of this book and comment was invited. These nine diseases are numbered 1 to 9 in the subsequent bibliography. Those with much clinical experience in Africa (Gelfand in Zimbabwe, Chapter 14; Williams and Williams in West

Nile, Uganda, Chapter 13, and Walker in South Africa, Chapter 18) have added a measure of agreement but offered limited data. A selected bibliography of recent publications in African journals is appended.

Some autoimmune diseases are organ specific, these are listed first in the appended list; those which are not organ specific are listed last, and an intermediate group appears in the middle. Certain genes, notably those of the HLA group, increase susceptibility in a varying degree to certain autoimmune diseases, notably ankylosing spondylitis. HLA gene frequency in the numerous African ethnic groups is seldom known. It is unlikely that genetic factors will explain the rarity of many of these autoimmune diseases, except perhaps ankylosing spondylitis in the South African Bantu (Chapter 6), for USA blacks and whites usually have similar rates of these diseases. One exception is systemic lupus erythematosus, commoner in US blacks than US whites, but of equal incidence in Cape Town blacks and whites (page 86). Environmental factors must therefore be considered in many of these diseases. Perhaps it should be added that although there is much evidence of the rarity and/or mildness of several of the commoner autoimmune diseases, there is less information about the incidence of many endocrine diseases, except with regard to those of the thyroid gland, in which there are much data.

Autoimmune diseases and endocrine diseases reported to be rare in sub-Saharal Africans

Organ-specific group
1. Thyrotoxicosis (Zoutendyk, 1970; Kungu, 1974; Kajubi, 1977; Oliech, 1977).
2. Hypothyroidism, adult (Taylor, 1968a, b; Gitau, 1975; Kajubi, 1977).
3. Hashimoto's thyroiditis (Taylor, 1968a, b; Kungu, 1974; Kajubi, 1977).
4. Pernicious anaemia (Hift et al., 1973; Nyame and Bruce-Tagoe, 1973; Adams, 1979).
5. Subacute combined degeneration (Mngola, 1968).
   Addison's disease, idiopathic (Bagshawe and Forrester, 1966).
   Hyperparathyroidism (Ancorn and Seedat, 1976).

Less organ-specific group
   Diabetes mellitus, type I[1] (Haddock, 1964; Marine et al., 1969; Adetuyibi, 1976; Scragg and Rubidge, 1978).
6. Multiple sclerosis (Shelley and Dean, Chapter 5; Adams, 1979).
7. Ulcerative colitis (Spencer and Nhonoli, 1972; Jones et al., 1977).
8. Crohn's disease (Davis et al., 1974; Masri and Satir, 1975; Novis et al., 1975; Trowell, 1975a).
   Myasthenia gravis (Singh, 1964; Geefhuysen et al., 1970).

[1] Especially under 14 years of age.

Non-organ-specific group
  9. Rheumatoid arthritis (Beighton and Solomon, Chapter 6).
     Still's disease (Greenwood, 1968).
     Ankylosing spondylitis (Beighton and Solomon, Chapter 6; Chalmers
     et al., 1977).
     Haemolytic anaemia (Esan, 1974).

References (Chapters 26 and 27)

Adadevoh, N. K. (1970). Endocrine patterns in the African. Clinical and
  biochemical assessment. *Tropical and Geographical Medicine*, **22**,
  125–141
Adams, E. B. (1979). *A Companion to Clinical Medicine in the Tropics and
  Subtropics*, 157–166. Oxford University Press, Oxford
Adetuyibi, A. (1976). The influence of age on onset on the pattern of diabetes
  mellitus in the Nigerian African. *Ghana Medical Journal*, **15**, 97–101
Ancorn, I. B. and Seedat, Y. K. (1976). Primary hyperparathyroidism in
  Black South Africans. *South African Medical Journal*, **50**, 1246–1248
Bagshawe, A. F. and Forrester, A. T. T. (1966). Addison's disease in Kenya.
  East African Medical Journal, **43**, 525–529
Bennett, F. J. (1971). Old age in rural Buganda. *East African Medical
  Journal*, **48**, 354–359
Bierman, E. L. (1976). Obesity, carbohydrate and lipid interactions in the
  elderly. In: *Nutrition and Aging*, 171–176. Editor M. Winick. Wiley and
  Sons, New York
Brothwell, D. and Brothwell, P. (1969). *Food in Antiquity*, 162. Thames and
  Hudson, London
Chalmers, I. M., Seedat, Y. K. and Mudaliar, M. Y. (1977). Ankylosing
  spondylitis in three Zulu men negative for the HLA B27 antigen. *South
  African Medical Journal*, **52**, 567–569
Davis, R., Schmaman, A. and Cosman, B. (1974). Crohn's disease in
  Transvaal Blacks. *South African Medical Journal*, **48**, 580–486
Drury, R. A. B. (1973). The cardiac pathology of elderly Ugandan Africans.
  East African Medical Journal, **50**, 566–573
Esan, G. J. F. (1974). Autoimmune haemolytic anaemia in Nigerians. *East
  African Medical Journal*, **51**, 701–709
Geefhuysen, J., Ronthal, M. and Rogers, M. A. (1970). Thymectomy for
  myasthenia gravis in Bantu children. *South African Medical Journal*,
  44, 239–241
Gitau, W. (1975). An analysis of thyroid disease seen at Kenyatta National
  Hospital. *East African Medical Journal*, **52**, 564–570
Gordon, H. L. (1936). An inquiry into the correlation of civilization and
  mental disorder in the Kenya native. *East African Medical Journal*, **12**,
  327–335
Greenwood, B. M. (1968). Autoimmune disease and parasitic infection in
  Africans. *Lancet*, **ii**, 380–382

Haddock, D. R. W. (1964). Diabetes mellitus and its complications in Dar-es-Salaam. *East African Medical Journal,* **41,** 145–155

Hift, W., Moshal, M. G. and Pillay, K. (1963). Pernicious-anaemia like syndromes in the non-White population of Natal. *South African Medical Journal,* **47,** 915–918

Jones, M. E., Bewes, P. C. and Hulme-Moir, A. B. (1977). Ulcerative colitis in an African. A fatal case in Tanzania. *East African Medical Journal,* **54,** 670–672

Kajubi, S. K. (1977). Thyroid disorders seen at the Mulago Radioisotope Laboratories. *East African Medical Journal,* **54,** 65–73

Kungu, A. (1974). The pattern of thyroid disease in Kenya. *East African Medical Journal,* **51,** 449–466

Marine, N., Vinik, A. S., Edelstein, B. A. and Jackson, W. P. U. (1969). Diabetes, hyperglycemia and glycosuria among Indians, Malays and Africans (Bantu) in Cape Town. *Diabetes,* **18,** 840–857

Masri, S. H. E. and Satir, A. A. (1975). Crohn's disease in three Sudanese patients. *East African Medical Journal,* **52,** 284–293

Mngola, E. N. (1968). Two cases of pernicious anaemia among Africans. *East African Medical Journal,* **45,** 669–672

Novis, B. H., Marks, I. N., Bank, S. and Louw, J. H. (1975). Incidence of Crohn's disease at Groote Schuur Hospital during 1970–74. *South African Medical Journal,* **49,** 693–697

Nyame, N. P. and Bruce-Tagoe, A. A. (1973). The first reported case of pernicious anaemia in a Ghanian. *Ghana Medical Journal,* **12,** 333–334

Oliech, J. S. (1977). Thyrotoxicosis at Kenyatta National Hospital, Nairobi. *East African Medical Journal,* **54,** 561–564

Page, L. B. (1979). Salt and hypertension: epidemiology and mechanisms. In: *Hypertension, Determinants, Complications and Intervention,* 3–11. Editors G. Onesti and C. R. Klimt. Grune and Stratton, New York

Painter, N. S. (1975). *Diverticular Disease of the Colon.* Heinemann, London

Scragg, J. N. and Rubidge, C. J. (1978). Patterns of disease in Black and Indian children in Natal. *South African Medical Journal,* **54,** 265–270

Singh, J. S. (1964). Myasthenia gravis in a Musoga girl. *East African Medical Journal,* **41,** 535–536

Spencer, S. S. and Nhonoli, A. M. (1972). Ulcerative colitis in East Africans. *East African Medical Journal,* **49,** 163–169

Taylor, J. R. (1968a). The thyroid in Western Nigeria. Part 1, Anatomy. *East African Medical Journal,* **45,** 383–389

Taylor, J. R. (1968b). The thyroid in Western Nigeria. Part 2, Pathology. *East African Medical Journal,* **45,** 390–398

Trowell, H. C. (1960). Endocrine and metabolic disease. In: *Non-infective Disease in Africa,* 276–319. Edward Arnold, London

Trowell, H. C. (1975a). Ulcerative colitis and Crohn's disease. In: *Refined Carbohydrate Foods and Disease,* 135–140. Editors D. P. Burkitt and H. C. Trowell. Academic Press, London

Trowell, H. C. (1975b). Auto-immune diseases: variations in endocrines. In: *Ibid.,* 320–331. Academic Press, London

Truswell, A. S. (1980). Historical and geographical perspectives. In: *Human Nutrition and Dietetics*, seventh edition, 2. Editors S. Davidson, R. Passmore, J. F. Brock and A. S. Truswell. Churchill-Livingstone, Edinburgh

United States Senate Select Committee on Nutrition and Human Needs (1977). *Dietary Goals for the United States,* second edition. US Government Printing Office, Washington

Walker, A. R. P. (1974). Survival rate at middle-age in developing and Western populations. *Postgraduate Medical Journal,* **50,** 29–32

Walker, A. R. P. (1975). The epidemiological emergence of ischemic arterial diseases. *American Heart Journal,* **89,** 133–136

Zoutendyk, A. (1970). Auto-antibodies in South African Whites, Coloured and Bantu. *South African Medical Journal,* **44,** 469–470

Index

Western diseases (*See* Preface xi) are marked with an asterisk (*)

(†indicates rates increase during
Westernization)